Care *of* Well Newborn

Edited by

B. J. Snell, PhD, CNM, FACNM

Professor Emeritus
Women's Health Care Concentration
School of Nursing
California State University, Fullerton
Fullerton, California

Sandra L. Gardner, MS, RN

Retired Clinical Nurse Specialist and Pediatric Nurse Practitioner
Director
Professional Outreach Consultation
Aurora, Colorado

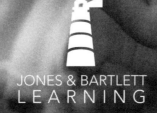

JONES & BARTLETT
LEARNING

World Headquarters
Jones & Bartlett Learning
5 Wall Street
Burlington, MA 01803
978-443-5000
info@jblearning.com
www.jblearning.com

Jones & Bartlett Learning books and products are available through most bookstores and online booksellers. To contact Jones & Bartlett Learning directly, call 800-832-0034, fax 978-443-8000, or visit our website, www.jblearning.com.

Substantial discounts on bulk quantities of Jones & Bartlett Learning publications are available to corporations, professional associations, and other qualified organizations. For details and specific discount information, contact the special sales department at Jones & Bartlett Learning via the above contact information or send an email to specialsales@jblearning.com.

The content, statements, views, and opinions herein are the sole expression of the respective authors and not that of Jones & Bartlett Learning, LLC. Reference herein to any specific commercial product, process, or service by trade name, trademark, manufacturer, or otherwise does not constitute or imply its endorsement or recommendation by Jones & Bartlett Learning, LLC and such reference shall not be used for advertising or product endorsement purposes. All trademarks displayed are the trademarks of the parties noted herein. *Care of the Well Newborn* is an independent publication and has not been authorized, sponsored, or otherwise approved by the owners of the trademarks or service marks referenced in this product.

There may be images in this book that feature models; these models do not necessarily endorse, represent, or participate in the activities represented in the images. Any screenshots in this product are for educational and instructive purposes only. Any individuals and scenarios featured in the case studies throughout this product may be real or fictitious, but are used for instructional purposes only.

The authors, editor, and publisher have made every effort to provide accurate information. However, they are not responsible for errors, omissions, or for any outcomes related to the use of the contents of this book and take no responsibility for the use of the products and procedures described. Treatments and side effects described in this book may not be applicable to all people; likewise, some people may require a dose or experience a side effect that is not described herein. Drugs and medical devices are discussed that may have limited availability controlled by the Food and Drug Administration (FDA) for use only in a research study or clinical trial. Research, clinical practice, and government regulations often change the accepted standard in this field. When consideration is being given to use of any drug in the clinical setting, the health care provider or reader is responsible for determining FDA status of the drug, reading the package insert, and reviewing prescribing information for the most up-to-date recommendations on dose, precautions, and contraindications, and determining the appropriate usage for the product. This is especially important in the case of drugs that are new or seldom used.

Production Credits

VP, Executive Publisher: David D. Cella
Executive Editor: Amanda Martin
Acquisitions Editor: Teresa Reilly
Editorial Assistant: Lauren Vaughn
Senior Production Editor: Amanda Clerkin
Marketing Communications Manager: Katie Hennessy
Product Fulfillment Manager: Wendy Kilborn
Composition: S4Carlisle Publishing Services

Cover Design: Kristin E. Parker
Rights & Media Specialist: Wes DeShano
Media Development Editor: Troy Liston
Cover Image: © Ramona Heim/Shutterstock, © monkeybusinessimages /iStockphoto
Printing and Binding: Edwards Brothers Malloy
Cover Printing: Edwards Brothers Malloy

Library of Congress Cataloging-in-Publication Data
Names: Snell, B. J., editor. | Gardner, Sandra L., editor.
Title: Care of the well newborn / edited by B.J. Snell and Sandra L. Gardner.
Description: Burlington, Massachusetts : Jones & Bartlett Learning, [2017] |
    Includes bibliographical references and index.
Identifiers: LCCN 2016013818 | ISBN 9781284093513
Subjects: | MESH: Infant, Newborn | Infant Care | Infant, Newborn, Diseases |
    Neonatal Screening | Evidence-Based Medicine
Classification: LCC RJ253 | NLM WS 420 | DDC 618.92/01--dc23
LC record available at https://lccn.loc.gov/2016013818

6048

Printed in the United States of America
20 19 18 17 16   10 9 8 7 6 5 4 3 2 1

Dedication

To the women with whom I have had the honor to share their birth, transition to motherhood, and getting my "baby fix" on a regular basis. There is nothing that inspires me more than the amazing gaze of a newborn baby. This book is dedicated to my mother, who shared her passion for nursing and the grace of being a mother; my husband, who shares his devotion to the work that I love; and my children, who allow me to continue to call them my babies!

B. J. S.

To all the families, newborns, and pediatric patients for whom I have cared in my 49 years of practice. You have been my mentors, my teachers, my joy, and my greatest accomplishment!

S. L. G.

Contents

Preface   xi

Foreword   xiv

Contributors   xvi

Reviewers   xviii

CHAPTER **1** | 1

Professional Responsibilities in the Provision of Newborn Care

Sandra L. Gardner and B. J. Snell

    Why Newborns Are Different   2

    Defining the Healthcare Provider's Practice   17

    Legal Issues   26

    Professional Practice and Care of the Neonate   29

    Conclusion   30

    References   30

CHAPTER **2** | 35

Perinatal History: Influences on Newborn Outcome

Pamela J. Reis and Amy Jnah

    Components of the Perinatal Health Record   36

    Perinatally Acquired Infections   49

    Perinatal Substance Abuse   51

    Intrapartum History   56

    Conclusion   61

    Student Practice Activities   62

    References   64

CHAPTER 3 | 69

Newborn Transition: The Journey from Fetal to Extrauterine Life

Jenna Shaw-Battista and Sandra L. Gardner

Epigenetics   70
The First Hour of Life   72
Labor and Birth in Water   81
Data Collection   82
Routine Care During Transition   89
Standards of Care   92
Cultural Considerations   94
Health Education   94
Conclusion   95
Student Practice Activities   95
References   97

CHAPTER 4 | 101

Physical Examination, Interventions, and Referrals

Nicole Boucher, Donna Marvicsin, and Sandra L. Gardner

Apgar Scoring and Gestational Age   101
Anthropometric Measurements   104
Physical Examination   104
Neurologic Examination   125
Student Practice Activities   133
References   134

CHAPTER 5 | 135

Newborn and Neonatal Nutrition

B. J. Snell and Sandra L. Gardner

Introduction   135
Influences on Breastfeeding Success: Prenatal, Intrapartal, and Postpartal   136
Physiology and Pathophysiology of Breastfeeding   139
Common Problems with Breastfeeding   146
Standard of Care/National Guidelines for Care   164
Teaching/Counseling About Breastfeeding   165
Formula Feeding   165

Normal Neonatal Physiology, Pathology, or Formula Intolerance?   176
Summary   182
Student Practice Activities 182
References   182

CHAPTER **6** | 191

Developmental Care of the Well Newborn

Barbara A. Overman and Dorinda L. Welle

Conceptual Foundations of Developmental Care
    of the Well Newborn   192
Developmental Care and Neonatal Behavioral Transition   198
The Predictable Behavioral Sequence   199
Newborn States: Co-regulation for Process Completion   201
"Co-regulation Boot Camp": Bringing in the Milk   205
Newborn Growth Spurt: Expanding and Maturing the Milk   207
Co-regulation for Conformity: Days, Nights, and Elimination   208
Saying Goodbye to the Neonatal Period: Colic, Fatigue, and Mother/Baby Blues   209
Conclusion   212
Student Practice Activities   213
References   214

CHAPTER **7** | 219

Newborn Discharge Timing

Katrina Wu and Rachel Stapleton

Introduction   219
Historical Perspective   220
Ethical Considerations   220
Data Collection   220
Teaching and Counseling   222
Standards of Care   223
Birth Center and Home Settings   225
Risk of Readmission   226
Cultural Considerations   228
Conclusion   229
Student Practice Activities   229
References   231

CHAPTER **8** | 235

Discharge Teaching

Cara Busenhart

Timing of Discharge   235
Standard of Care/National Guidelines for Care   236
Preparation for Discharge   238
Follow-Up Care   247
Student Practice Activities   248
References   250

CHAPTER **9** | 253

Hyperbilirubinemia of the Newborn Born After 35 Weeks' Gestation

Susan Dragoo

Incidence   255
Bilirubin Metabolism   256
Current Guidelines for Management   259
Pathologic Jaundice   268
Student Practice Activities   271
References   272

CHAPTER **10** | 275

Infection in the Neonate

Sandra L. Gardner and B. J. Snell

Definition and Etiology   275
Prevention   278
Data Collection   278
Differential Diagnoses   301
Standard of Care for Treatment   302
Cultural Considerations   304
Parent Education   305
Student Practice Activities   306
References   308

CHAPTER 11 | 313

General Considerations of the Newborn with Complications

Sheron Bautista and Curry J. Bordelon

    Factors Affecting the Developing Fetus   313
    Fetal Growth   316
    Delivery Complications   319
    Genetic Complications   321
    Structural Complications   323
    Conclusion   326
    Student Practice Activities   327
    References   329

CHAPTER 12 | 331

Health Maintenance Visits in the First Month of Life

Karla Reinhart and Sandra L. Gardner

    Introduction   331
    Outpatient Visits   332
    Newborn Development   333
    Health Maintenance Visits   336
    Standard of Care/National Guidelines for Care   348
    Cultural Considerations   348
    Conclusion   350
    Student Practice Activities   351
    References   353

Appendix A: Answers to Student Practice Activities   355
Appendix B: Resources for Parents   363
Index   371

Preface

Forty years ago, B. J. Snell and Sandy Gardner became colleagues and friends while working on the first March of Dimes grant that funded perinatal outreach education in Colorado and the seven surrounding states. As the Perinatal Education Coordinator, Sandy recognized that a maternal/obstetric nurse was needed on the team, so she interviewed and hired B. J., who brought her passion and knowledge of the maternal/obstetric field to the perinatal outreach program. The concept of a team approach to provision of perinatal care has informed both of our practices. In 2014, when B. J. was in Denver attending the American College of Nurse–Midwives (ACNM) annual meeting, we met for lunch. During that conversation, we discussed the lack of a textbook for midwifery students about care of the well newborn from birth through the first month of life. When B. J. asked, "Want to write a book with me?" Sandy jumped at the chance to co-edit and co-author another book about our favorite topic: the newborn baby!

Together we bring more than 90 years of clinical practice, writing, teaching, and consulting in maternal, obstetric, midwifery, neonatal, and pediatric care to this project. Before describing the goals and focus of *Care of the Well Newborn*, this is our opportunity to introduce ourselves to you, our readers.

Dr. B. J. Snell is owner and clinical director of Beach Cities Midwifery and Women's Health Care and the Beach Side Birth Centers in Laguna Hills, Long Beach, and Corona, California. In addition to specializing in out-of-hospital/birth center practice, she has privileges at Saddleback Memorial Medical Center, where she manages women who require hospital-based care. B. J. works collaboratively with obstetric, pediatric, and primary care physicians and nurse practitioners to provide the wide variety of services needed. She is Professor Emeritus at the School of Nursing at California State University, Fullerton. B. J. is the founder of the Women's Health Care Concentration at California State University, Fullerton, and continues teaching in the midwifery and women's health nurse practitioner specialties. She received her BSN from the University of Alabama, Birmingham, in 1974; her MSN and women's health nurse practitioner education from the University of Colorado, Denver, in 1976; and her nurse–midwifery education and PhD from Oregon Health Science University (OHSU) in Portland, Oregon, in 1987 and 1991, respectively. She is nationally certified by the American Midwifery Certification Board. B. J. is recognized nationally as a Fellow in the American College of Nurse–Midwives and is active in health policy advocacy both nationally and in California. She is a strong advocate for women's health issues and has worked to decrease barriers to midwifery care and improve access to safe pregnancy and childbirth. B. J. provides significant community leadership through invited presentations and publications and continues to work with the March of Dimes.

Sandy Gardner is currently Editor of *Nurse Currents*, *NICU Currents*, and *Pediatric Currents* (http://www.anhi.org) and the Director of Professional Outreach Consultation (http://www.professionaloutreachconsultation.com), a national and international consulting firm established in 1980. Sandy plans, develops, teaches, and coordinates educational workshops on perinatal/neonatal/pediatric topics. She graduated from a hospital school of nursing in 1967 with a diploma, obtained her BSN at Spalding College in 1973 (magna cum laude), and completed her MS at the University of Colorado School of Nursing in 1975 and her PNP in 1978. Sandy has worked in perinatal/neonatal/pediatric care since 1967 as a clinician (37 years in direct bedside care), practitioner, teacher, author, and consultant. In 1974, she was the first Perinatal Outreach Educator in the United States funded by the March of Dimes. In this role, she taught nurses and physicians in Colorado and the seven surrounding states how to recognize and stabilize at-risk pregnancies and sick neonates. She consulted with numerous March of Dimes grantees to help them establish perinatal outreach programs. In 1978, Sandy was awarded the Gerald Hencmann Award from the March of Dimes for "outstanding service in the improvement of care to mothers and babies in Colorado." For 30 years, Sandy has co-edited *Merenstein and Gardner's Handbook of Neonatal Intensive Care*; of the eight editions, the first (1985), fifth (2002), seventh (2010), and eighth (2015) have all won Book of the Year Awards from the *American Journal of Nursing*. Sandy is a founding member of the Colorado Perinatal Care Council (now the Colorado Perinatal Care Quality Collaborative), its treasurer, and a member of the Executive Committee. She is also an active member of the Colorado Nurses Association/American Nurses Association, the Academy of Neonatal Nurses, and the National Association of Neonatal Nurses.

Care of the Well Newborn focuses on care at birth and through the first month of life. It is written by teams of advanced practice nurses (nurse–midwives and nurse practitioners) and is intended to be a comprehensive text for midwifery and nurse practitioner students and providers. A secondary group of students (physician assistants; medical interns and residents) and providers will find that *Care of the Well Newborn* also enables them to provide evidence-based care to this resilient yet fragile population.

While concentrating on care of the well newborn, this text presents the reader with assessment criteria for recognition of deviations from normal and strategies for management based on national recommendations, guidelines, and the standards of care in the literature. Following a format that includes description of physiology and pathophysiology, data collection, differential diagnosis, cultural considerations, and parent education, each chapter presents the latest evidence-based practice. Each chapter also clearly identifies the necessity of consultation, collaboration, and transfer of care to medical colleagues and specialists when the "well newborn" develops a complication or becomes "at risk" for a compromised outcome.

Most chapters include activities intended to augment learning and assist faculty in evaluating learning. These activities include multiple choice questions, case studies, and student activities. The content is influenced by the core competency requirements for advanced practice nursing programs and medical education programs. An appendix listing available parent-education information is also provided.

In the introduction to the sixth edition of *Handbook of Neonatal Intensive Care*, one of our medical colleagues, Brian Carter, MD, wrote:

> The goals of care should be patient-and-family centered. It is the patient we treat, but it is the family, of whatever construct, with whom the baby will go home. Indeed, it is the family who must live with the long-term consequences of our daily decisions in caring for their baby.

Provision of skilled professional care is included in these goals. An effective perinatal care team consists of educated, skilled professionals of many disciplines. Our hope is that *Care of the Well Newborn* becomes the text that many disciplines use for evidence-based care.

It has been our honor and privilege to work with our co-authors, all of whom are patient-and-family centered. We also deeply appreciate our amazing editing team of Danielle Bessette and Teresa Reilly, who have produced this text in 9 months, an appropriate time frame for the birth of this effort!

B. J. Snell and Sandy L. Gardner
Co-editors

Foreword

This book is designed to facilitate the efforts of students to learn about the care of the well newborn. It differs from textbooks in which the newborn is just one part of the totality of the practice of a specialty (e.g., midwives and family nurse practitioners), and even from textbooks that address all aspects of care of the newborn, including the critically ill newborn. *Care of the Well Newborn* is a comprehensive text that focuses exclusively on the well newborn.

Care provided by nurse–midwives has always included care of the well newborn, but the scope of this care has greatly evolved over the years. Nurse–midwives from the mid-1920s to the early 1950s were also public health nurses; thus, they provided health care for the entire family. The move of nurse–midwives into the hospital for births began during the mid-1950s. In the hospital setting, nurse–midwifery care of the newborn was limited to immediate evaluation to determine the need for resuscitation and to the provision of whatever care was needed. Once in the nursery, the baby was under the care of a pediatrician.

The education of a nurse–midwife regarding the care of the newborn needed to cover more than this immediate resuscitation evaluation and provision, however, because of the expanded care provided for babies born out-of-hospital and the extended care determined by the needs of the population served. For example, nurse–midwives in Mississippi during the early 1970s were able to cut the infant mortality by nearly half in the population they served. The babies were born in the hospital with nurse–midwives in attendance, but the nurse–midwives then continued to provide well-baby evaluation and care combined with parental education through an intensive postpartal/neonatal/infant home-visiting program for the first year of life. In addition, midwifery care has always emphasized facilitation of breastfeeding regardless of locale of birth.

When the first American College of Nurse–Midwives (ACNM) *Core Competencies* document was published in 1978, it included expected competencies in the care of the newborn. The 2002 revision of the *Core Competencies* made it clear that nurse–midwifery care of the newborn was specifically care during the first 28 days of life.

The creators and editors of this text are two deeply committed and highly experienced expert clinicians and educators who have lived much of the history of the early movement of nurse practitioners and their professional organizations, as well as that of the involvement of the March of Dimes in perinatal outreach and education. The nurse practitioner movement started in 1965 at the University of Colorado. Women's healthcare nurse practitioners followed the path first tread by family planning nurse practitioners during the 1970s and the obstetric and gynecologic nurse practitioners of the 1980s. In addition to the emergence of the nurse practitioner, the evolution of neonatal nurse practitioners was influenced by developments in the care of the neonate, changes in pediatric residency requirements, and expansion of the role of the neonatal clinical nurse specialist in the neonatal intensive care unit. The Nurses Association of the American College of Obstetricians and Gynecologists (NAACOG) was founded in 1969 and provided a home for nurses specializing in maternity care, including care of the newborn. In 1993 NAACOG separated from the American Congress of Obstetricians and Gynecologists (ACOG) as an independent organization and renamed itself the Association of Women's Health, Obstetric, and Neonatal Nursing (AWHONN). The evolving specialty of neonatal nursing led to the founding of the National Association of Neonatal Nurses (NANN) in 1984. The National Association of Neonatal Nurse Practitioners became a membership division of the NANN in 2007. All of these professional organizations (NAACOG/AWHONN, NANN), the ACNM, and others have developed standards of care, written guidelines, identified expected competencies, and provided standards for education for the care of the newborn.

The editors, and their expert chapter authors, have written a text that incorporates both their experience and the current best evidence underlying the care advocated. In addition, they have made effective use of their experience in teaching and educational principles through their provision of learning activities such as case studies, multiple choice questions, boxes and tables that organize and summarize content, illustrative figures, and references. Through all of these efforts, they have produced an enormously useful text for students and practitioners alike in the care of the well newborn.

Helen Varney Burst, CNM, MSN, DHL (Hon.), FACNM
Professor Emeritus
Yale University School of Nursing

Contributors

Sheron A. Bautista, MSN, NNP-C
Neonatal Nurse Practitioner
Parkland Health & Hospital Systems
Children's Health Children's Medical Center
Allen, TX

Curry J. Bordelon, NNP-BC,
  CPNP-AC, MBA
Lead Practitioner
Mednax Medical Group
Piedmont Healthcare
Atlanta, GA

Nicole Boucher, PhD, RN, CPNP-PC
Clinical Assistant Professor
Department of Health Behavior and
  Biological Sciences
School of Nursing
University of Michigan
Ann Arbor, MI

Cara A. Busenhart, PhD, CNM, APRN
Program Director, Nurse-Midwifery
  Education
Clinical Assistant Professor
School of Nursing
University of Kansas Medical Center
Kansas City, KS

Susan Dragoo, DNP, WHNP
St. Joseph Hospital Women's Services
Orange, CA
Lecturer
School of Nursing
California State University, Fullerton
Fullerton, CA

Amy Jnah, BSN, MSN, DNP, NNP-BC
Clinical Assistant Professor
East Carolina University
Greenville, NC

Donna J. Marvicsin, PhD, PPCNP-BC, CDE
Clinical Associate Professor
Health Behavior and Biological Sciences
School of Nursing
University of Michigan
Ann Arbor, MI

Barbara A. Overman, CNM, PhD
Associate Professor
College of Nursing
University of New Mexico
Albuquerque, NM

Karla Reinhard, DNP, FNP-C, ARNP
Clinical Assistant Professor
School of Nursing
Oregon Health and Science University
Ashland, OR

Pamela J. Reis, PhD, CNM, NNP-BC
College of Nursing
East Carolina University
Greenville, NC

Jenna Shaw-Battista, RN, NP, CNM, PhD
Associate Health Sciences Clinical Professor
Director
Master's Entry Program in Nursing
Betty Irene Moore School of Nursing
University of California, Davis
Sacramento, CA

Rachel Stapleton, BSN, RN
Student Nurse-Midwife
Minneapolis, MN
Adjunct Faculty
Nursing Department
Bethel University
Saint Paul, MN

Dorinda L. Welle, PhD
Assistant Professor
College of Nursing
University of New Mexico
Albuquerque, NM

Katrina Wu, CNM, MSN
Nursing Faculty
Nurse-Midwifery Program
Bethel University
Health Foundations Birth Center
Saint Paul, MN

Reviewers

Becky Bagley, DNP, CNM
Associate Clinical Professor, Program
   Director
East Carolina University College of Nursing

Claudia Beckmann, PhD, APN
Associate Dean and Associate Professor
Rutgers University School of Nursing,
   Camden

Melissa Davis, MSN, CNM, FNP
Instructor of Clinical Nursing
Vanderbilt University School of Nursing

Barbara Lester, PhD
Professor
Northwest Nazarene University

**Steadman McPeters, DNP, CPNP-AC,
   CRNP, RNFA**
Dual Option Pediatric Nurse Practitioner
   Specialty Track Coordinator
University of Alabama, Birmingham

Gretchen G. Mettler, PhD
Assistant Professor
Director, Nurse–Midwife Education
   Program
Frances Payne Bolton School of Nursing,
   Case Western Reserve University

Pamela J. Reis, PhD, CNM, NNP-BC
Assistant Professor
East Carolina University College of Nursing

Tedra S. Smith, DNP, CPNP-PC
Assistant Professor
University of Alabama, Birmingham

CHAPTER 1

PROFESSIONAL RESPONSIBILITIES IN THE PROVISION OF NEWBORN CARE

Sandra L. Gardner and B. J. Snell

Newborn care is provided by a wide variety of providers, ranging from nurse practitioners, certified nurse–midwives, certified midwives, and certified professional midwives, to clinical nurse specialists, physicians, and physician assistants. Education with a focus on the newborn and initial month of life ensures the stabilization and ongoing transition of the baby from birth. Care of the newborn requires the provider to not only have current expertise but also be cognizant of and meet the standards of care.

The purpose of such standards is to assist clinicians in providing effective neonatal health services, and to encourage them to use resources appropriately to achieve optimal healthcare outcomes. The term newborn resulting from an uncomplicated pregnancy and birth requires more surveillance—rather than intervention—after the initial stabilization. Neonatal resuscitation guidelines label this practice "routine care." Early surveillance and development of a plan of care provides a foundation for the baby to make the transition to extrauterine life and thrive in the first month of life.

While the information included in this text is addressed to nonphysician providers, the content is not specific to any particular profession. In 1980, the American Nurses Association (ANA, 1980) defined nursing as "the diagnosis and treatment of the human response to actual or potential health problems." In 2003, the ANA updated the definition of nursing to include the following elements:

- The protection, promotion, and optimization of health and abilities
- Prevention of illness and injury

- Alleviation of suffering through the diagnosis and treatment of the human response to actual or potential health problems
- Advocacy in the care of individuals, families, communities, and populations

A newer definition of nursing includes important components of the ANA's (2015a) *Code of Ethics for Nurses.*

In addition, advanced clinicians (i.e., certified nurse–midwives [CNM], certified midwives [CM], certified professional midwives [CPM], nurse practitioners [NP], clinical nurse specialists [CNS], and certified registered nurse anesthetists [CRNA]) are responsible for taking medical histories, performing physical examinations, performing diagnostic testing, establishing diagnoses, and providing treatments. Consultation, collaboration, co-management, and referral of the patient to medical colleagues and other health professionals, when necessary, are other responsibilities of the advanced practice provider.

The newly born human infant and the neonate (defined as an infant from birth through the first 28 days of life) rely on nurses and advanced practice providers to render care that meets national, state, and local standards. This chapter outlines the professional responsibilities of such healthcare providers, including an overview of why newborns are different; professional practice including standards of care, scope of practice, and evidence-based practice; and ethical and legal guidelines that apply to all providers of care to newborns and neonates.

Why Newborns Are Different

The newborn/neonate is a unique patient who, although unable to communicate with language, communicates with astute, observant, and educated care providers through his or her behavior. Newborns/neonates rely on their care providers, both professional and parental, for prompt, safe, and effective interpretation of their behaviors so that the correct care is provided. Delay in action or misinterpretation of behaviors or signs and symptoms of illness may result in lifelong morbidity, and sometimes even mortality.

Newborns/neonates are anatomically, physiologically, and developmentally different from older infants, children, and adults (**Table 1-1**). Pediatrics—that is, the care of children and their families—is a subspecialty in health care that requires specialized knowledge, skills, and expertise. Pediatric patients are *not* miniature adults, and newborns are *not* miniature infants or adults. Expertise in care of older infants, children, and adults does not enable a care provider to be competent (i.e., safe) in the care of newborns or neonates.

Neonatology—that is, care of newborns from birth through the first 28 days of life—is a subspecialty of pediatric medicine and nursing. Although care of sick children and their parents is part of the curriculum in most health care (medicine, nursing, and midwifery)

Table 1-1: Why Newborns/Neonates Are Different

System	Anatomic/Physiologic Difference	Developmental Immaturity
Respiratory (Gardner, Enzman, & Nyp, 2016)	22–24 weeks' gestation: Differentiation into type I and type II cells (type II create and store surfactant).	Lung development related to gestational age. Surfactant deficiency causes alveolar collapse and is the cause of respiratory distress syndrome in premature lungs.
	24–40 weeks' gestation: Lung differentiates into alveolar ducts and alveoli; decreased mesenchyme and pulmonary capillaries approximate alveoli for gaseous exchange.	Prior to 24–40 weeks, the fetal lungs are incapable of supporting adequate gaseous exchange.
	At term, the number of airways is complete, sufficient for gaseous exchange, and the pulmonary capillary bed is sufficient to carry the gases exchanged.	Continues to develop from birth to about 8 years of age. Ongoing lung development enables infants who suffer severe lung disease at birth to "outgrow" their disease.
	Smaller size, number, and shape of alveoli; smaller diameter of airways.	
	The first breath of life occurs as a result of changes in temperature, handling, and changes in PaO_2 and $PaCO_2$. Exposure of the lung to oxygen decreases pulmonary vascular resistance, increases pulmonary blood flow from 10% in fetal life to 100% in neonatal life, and results in increased pulmonary perfusion and oxygenation.	
	The closer an infant is to term gestation, the more musculature there is around the pulmonary capillary bed. Sudden increases or decreases in oxygen concentration	Adjusting supplemental oxygen, especially lowering the concentration, must be done slowly and in small increments (i.e., 2% to 5%) to avoid the *flip-flop*

(Continued)

Table 1-1: Why Newborns/Neonates Are Different (*Continued*)

System	Anatomic/Physiologic Difference	Developmental Immaturity
	may result in a disproportionate increase or decrease in PaO_2 caused by vasodilation or vasoconstriction.	*phenomenon*. Lowering oxygen concentration, or any hypoxic insult, initiates pulmonary vasoconstriction, which causes hypoperfusion and increased pulmonary vascular resistance.
Cardiac (Gardner, Enzman, & Nyp, 2016)	The first breath of life initiates the change from fetal to adult cardiac circulation as the ductus arteriosus closes in the presence of oxygen and the foramen ovale closes in the presence of increased left-sided heart pressure.	The ductus arteriosus is functionally closed at birth, but is anatomically closed only at around 3 months of age. Any hypoxia event occurring before anatomic closure results in opening of the ductus arteriosus.
	The ductus venosus in the liver is an anatomic shunt that also closes at birth.	The combination of pulmonary hypoperfusion and increased pulmonary vascular resistance in the lungs and the opening of the ductus arteriosus is a return to fetal circulation, a pathologic condition called persistent pulmonary hypertension of the newborn (PPHN).
Central Nervous System (CNS) Thermoregulation (Altimier, 2012; Gardner & Hernandez, 2016a)	Humans are homeotherms—able to increase and decrease body temperature so as to maintain normal core temperature over a wide range of environmental temperatures.	At birth neonates are able to respond as homeotherms, but within a narrower body temperature range than an adult.
	The first neonatal organ that responds to cold stress is the skin. A skin temperature of 36.5°C (97.7°F) is the temperature at which a newborn is thermal neutral or is in a thermal neutral environment (i.e., the	The basal metabolic rate of a newborn is twice that of an adult, so more energy is necessary to maintain normal body temperature.

System	Anatomic/Physiologic Difference	Developmental Immaturity
	temperature at which oxygen consumption and basal metabolic rate are minimal). Waiting for the core temperature (i.e., rectal temperature) to fall is too late for intervention.	
	Skin-to-skin care with parents at and after birth maintains thermal neutrality in newborns. In response to a drop in the newborn's temperature, mothers automatically raise their body temperature (a process called thermal synchrony) to warm their infant.	Lack of subcutaneous fat for insulation, lack of brown fat for nonshivering thermogenesis, and lack of the ability to flex to conserve heat compromise the preterm infant's ability to maintain thermal neutrality. In addition, the hypothalamus of a preterm infant is immature and unable to maintain temperature. The ability to maintain normal body temperature is related to gestational age. Younger, smaller neonates, including late-preterm infants (34 0/7 to 36 6/7 weeks' gestation), are unable to maintain their own body temperature and may need assistance.
	Term newborns may be able to sweat, first on their foreheads, then on their chest, upper arms, and lower body.	Infants less than 36 weeks' gestation do not have the ability to sweat, so they are unable to cool themselves if they are environmentally overheated or if they are febrile.
Pain (Gardner, Enzman, & Agarwal, 2016)		Myelination of pain pathways occurs between 30 and 37 weeks' gestation. Unmyelinated fibers carry pain stimuli more slowly, but in the neonate this is offset by the shorter distance the impulse must travel.

(Continued)

Table 1-1: Why Newborns/Neonates Are Different (*Continued*)

System	Anatomic/Physiologic Difference	Developmental Immaturity
Sensory (Gardner, Goldson, & Hernandez, 2016)	Neonates, including preterm infants, have a CNS that is mature enough to carry and interpret pain stimuli.	Pain perception is well developed in the premature infant, but the inhibitory ability of the CNS to pain is not well developed. Therefore, neonates of younger gestational ages experience more—rather than less—pain. With decreasing gestational age, behavioral pain responses are less robust because of the immaturity of the CNS.
	Pain responses include behavioral, physiologic, and metabolic/ hormonal changes.	
	At birth, term newborns have fully developed and functional sensory perception:	
	• Hearing: Have been hearing since 20–22 weeks in utero; react to loud noises; able to distinguish parents' voices from those of strangers; turn toward auditory stimuli; able to turn toward preferred story heard in utero.	
	• Vision: Able to see light/dark in utero; able to see 8–10 inches from face; able to distinguish/prefer parents' faces; able to follow objects horizontally/ vertically; prefer human face and patterns; recoil from bright light.	Eyes are fused until approximately 26 weeks' gestational age.
	• Smell/taste: Able to taste flavors in utero and know mother's scent from scent in amniotic fluid; able to find maternal nipple by smell; by 5 days of age, term babies are able to turn toward own mother's nursing pad and start sucking; recoil from unpleasant smells	Unable to differentiate salty solution.

System	Anatomic/Physiologic Difference	Developmental Immaturity
	(vinegar, ammonia) and tastes (bitter, acid, sour); prefer sweet taste. • Tactile/kinesthetic: Major method of communication and highest developed sense. Touch is especially well developed in face, around lips (root reflex), and in the hands (grasp reflex). Able to "read" an adult by the manner in which the adult handles and cares for the infant. • Communication: Crying is the language newborns and infants use to communicate their needs. Crying may also be a response to a noisy, cold, boring, or over-stimulating environment. The more responsive adults are to the infant's cries and needs, the less crying is necessary. Infants learn to associate comfort with the responsive caregiver.	Noxious smells cause apnea in younger gestational-age infants.
Circadian rhythm/ sleep–wake cycles (Gardner, Goldson, & Hernandez, 2016)	Humans cycle body functions (i.e., blood pressure, temperature, hormonal changes, urine volume, and sleep–wake) in a 24-hour period.	Development of circadian rhythms in infants is influenced by genetic factors, gender, brain maturation, and the environment.
	Active sleep: Rapid eye movements (REM) and muscle activity such as sucking, rooting, and startles. Adults dream in REM sleep.	At birth and in the first few weeks of life, term newborns begin sleep in active (rather than quiet) sleep, spend more time in active sleep than do adults, sleep 16–19 hours/ day, and distribute their sleep over a 24-hour period.
	Quiet sleep: No rapid eye movement (non-REM).	Infant sleep-cycle duration: 50–60 minutes.

(Continued)

Table 1-1: Why Newborns/Neonates Are Different (*Continued*)

System	Anatomic/Physiologic Difference	Developmental Immaturity
	Adult sleep-cycle duration: 90–100 minutes. Maturation of infant sleep: Better organization of sleep states, decrease in total sleep time, increased quiet sleep, decrease in active sleep, and increase in active and quiet waking. Term newborns develop day–night cycling that is similar to adult cycles of wakefulness and sleep by 9 months of age.	At birth, newborns may still be operating on their "in utero" clock: More active/more quiet behaviors correspond to activity/quiet cycles as a fetus. Gradually, through caregiving, parents teach the infant synchronization with family rhythms.
Neurologic conditions/ presentations (Gardner, Enzman, & Nyp, 2016; Gardner, Goldson, & Hernandez, 2016; Parsons, Seay, & Jacobson, 2016)	At birth newborns display reflexive, unlearned behaviors : • Survival behaviors: Root reflex—finding food	Reflex behaviors are influenced by gestational age: Begins at 28 weeks' gestation; integrates at 3 months of age. Response is less if the baby is sleepy or satiated.
	Sucking—removing food	Begins at 26–28 weeks' gestation.
	Swallowing—ingesting food	Begins at 12 weeks' gestation.
		Not effectively coordinated for oral feedings before 32–34 weeks' gestational age. Coordination of respiration with sucking/ swallowing is consistently achieved by infants more than 37 weeks' postconceptual age.
	• Protective behaviors:	
	Moro reflex	Begins at 28 weeks' gestation.
	Palmar grasp	Begins at 28 weeks' gestation.
	Plantar grasp	Begins at 28 weeks' gestation.
	Babinski reflex	Begins at 28 weeks' gestation.
	Tonic neck reflex	Begins at 35 weeks' gestation.

System	Anatomic/Physiologic Difference	Developmental Immaturity
	Gag reflex	Begins at 36 weeks' gestation. Protects against aspiration and never disappears.
	Blink reflex	Begins at 25 weeks' gestation. Does not disappear.
	Crossed extension	Begins at 28 weeks' gestation.
	Pulmonary ventilation:	
	Breathing is controlled by the neural and chemical systems. The cerebral cortex and brain stem regulate respiratory rate and rhythm. The medulla contains the chemical control system that is sensitive to changes in oxygen and carbon dioxide levels.	In response to hypoxemia, newborns have a brief period of increased ventilation, followed by respiratory depression and even apnea.
	In response to hypoxemia, adults have a sustained increase in ventilation.	Neuronal immaturity is a cause of apnea because respiratory efforts are more unstable at younger gestational ages. Primary apnea or apnea of prematurity occurs when premature infants (including the late-preterm infant) cease respirations for more than 20 seconds and have no other cause for their apnea.
		Because primary apnea or apnea of prematurity is a diagnosis of exclusion, secondary apnea due to other causes must be ruled out. Other causes of secondary apnea may include infection, seizures, airway obstruction, respiratory/cardiac diseases, vomiting/aspiration, drugs, hypoglycemia, hypocalcemia, hypothermia, stooling, position, pain, and anemia.
	Neonatal seizures are among the most frequent signs, and occasionally the only sign, that there is CNS dysfunction.	Clinical presentation of neonatal seizure is more subtle and less organized than seizure presentations in older children and adults. This subtle presentation of seizures depends on gestational

(Continued)

Table 1-1: Why Newborns/Neonates Are Different (*Continued*)

System	Anatomic/Physiologic Difference	Developmental Immaturity
	Seizures occur more frequently in the neonatal period than at any other period of life (Volpe, 2008). Neonatal seizures may be caused by acute or chronic disorders of the brain, including metabolic conditions, genetic metabolic conditions, infections, hemorrhage, and hypoxic-ischemic encephalopathy. Congenital malformations, drug withdrawal, kernicterus, local anesthetic intoxication, and familial and idiopathic seizures are also possible causes.	age, so that premature infants present with even less organized seizure activity than term infants (Volpe, 2008).
Immune System		
Antiallergenic	Maternal intake of cow and/or soy protein may sensitize the fetus.	Newborns sensitized in utero to cow and/or soy protein (Kattan, Cocco, & Jarvinen, 2011; Klemola et al., 2002; Martinez & Ballew, 2011).
Anti-inflammatory/ anti-infective (Gardner, 2008, 2009; Gardner & Lawrence, 2016)	Maternal antibodies are passed through the placenta to the fetus. Colonized with maternal flora if born vaginally; colonized with institutional flora if born by cesarean section. Antibodies to all infections that the mother has had or been immunized against are passed through maternal breastmilk. Breastmilk has anti-infective and anti-inflammatory properties, as well as nucleotides, that protect newborns/neonates from inflammation and infection.	Immature immune system that is gestational age-specific: • Less nonspecific (inflammatory) immunity • Less specific (humoral) immunity • Less passive immunity • No local inflammatory reaction to portal of entry of infection Undernourished/growth-restricted infants of any gestational age are more prone to infections because of the effect of under-nutrition on the immune system.

System	Anatomic/Physiologic Difference	Developmental Immaturity
Hematologic		
Hyperbilirubinemia (Kamath-Rayne, Thilo, Deacon, & Hernandez, 2016)	Red blood cells' (RBC) life span in adults: 120 days. Neonates have higher RBC mass per kilogram weight when compared to adults.	RBCs' life span in neonates: 70–90 days.
	Neonates' rate of bilirubin production (8–10 mg/kg/h) is 2–2.5 times higher than that in adults. Accelerated RBC breakdown accounts for 75–85% of increased bilirubin levels in newborns.	Ability of liver to handle bilirubin production related to gestational age: The younger the gestational age, the more problems the infant will have in managing bilirubin.
	Enterophepatic circulation of bilirubin results when conjugated bilirubin (in the meconium in the large intestine) is converted by beta-glucuronidase back into glucuronic acid and unconjugated bilirubin and is reabsorbed.	Compared to full-term newborns, late-preterm newborns: • Have peak bilirubin levels later (5–7 days of life) • Are 2.4 times more likely to develop significant hyperbilirubinemia • Are readmitted to the hospital for treatment of bilirubin 2–2.5 times more often
		Developmental immaturity of the glucuronyl-transferase system causes hyperbilirubinemia in late-preterm infants.
	Physiologic jaundice in normal full-term newborns: • Phase I: Mean peak total serum bilirubin (TSB) of 5–6 mg/dL between 3 and 4 days of life. • Phase II: Rapid decline in TSB to 3 mg/dL by the end of first week of life, until the normal adult level of 2 mg/dL is reached at the end of the second week of life.	Physiologic jaundice excluded in full-term newborn: • Clinical jaundice in first 24 hours of life. • TSB concentration increases more than 0.2 mg/dL/h. • TSB concentration exceeds 95th percentile for age in hours. • Direct serum bilirubin level is more than 1.5–2 mg/dL. • Clinical jaundice persists more than 2 weeks.

(Continued)

Table 1-1: Why Newborns/Neonates Are Different (*Continued*)

System	Anatomic/Physiologic Difference	Developmental Immaturity
Gastrointestinal (GI)	GI tract is anatomically complete by 20–22 weeks' gestation. Functional development begins in utero and continues into infancy (Brown et al., 2016). GI functions that are activated at birth, regardless of the length of gestation: • Decreased intestinal permeability • Increased mucosal lactase activity GI functions that are intrinsically programmed to occur at a specific postconceptual age: • Onset of peristalsis at 28–30 weeks • Coordination of suck, swallow, and breathing at 33–36 weeks GI functions that are influenced by the environment: • Colonization by bacteria at birth • Introduction of enteral nutrients into the GI tract, which promotes ongoing maturation and development of the GI tract Colic, excessive air in the GI tract, and/or gastroesophageal reflux disease (GERD) may present with fussiness/irritability, gassiness, and crying. Other symptoms of GERD include distress with regurgitation, refusal to feed, painful swallowing, arching of the back, aspiration, apnea/bradycardia, and emesis, resulting in complications or decreased quality of life for the	Infants born before term gestation, including late-preterm infants, have anatomic and functional limits to the tolerance and digestion of enteral nutrition (Brown et al., 2016): • Neurologic immaturity influences coordination of suck, swallow, and breathing and GI motility. • Peristalsis that is bidirectional with forward movement toward the stomach develops near term gestation. • Intermittent relaxation of the lower esophageal sphincter muscle, combined with abnormal peristalsis, contributes to GERD. • Immature, disorganized intestinal motor activity compared to term infants; maturation of motor activity occurs between 33 and 40 weeks' gestation • Increased lactase activity with enteral feeding approaches full-term infant levels by 10 days after birth.

System	Anatomic/Physiologic Difference	Developmental Immaturity
	infant and family (Bhatia & Parish, 2009; Neu et al., 2012; Vandenplas & Alarcon, 2015).	
	Nearly 73% of term infants experience at least one episode of regurgitation/day, with the highest rate in the first month of life (Hegar et al., 2009). No symptoms of irritability or discomfort accompanying regurgitation results in these infants being called "happy spitters" (Hegar et al., 2009).	Regurgitation—the involuntary return of previously swallowed formula or secretions into or out of the mouth—is a benign, normal process due to (Hegar et al., 2009; Hyman et al., 2006): • Shortened esophagus • Immaturity of the esophagus and stomach • The obtuse angle of His • Reduced esophageal pressure • A diet of liquids
Glucose Homeostasis (Rozance, McGowan, Price-Douglas, & Hay, 2016)	At birth, both glucose supply and serum glucose concentrations fall. After birth, catecholamine levels increase, as do glucagon concentrations and receptor sensitivity. Increased glucagon and norepinephrine levels induce glycogenolysis, and hepatic glucose is released. Increased levels of catecholamines release fatty acids that are metabolized into precursors for gluconeogenesis.	Causes of hypoglycemia: • Inadequate substrate supply • Abnormal endocrine regulation of glucose metabolism • Increased rate of glucose utilization
	Glucose homeostasis is the result of the balance between hepatic glucose output (rate of glycogenolysis and gluconeogenesis) and glucose utilization by the brain and peripheral tissues.	Peripheral glucose utilization varies depending on the metabolic demands placed on the newborn. Normal term newborns' steady-state glucose production/utilization rate is 4–6 mg/min/kg—twice the weight-specific rate of adults.

(Continued)

Table 1-1: Why Newborns/Neonates Are Different (*Continued*)

System	Anatomic/Physiologic Difference	Developmental Immaturity
	Perinatal glucose utilization increases in: • Hypoxia, due to inefficiency of anaerobic glycolysis • Hyperinsulinemia, which increases glucose uptake by insulin-sensitive tissues • Respiratory distress, due to increased muscle activity • Cold stress, which leads to increased sympathetic nervous system activity with release of norepinephrine, epinephrine, and thyroid hormones, which increase metabolic rate	
Nephrology/Renal (Cadnapaphornchai, Schoenbein, Woloschuk, Soranno, & Hernandez, 2016)	The fetal kidney regulates amniotic fluid balance. By 34–35 weeks' gestation, the kidney contains the adult complement of 600,000 nephrons. Extracellular fluid (ECF) volume of the term newborn is 40%. The newborn kidney reduces ECF during the first week of life, so that body weight may decrease by 10%. A marked increase in the glomerular filtration rate (GFR) occurs after term birth. Newborns have a limited capacity to concentrate urine.	Preterm birth decreases the number of nephrons compared to the number in full-term newborns. Undernourished/growth-restricted and extremely low-birth-weight newborns may never achieve a normal number of nephrons. Risk of intravascular volume depletion is higher when fluid intake is limited; infants become dehydrated more quickly if intake is inadequate.

System	Anatomic/Physiologic Difference	Developmental Immaturity
Skin	Skin receptors sense environmental temperature and the rate of temperature change. Skin receptors, located throughout the body, are especially concentrated in the trigeminal area of the face. Both peripheral and central receptors send messages to the hypothalamus of the brain, which controls conservation, dissipation, and production of body heat.	A decrease in core temperature in adults is the impetus for heat production, whereas a decrease in skin temperature is the impetus for heat production in the neonate. In the first week of life, the immaturity of a newborn's skin—even a term baby's skin—is the largest contributor to heat loss through evaporation.
Hormonal	Response to cold stress (Altimier, 2012). Hormonal/catabolic stress response to uncontrolled pain (Gardner, Enzman, & Agarwal, 2016): • Increased: plasma renin levels; catecholamine levels (epinephrine/norepinephrine); cortisol levels; nitrogen excretion/ protein catabolism; release of growth hormone, glucagons, and aldosterone; serum levels of glucose, lactate, pyruvate, ketones, and nonesterified fatty acids • Decreased: insulin secretion, prolactin, immune responses	Insufficient amounts of epinephrine and norepinephrine may dampen the newborn's response to cold stress. Decompensatory phase in which the body is unable to maintain "fight or flight" response: Vital signs return to normal, complicating the assessment for pain, but the newborn is still in pain (Gardner, Enzman, & Agarwal, 2016).

programs, care of well newborns is usually relegated to a few days of caring for normal term newborns and their mothers. The subspecialty of neonatal nursing is learned on the job and in graduate and doctoral advanced practice preparation. *All* advanced practice providers—CNMs, CMs, CPMs, NPs (i.e., family, pediatric, and neonatal), and CNSs—who care for newborns and neonates must be educated to care for this special, resilient, yet fragile pediatric population.

The following principles of neonatal assessment govern care of the newborn and neonate, regardless of the type of provider:

- *The younger the child, the more quickly care providers need to diagnose and treat the child.* For example, when considering postnatal age, a 4-hour-old infant needs care faster than a 4-day-old infant, who needs care faster than a 4-week-old infant. Postconceptual age also needs to be considered. Late-preterm infants, defined as those from 34 6/7 to 36 6/7 weeks' gestation (Engle, 2006), have increased morbidity and mortality when compared to full-term (39–40 weeks' gestation) infants.

- *Care of a newborn or neonate involves care of the whole family.* Parents must be taught how to read and interpret infant cues, how to know if their infant is acting differently, and who to contact if they have concerns about their infant. Newborns and neonates cannot verbalize that they are having a "hard time breathing" or "it hurts here"—parents and caregivers need to be able to objectively discern this information, know the significance, and take immediate action. A change in feeding behavior is often the earliest symptom perceived by parents. An 8-day-old full-term baby with a history of demanding and feeding every 1 to 3 hours who is now not demanding, is difficult to awaken, or refuses to feed needs to be evaluated immediately by the care provider. Normal, healthy, full-term 8-day-old babies do not change their feeding behavior for no reason!

- *Neonatal signs and symptoms of illness are subtle and may be caused by numerous etiologies that have to be ruled in and out.* For example, the full-term newborn who shows the change in feeding behaviors mentioned previously needs to be assessed for all of the following:

  - Hypoglycemia: This condition is not as common in full-term infants, but hypoglycemic infants feed poorly. A point-of-care (POC) glucose screening test can quickly rule hypoglycemia in or out of the differential diagnosis.

  - Hyperbilirubinemia: Is this baby visibly jaundiced? Jaundice can be a symptom of neonatal infection. Hyperbilirubinemia makes babies sleepy and can be a cause of poor feeding.

  - Dehydration: Is this baby's intake sufficient to maintain adequate intake of fluids (and calories)? By the end of the first week of life, a neonate should be gaining weight at the rate of ½–1 oz/day. Weigh the baby and compare the result to the last weight.

  - Neonatal infection/sepsis: Is this baby infected? Besides feeding changes, how are the vital signs (temperature, pulse, respirations, blood pressure, pain) and perfusion (capillary refill time, mottling, cyanosis, pallor)? Are there any obvious sites of infection on physical examination, such as an erythematous, indurated area around the umbilicus or the baby's mouth coated with oral thrush? In infants with infection, physical examination of the abdomen may show distention, pain with palpation, and a bloody stool. A pulse oximetry evaluation of 85% saturation in room air is worrisome. A hypotonic, floppy baby who does not respond to the physical examination with crying or respond to the heel stick may have sepsis.

Defining the Healthcare Provider's Practice

Professional Nursing and Midwifery Practice

Standards of Care and Practice From a legal standpoint, professional nursing care providers are responsible and accountable to provide the standard of care to their patients. The standard of care is defined as care given by a reasonably prudent provider, advanced practice nurse, or midwife (or physician assistant or physician) in the same or similar circumstances (Meissner-Cutler & Gardner, 1997). Professionals are responsible and accountable to provide their patients with the national, state, and local standard of care. The standard of care for specialty practice (e.g., families, newborns, and neonates) constantly changes based on research and technology. Professional nurses and advanced practice nurses are required by the *Code of Ethics for Nurses* (ANA, 2015a) and their state nurse practice acts to remain competent. Likewise, midwives are required by the American Midwifery Certification Board (AMCB), the International Confederation of Midwives (ICM), and their respective state laws and regulations to maintain competency in the care of newborns.

Standards of nursing care and practice are promulgated by professional nursing organizations, regulatory agencies, and legislative bodies (Enzman Hines, 2012). The American Nurses Association creates and publishes standards that apply to all professional nursing practitioners and provides the template, based on nursing process and diagnosis, for specialty nursing standards (ANA, 2015b). **Table 1-2** outlines these universal standards as well as specialty practice standards for nurses and advanced practice nurses caring for mothers, newborns, and neonates. In addition to standards created by nursing and midwifery organizations, standards, guidelines, and position statements for care are promulgated by midwifery, neonatal, and pediatric organizations that must also be considered and followed by healthcare practitioners (Table 1-2).

The standard (scope) of practice is defined in each state's nurse (or medical) practice act. In a few instances, independent boards regulate the practice of midwives. State practice acts outline and define the activities within the scope of practice for a given type of provider. The standard of care is also defined and delineated in institutional policies, procedures, and protocols.

A birth center or hospital maternal–newborn service must have policies, procedures, guidelines, and protocols that meet the following criteria:

- Reflect the national and state standard of care
- Are periodically updated and dated

Table 1-2: Standards of Care and Practice for Specialty Care Providers for Families, Newborns, and Neonates

Organization	Standards	Description
American Nurses Association (ANA) • First nursing organization (1911) • First definition of professional nursing (1932) • First standards of nursing practice (1973)	1980: *Nursing: A Social Policy Statement*	Defines basic standards of professional nursing practice; differentiates between standards of care and standards of professional practice. Defines nursing and clarifies the nature and scope of nursing practice.
	2015: *Nursing: Scope and Standards of Practice,* 3rd ed.	Defines basic standards for all types of nursing practice; encompasses minimally acceptable levels of nursing care and nursing performance.
	2015: *Code of Ethics for Nurses with Interpretive Statements*	Defines nine components of nursing's ethical code of conduct and establishes the ethical standard for the nursing profession. The code is not negotiable in any setting, nor is it subject to revision or amendment except by the ANA.
American Nurses Association (ANA) and National Association of Neonatal Nurses (NANN)	2013: *Scope and Standards of Practice for Neonatal Nursing,* 2nd ed.	Defines the responsibilities and accountability to the public and the nursing profession of all registered nurses who care for high-risk neonates and their families.
American College of Nurse–Midwives (ACNM) • Roots dating to 1929 • Professional organization of certified nurse–midwives (CNM) and certified midwives (CM)	2011: *Standards for the Practice of Midwifery*	Presents 8 standards of CNM and CM practice related to qualifications and a safe environment; supports individual rights and self-determination

Organization	Standards	Description
		within the boundaries of safety, culturally competent care, with written practice guidelines, documented completely and in an accessible form, evaluated for quality management that includes a plan to identify and solve problems, and expansion beyond ACNM core competencies.
	2012: *Definition of Midwifery and Scope of Practice for Certified Nurse–Midwives and Certified Midwives*	Defines CNMs and CMs who, after their midwifery education, must demonstrate that they meet the *Core Competencies for Basic Midwifery Practice* of the ACNM (2012a) and must practice within the ACNM's *Standards for the Practice of Midwifery* (2011).
Provides standard setting documents to articulate Women's Health and Newborn Care	2015: *Code of Ethics with Explanatory Statements*	Describes midwifery code of conduct.
	2011: *Position Statement Breastfeeding*	Provides midwifery support for and involvement with breastfeeding to ensure success.
	2012: *Core Competencies for Basic Midwifery Practice, VI. Newborn Care Core Competencies*	Articulates the specialized knowledge, skills, and basic competencies of midwifery practices attained in formal education program.
Association of Women's Health, Obstetric, and Neonatal Nurses (AWHONN) • Founded in 1969 • Published first standards in 1974 • Became an independent organization in 1993	2006: *Hyperbilirubinemia: Identification and Management in Healthy Term and Late Preterm Infants*, 2nd ed.	Clinical practice monograph for nurses about hyperbilirubinemia that supports the 2004 AAP guideline on universal screening of all neonates before discharge from the hospital.

(Continued)

Table 1-2: Standards of Care and Practice for Specialty Care Providers for Families, Newborns, and Neonates (*Continued*)

Organization	Standards	Description
	2007: *Neonatal Nursing Clinical Competencies and Education Guide*, 6th ed.	A framework for the specialized knowledge, skills, and competencies necessary for evidence-based neonatal nursing practice. Used for orientation and continuing education for all levels of neonatal nurses.
	2009: *Standards for Professional Nursing Practice in the Care of Women and Newborns*, 7th ed.	Describes specialty-specific practice standards for inpatient and outpatient care.
	2013: *Evidence-Based Clinical Practice Guideline: Neonatal Skin Care*, 3rd ed.	Clinical practice guideline on care of neonatal skin based on the latest research evidence.
	2014: *Assessment and Care of the Late Preterm Infant*	Evidence-based clinical practice guidelines for nursing care and advanced practice nursing care of the late-preterm infant.
	2015: *Breastfeeding*	Position statement about the importance of supporting, protecting, and promoting breastfeeding as the optimal nutrition for human newborns.
National Association of Neonatal Nurses (NANN) • Founded in 1984 • Consists of subspecialty interest groups (i.e., clinicians, practitioners, clinical nurse specialists, transport nurses, and educators) • Promulgates standards on practice and education	2010: *Prevention of Acute Bilirubin Encephalopathy and Kernicterus in Newborns*	Position statement #3049 recommends universal screening of all newborns with either serum or transcutaneous bilirubin levels, parent education, and follow-up after discharge.
	2013: Walden & Gibbens: *Newborn Pain Assessment and Management Guideline for Practice*, 3rd ed.	Clinical practice guideline on best evidence-based practices in pain assessment and management for full-term and premature newborns.

Organization	Standards	Description
National Association of Pediatric Nurse Practitioners (NAPNAP) • Established in 1973	2010: *PNP's Role in Supporting Infant and Family Well-Being in the First Year of Life*	Position statement about the PNP's role and skills in providing care for newborns and infants and their families.
• Dedicated to improving the quality of health care for infants, children, and adolescents by advancing the pediatric nurse practitioner's (PNP) role in providing pediatric care	2012: *Breastfeeding*	Position statement about the importance of PNPs in educating, promoting, and supporting breastfeeding as optimal infant nutrition.
American Academy of Pediatrics (AAP) and American College of Obstetrics and Gynecology (ACOG) (with a liaison representative from NANN)	2012: *Guidelines for Perinatal Care*, 7th ed.	Evidence-based recommendations to improve pregnancy outcomes, reduce maternal and perinatal mortality and morbidity, ensure safe and effective diagnostic and therapeutic interventions in maternal–fetal and neonatal care. Revised definitions of levels of care.
American Academy of Pediatrics (AAP), Committee on Fetus and Newborn	2012: "Circumcision Policy Statement"	Policies and position statements about the need to relieve the pain of male infants while being circumcised as well as after the procedure.
American College of Obstetricians and Gynecologists (ACOG)	2001: "Committee Opinion #260: Circumcision"	
American Society of Pain Management Nurses	2011: *Position Statement: Male Infant Circumcision Pain Management*	
American Academy of Pediatrics (AAP) and American Heart Association (AHA)	2011: Neonatal Resuscitation Program (NRP) (Kattwinkel, 2011)	Provides training for care providers in the equipment and skills necessary and the evidence to support the scientific consensus of the International Liaison Committee on Resuscitation (ILCOR).

(Continued)

Table 1-2: Standards of Care and Practice for Specialty Care Providers for Families, Newborns, and Neonates (*Continued*)

Organization	Standards	Description
Adamkin and American Academy of Pediatrics (AAP), Committee on Fetus and Newborn	2011: *Postnatal Glucose Homeostasis in Late-Preterm and Term Infants*	Guideline for the screening and management of neonatal hypoglycemia in asymptomatic late-preterm and term infants born to mothers with diabetes, as well as newborns who are small or large for gestational age.
American Academy of Pediatrics (AAP), Subcommittee on Hyperbilirubinemia	2004: "Clinical Practice Guideline: Management of Hyperbilirubinemia in the Newborn Infant 35 or More Weeks' of Gestation"	Guidelines for phototherapy and exchange transfusion and stratification of infants 35 or more weeks' gestation as being at low, medium, or higher risk to develop significant hyperbilirubinemia.
	2009: Maisels et al.: "Hyperbilirubinemia in the Newborn Infant 35 or More Weeks' Gestation"	Algorithm of recommendations for management and follow-up according to predischarge transcutaneous or serum bilirubin levels, gestation, and risk factors for hyperbilirubinemia.
American Academy of Pediatrics (AAP), Task Force on Sudden Infant Death Syndrome (SIDS)	2011: "SIDS and Other Sleep Related Infant Deaths: Expansion of Recommendations for a Safe Infant Sleep Environment"	Recommendations for safe sleep, such as supine rather than prone sleeping, no bed sleeping with parents or siblings, and no soft bedding, toys, or blankets.
Anand and International Evidence-Based Group for Neonatal Pain	2001: "Consensus Statement For the Prevention and Management of Pain in the Newborn"	Evidence-based guidelines for prevention, assessment, and management of neonatal pain regardless of gestational age or severity of illness.
AWHONN statement endorsed by American Academy of Family Physicians, American Academy of Pediatrics, American College of Nurse–Midwives, American College of Obstetricians and Gynecologists, and Society for Maternal–Fetal Medicine	2012: "Quality Patient Care in Labor and Delivery: A Call to Action"	Call to action for all who provide perinatal care to optimize maternal health outcomes through effective communication, shared decision making, teamwork, and data-driven quality improvement initiatives.

Organization	Standards	Description
Academy of Breastfeeding Medicine	2010: "Protocol #23: Non-pharmacologic Management of Procedure-Related Pain in the Breastfeeding Infant"	Recommendations about the use of breastfeeding and other nonpharmacologic interventions for procedural pain in the breastfeeding infant.
Centers for Disease Control and Prevention (CDC)	2010: "Prevention of Perinatal Group B Streptococcal (GBS) Disease Among Newborns" (revised guidelines from CDC, 2010)	Algorithm for secondary prevention of early-onset group B streptococcal (GBS) disease in newborn infants.
Engle, Tomashek, Wallman, and Committee on Fetus and Newborn of the American Academy of Pediatrics	2007: "'Late-Preterm' Infants: A Population at Risk"	18 discharge criteria for the late-preterm infant.

- Are prepared by a qualified committee through the collaboration of nurses, midwives, and physicians who practice in the area
- Reflect evidence-based care from the professional literature
- Are archived by the institution for the length of liability
- Are accessible and familiar to the staff

Institutional policies, procedures, and protocols *are* the standard of care for an institution, and their existence creates a presumption that the policies, procedures, guidelines, and protocols of the institution *will be* followed.

Scope of Practice The scope of practice for nurses and midwives is defined by professional nursing and midwifery organizations, regulatory agencies, and legislative bodies (Enzman Hines, 2012). Scope of practice addresses the "who, what, where, why and how of nursing practice" (ANA, 2015b). The depth and breadth of practice (in nurses and midwives with experience ranging from newly graduated to advanced practice) depends on the practitioner's education, experience, roles, and population(s) served (ANA, 2015b).

The scope of professional nursing practice encompasses three functions or actions, as outlined in **Table 1-3**. Independent nursing functions, such as the provision of a safe physical environment, apply to patient care in acute- and chronic-care settings, in clinics, in birth centers, and at home. Collaboratively written practice protocols and guidelines are examples

Table 1-3: Scope of Professional Nursing Practice

Functions/Actions	Definitions
Independent	Aspects of nursing practice contained in state nurse practice acts that require no supervision or direction. Formulation of nursing diagnoses and application of the nursing process are independent nursing functions required by statute of the licensed professional nurse.
Interdependent	Aspects of nursing practice performed in collaboration with other healthcare professionals. Collaboratively written institutional protocols delineate the conditions and treatments the nurse is permitted to administer.
Dependent	Aspects of nursing practice dependent on the written order of another professional. The advanced practice nurse or physician prescribes medications; the nurse administers the prescribed medication. The nurse is also responsible for independent actions: (1) knowing the proper medication, dosage, and route; (2) safe administration; (3) monitoring effects and adverse responses; and (4) advocating for the patient regarding proper administration, dosage, and route.

Reproduced from Meissner-Cutler, S., & Gardner S., L. (1997). Maternal–child nursing and the law. In S. L. Gardner & M. Enzman Hagedorn (Eds.), *Legal aspects of maternal–child nursing practice*. Menlo Park, CA: Addison-Wesley. ©1997. Reprinted by permission of Pearson Education, Inc., New York, New York.

of documents specifying interdependent nursing functions. Practice protocols and guidelines should be periodically reviewed, revised, and updated according to the schedules of accrediting or licensing agencies (such as The Joint Commission, the Commission for the Accreditation of Birth Centers, or the State Board of Nursing) (Enzman Hines, 2012). Dependent functions require the order of another professional, but also necessitate that the nurse or midwife carries out orders within her or his scope of practice, carries out orders safely and properly using independent knowledge, and uses competence to advocate for and protect patients (Meissner-Cutler & Gardner, 1997).

Professional Medical Practice

Physicians and physician assistants are required to provide their patients with the standard of care and to adhere to the standards of practice of their professions as promulgated by their professional organization(s) and defined by their state practice acts. In addition, their scope of practice is defined by their professional organizations, regulatory agencies, and legislative bodies. Medical practice and the standards of medical practice are beyond the scope of this text; instead, readers are referred to their professional organizations and the medical practice acts of the states in which they work.

Evidence-Based Practice

Evidence-based practice (EBP) requires integration of the best and highest-quality research evidence with clinical expertise and each patient's unique values and circumstances (Pantoja & Enzman Hines, 2016; Straus, Glasziou, Richardson, & Haynes, 2011). All too often, clinicians fail to use evidence in an optimal manner—that is, evidence-based therapies may be underused, overused, or misused, or system failures occur (Pantoja & Enzman Hines, 2016). Best care for patients, however, demands true EBP.

All research is not equal. Quantitative clinical research to evaluate the safety and efficacy of therapies has been divided by Sinclair and Bracken (1992) into four levels:

- Highest level: Randomized controlled trials (RCTs)
- Nonrandomized studies with concurrent controls
- Nonrandomized studies with historical controls
- Lowest level: Single case or case series reports without controls

From an international collaboration, the GRADE system was developed for grading evidence and the strength of recommendations. GRADE classifies evidence into one of four levels—high, moderate, low, or very low—with the strength of the evidence rated as strong or weak (**Table 1-4**). Values, preferences, economic implications, and desirable and undesirable effects are factors that influence the strength of the recommendations within this

Table 1-4: Levels of Evidence

Level of Evidence	Therapy/Prevention/Etiology/Harm
1a	Systematic reviews
1b	Individual RCT with narrow confidence intervals
1c	All or none
2a	Systematic review of cohort studies
2b	Individual cohort study (including low-quality RCT [less than 80% follow-up])
3a	Systematic review of case-control study
3b	Individual case-control
4	Case-controlled studies
5	Expert opinion without critical appraisal

Abbreviation: RCT, randomized controlled trial.
Reproduced from Straus, S. E., Glasziou, P., Richardson, W. S., & Haynes, R. B. (2011). Evidence-based medicine: How to practice and teach it (4th ed.). London, UK: Harcourt. Copyright Harcourt Publishers 2011. Reprinted by permission of Elsevier.

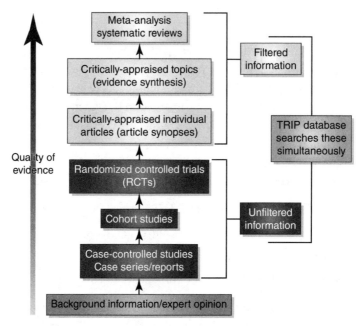

Figure 1-1: Evidence appraisal.
Data from Pantoja, A. F., & Enzman Hines, M. (2016). Evidence-based clinical practice. In S. L. Gardner, B. S. Carter, M. Enzman Hines, & J. A. Hernandez (Eds.), *Merenstein and Gardner's handbook of neonatal intensive care* (8th ed., pp. 1–10). St. Louis, MO: Mosby-Elsevier.

system (**Figure 1-1**). RCTs, for example, test hypotheses by randomly assigning treatment and control groups of adequate size to examine the safety and efficacy of new therapies. A meta-analysis is a systematic review of the highest-quality research (generally RCTs) from the current literature that uses statistical methods to combine the results of individual studies and summarize the results (e.g., Cochrane Neonatal Review Group, http://neonatal .cochrane.org).

Qualitative research facilitates an understanding of the lived experiences and values of patients being studied. It guides decision making as to whether the findings of quantitative research are replicable in other, different populations (Pantoja & Enzman Hines, 2016).

Legal Issues

Statute of Limitations

All states have legislation defining a specific time frame in which a person who is injured or harmed due to professional negligence may file a lawsuit. This time limit for filing a lawsuit is called the statute of limitations. The statute of limitation varies by state but generally ranges from 2 to 7 years from the date of the negligence resulting in injury or harm

(Meissner-Cutler & Gardner, 1997). In the case of a minor (most often defined as a child younger than the age of 18 years), however, the term of the statute of limitations may not begin to run until the child reaches the age of majority (i.e., 18 to 21 years depending on state law). Therefore all providers caring for minors have a protracted period of liability.

Not only does the term of the statute of limitations vary by state, but the application differs by state. The time period for the statute may be designated as beginning to run from any one of the following:

- The date of the act causing the injury (*Olsen v. St. Croix Valley Memorial Hospital*, 1972)
- The date of last treatment by the particular care provider
- The "date of the discovery" of the injury (*Teeters v. Currey*, 1974)

The date of discovery is the date that the patient knew or should have known of the injury (*Renslow v. Mennonite Hospital*, 1977). The following maternal–child nursing example illustrates the possibility of delay in knowing of the injury one has suffered from professional negligence.

Suppose a nurse caring for a postpartum woman fails to administer an ordered RhoGAM injection to an Rh-negative patient who delivered an Rh-positive baby, or a midwife caring for a postpartum woman fails to order a RhoGAM injection for an Rh-negative patient who delivered an Rh-positive baby. Four years later, this same woman becomes pregnant. Because of the prior development of antibodies, her new Rh-positive fetus is affected, causing injury to the child's brain, nervous system, and other organs. Even though more than 2 years has passed since the failure to order or administer RhoGAM, the woman did not and reasonably would not have learned of the omission until she again became pregnant and delivered a sensitized Rh-positive newborn. In this case, the 2-year discovery rule stipulates that the term of the statute of limitations commences at the time the patient knew or should have known of the failure to receive RhoGAM—that is, when she delivered her second child (Meissner-Cutler & Gardner, 1997).

Professional Negligence

Professional negligence, or malpractice, occurs when a provider, regardless of type, who is caring for mothers and their newborns fails to possess the same or similar skill and knowledge that is customary in other providers in the same or similar circumstances. Professional negligence occurs when there is a lack of "ordinary" or "reasonable" care, which results in injury/harm to a patient. Any professional caring for a newborn can be found liable of negligence when there is a failure (1) to possess the requisite skill and knowledge, (2) to exercise reasonable care, or (3) to use best judgment (Meissner-Cutler & Gardner 1997). A professional must not only possess the requisite skill and knowledge, but also use best judgment in exercising that skill and applying that knowledge (*Pike v. Honsinger,* 1898). A practitioner may be liable for (1) not knowing what to do when a reasonably prudent practitioner would have known what to do; (2) knowing what to do, but not doing it; or (3) knowing what to do but doing it carelessly.

Professional negligence is proved by establishing that the caregiver met four criteria:

+ Had a duty to the patient
+ Breached the duty to the patient
+ Injured or harmed the patient
+ The breach of duty caused the injury/harm

All care providers are professionally accountable for their practice, which is premised on the concept of duty—an obligation to another to comply with particular standards of conduct. According to the *Code of Ethics for Nurses* (ANA, 2015a), nurses are duty-bound to themselves, their patients and the public, their employer, and the nursing profession.

All providers are expected to perceive a patient's needs and risks to a degree that the average layperson would not perceive them. Providers are expected to exercise reasonable care to avoid conduct that can foreseeably cause injury to the patient. As an example, the legal precedent for the nurse's duty to the patient was determined in *Darling v. Charleston Community Memorial Hospital* (1966); in this ruling, such duty was defined to include affirmative action, notification of the chain-of-command, advocacy, and disclosure. A breach of duty to the patient can result in liability for any subsequent harm resulting from that breach (Meissner-Cutler & Gardner, 1997).

Care providers owe a duty to their employer to practice within the standards set forth in the institution's policies, procedures, guidelines, and protocols. When a provider fails to perform the duty to an employer, the institution can be held liable for acts of omission or commission of the employee that injured or harmed a patient. An institution can also be held independently negligent under the doctrine of corporate liability. A birth center or hospital has a responsibility to patients to screen, select, educate, and retain only qualified and competent staff (*Bleiler v. Bodnar*, 1985; *Darling v. Charleston Community Memorial Hospital*, 1966). A birth center or hospital also has a responsibility to have and enforce written, relevant, current, evidence-based policies, procedures, and protocols as the standard of care for that institution.

Before a caregiver can be found liable of professional negligence, the patient's attorney must prove that the negligent act (commission) or failure to act (omission) actually caused the patient injury or harm. A professional cannot be held responsible for a patient's injury or harm if the damages were not sustained as a result of the act of negligence forming the basis for the claim (Meissner-Cutler & Gardner 1997). Causation of the injury or harm must be established to a reasonable degree of medical probability (defined as more than 50%) by an expert witness who is competent and qualified to render such opinion.

Although professional negligence is generally not a crime, acts of negligence that are wanton or done with malice may be considered criminal. In particular, gross negligence—an aggravated form of negligence "usually accompanied by a conscious indifference to the consequences" or with reckless disregard for the rights and safety of others—can be a crime (Prosser, 1984, p. 213). Generally, for an individual to be convicted of a crime, it must be proved that the person had a state of mind and intent to do harm, as well as criminal conduct.

Professional Practice and Care of the Neonate

Professional practice related to care of the newborn or neonate is defined by the professional associations using the best evidence for optimal outcomes. The American College of Nurse–Midwives defines the components of midwifery care of the newborn. The midwife independently manages the care of the newborn immediately after birth and continues to provide care to well newborns up to 28 days of life using consultation, collaboration, and/or referral to appropriate healthcare services as indicated. The National Organization of Nurse Practitioner Faculty (NONPF, 2014) identifies core competencies for neonatal nurse practitioners, pediatric nurse practitioners, and family nurse practitioners. The competencies recognize the independent practice of NPs in caring for newborns. The AAP has identified guidelines for hospital care of late-preterm and term newborns and includes criteria for early discharge (Benitz & AAP, Committee on Fetus and Newborn, 2015; Engle, Tomashek, Wallman, & AAP, Committee on Fetus and Newborn, 2007). These guidelines apply to nurse practitioners, certified nurse–midwives, certified midwives, certified professional midwives, and all providers of care to newborns. Medical care providers, including medical students, residents, and physician assistants, must be familiar with their own practice requirements.

An example of how evidence influences practice can be seen in the recent changes in care of the late-preterm infant. The "epidemic" of births before 39 weeks' gestation prompted professional and public education on the importance of maintaining pregnancy to term and the increased morbidities and mortalities experienced by late-preterm infants. In keeping with this campaign, beginning in 2011, one of the five perinatal core measures for The Joint Commission (TJC, 2011) became reduction of elective deliveries prior to the 39th week of pregnancy.

Because of their anatomic and physiologic differences and the developmental immaturity (Table 1-1) of even healthy full-term infants, quick action and a high index of suspicion are necessary to provide safe, efficacious care to these babies. Even early term newborns with a gestational age of 37 to 38 weeks have been found to be 120 times more likely to require ventilator support for surfactant deficiency (the physiologic cause of respiratory distress syndrome, a condition of the immature lung) than newborns of 39 to 41 weeks' gestation (Madar, Richmond, & Hey, 1999). The risks of iatrogenic respiratory distress syndrome are greatly reduced if delivery occurs at 39 weeks' gestation (Minkoff & Chervenak, 2003; Morrison, Rennie, & Milton, 1995; Zanardo et al., 2004). Research has consistently associated increased respiratory morbidity with delivery (including elective cesarean section) prior to

39 weeks' gestation (Barrington, Vallerand, & Usher, 2004; Boyle et al., 2015; Chioukh et al., 2014; Clark, 2005; Escobar, Clark, & Greene, 2006; Hansen, Wisborg, Uldbierg, & Henriksen, 2007; Haroon, Ali, Ahmed, & Maheen, 2014; Horgan, 2015; Kashu, Narayanan, Bhargava, & Osiovich, 2009; Mahoney & Jain, 2013; Mally, Hendricks-Munoz, & Bailey, 2013; Morrison et al., 1995; Rubaltelli, Bonafe, Tangucci, Spagnolo, & Dani, 1998; Tita et al., 2009: Van Den Berg, Van Elburg, Van Geijn, & Fetter, 2001; Zanardo et al., 2004). The mortality rate for infants born at 37 to 38 weeks' gestation is 3.01 deaths per 100,000 births—63% higher than the rate for full-term infants (Mathews, MacDorman, & Thoma, 2015).

This text is written for students and clinicians (i.e., certified nurse–midwives, certified midwives, certified professional midwives, nurse practitioners, physician assistants, medical students/residents, and family practice physicians) who care for late-preterm and term newborn infants at birth and through the neonatal period (i.e., the first 28 days of life). Each chapter contains the latest evidence-based practice as well as published standards of care, position statements, guidelines, and recommendations for care of the well newborn.

Conclusion

Normal newborns are unique in their anatomy and physiology. Because of their uniqueness, the standards of care focus on the needs for the transition from birth through the first 28 days of life. The neonatal care provider must keep abreast of the practices that are specific to these unique humans. This text provides content for provision of care that meets the standards of professional associations, reflects national guidelines, and represents current evidence-based practice.

References

Academy of Breastfeeding Medicine Protocol Committee. (2010). ABM protocol #23: Non-pharmacologic management of procedure-related pain in the breastfeeding infant. *Breastfeeding Medicine, 5*, 315–319.

Adamkin, D. H., & American Academy of Pediatrics (AAP), Committee on Fetus and Newborn. (2011). Postnatal glucose homeostasis in late-preterm and term infants. *Pediatrics, 127,* 575–579.

Altimier, L. (2012). Thermoregulation: What's new? What's not? *Newborn and Infant Nursing Reviews, 12*(1), 51–63.

American Academy of Pediatrics (AAP), Committee on Fetus and Newborn. (2012). Circumcision policy statement. *Pediatrics, 130,* 585–586.

American Academy of Pediatrics (AAP), Subcommittee on Hyperbilirubinemia. (2004). Clinical practice guideline: Management of hyperbilirubinemia in the newborn infant 35 or more weeks' of gestation. *Pediatrics, 114,* 297–316.

American Academy of Pediatrics (AAP), Task Force on Sudden Infant Death Syndrome. (2011). SIDS and other sleep related infant deaths: Expansion of recommendations for a safe infant sleep environment. *Pediatrics, 128,* e1341–e1367.

American Academy of Pediatrics (AAP) & American College of Obstetricians and Gynecologists (ACOG). (2012). *Guidelines for perinatal care* (7th ed.). Washington, DC: AAP.

American College of Nurse–Midwives (ACNM). (2011). *Standards for the practice of midwifery.* Silver Springs, MD: ACNM Board of Directors.

American College of Nurse–Midwives (ACNM). (2012a). *Core competencies for basic midwifery practice.* Silver Spring, MD: ACNM Board of Directors.

American College of Nurse–Midwives (ACNM). (2012b). *Definition of midwifery and scope of practice for certified nurse–midwives and certified midwives.* Silver Springs, MD: ACNM Board of Directors.

American College of Obstetricians and Gynecologists (ACOG). (2001). Committee opinion #260: Circumcision. *Obstetrics & Gynecology, 98,* 707–708.

American Nurses Association (ANA). (1980). *Nursing: A social policy statement.* Kansas City, MO: Author.

American Nurses Association (ANA). (2003). *Nursing: A social policy statement.* Washington, DC: Author.

American Nurses Association (ANA). (2015a). *Code of ethics for nurses with interpretive statements.* Washington, DC: Author.

American Nurses Association (ANA). (2015b). *Nursing: Scope and standards of practice* (3rd ed.). Washington, DC: Author.

American Nurses Association (ANA) & National Association of Neonatal Nurses (NANN). (2013). *Scope and standards of practice for neonatal nursing* (3rd ed.). Washington, DC: Authors.

American Society of Pain Management Nurses. (2011). *Position statement: Male infant circumcision pain management.* Lenexa, KS: Author.

Anand, K. J., & International Evidence-Based Group for Neonatal Pain. (2001). Consensus statement for the prevention and management of pain in the newborn, *Archives of Pediatric and Adolescent Medicine, 155,* 173–180.

Association of Women's Health, Obstetric, and Neonatal Nurses (AWHONN). (2006). *Hyperbilirubinemia: Identification and management in healthy term and late preterm infants* (2nd ed.). Washington, DC: Author.

Association of Women's Health, Obstetric, and Neonatal Nurses (AWHONN). (2007). *Neonatal nursing clinical competencies and education guide* (6th ed.). Washington, DC: Author.

Association of Women's Health, Obstetric, and Neonatal Nurses (AWHONN). (2009). *Standards for professional nursing practice in the care of women and newborns* (7th ed.). Washington, DC: Author.

Association of Women's Health, Obstetric, and Neonatal Nurses (AWHONN). (2012). Quality patient care in labor and delivery: A call to action. *Journal of Obstetric, Gynecologic and Neonatal Nursing, 41,* 151–153.

Association of Women's Health, Obstetric, and Neonatal Nurses (AWHONN). (2013). *Evidence-based clinical practice guideline: Neonatal skin care* (3rd ed.). Washington, DC: Author.

Association of Women's Health, Obstetric, and Neonatal Nurse (AWHONN). (2014). *Assessment and care of the late preterm infant.* Washington, DC: Author.

Association of Women's Health, Obstetric, and Neonatal Nurses (AWHONN). (2015). *Breastfeeding.* Washington, DC: Author.

Barrington , K., Vallerand, D., & Usher, R. (2004). Frequency of morbidities in near-term infants. *Pediatric Research, 55,* 372A.

Benitz, W. E., & American Academy of Pediatrics (AAP), Committee on Fetus and Newborn. (2015). Hospital stay for healthy term newborn infants. *Pediatrics, 135*(5), 948–953.

Bhatia, J., & Parish, A. (2009). GERD or not GERD: The fussy infant. *Journal of Perinatology, 29,* S7–S11.

Bleiler v. Bodnar, 65 N.Y. 2d,65,479 N.E.2d 230,489 N.Y.S. 2d 885 (1985).

Boyle, E. M., Johnson, S., Manktelow, B., Draper, E. S., et al. (2015). Neonatal outcomes and delivery of care for infants born late preterm or moderately preterm: A prospective population-based study. *Archives of Disease in Childhood—Fetal and Neonatal Edition.* [Epub ahead of print]. doi: 10.1136/archdischild-2014-307347

Brown, L. D., Hendrickson, K., Evans, R., Davis, J., Anderson, M. S., & Hay, W. W. (2016). Enteral nutrition. In S. L. Gardner, B. S. Carter, M. Enzman Hines, & J. A. Hernandez (Eds.), *Merenstein and Gardner's handbook of neonatal intensive care* (8th ed., pp. 377– 418). St. Louis, MO: Mosby-Elsevier.

Cadnapaphornchai, M. A., Schoenbein, M. B., Woloschuk, R., Soranno, D. E., & Hernandez, J. A. (2016). Neonatal nephrology. In S. L. Gardner, B. S. Carter, M. Enzman Hines, & J. A. Hernandez (Eds.), *Merenstein and Gardner's handbook of neonatal intensive care* (8th ed., pp. 689–726). St. Louis, MO: Mosby-Elsevier.

Centers for Disease Control and Prevention (CDC). (2010). Prevention of perinatal group B streptococcal (GBS) disease among newborns. *Morbidity and Mortality Weekly Report, 59*(RR-10), 1–36.

Chioukh, F. Z., Skalli, M. I., Laajili, H., Hmida, B. H., Ameur, B. K., & Bizid, M. (2014). Respiratory disorders among late-preterm infants in a neonatal intensive care unit. *Archives of Pediatrics, 21,* 157–161.

Darling v. Charleston Community Memorial Hospital, 33 IL, 2d 326,211 N.E. 2d 253 (1966).

Engle, W. (2006). A recommendation for the definition of "late preterm" (near-term) and the birth weight– gestational age classification system. *Seminars in Perinatology, 30,* 2–7.

Engle, W., Tomashek, K. M., Wallman, C., & American Academy of Pediatrics (AAP), Committee on Fetus and Newborn. (2007). "Late-preterm": A population at risk. *Pediatrics, 120*(6), 1390–1401.

Enzman Hines, M. (2012). The scope and standards of professional nursing practice. *NICU Currents, 3*(3), 6–11, 14.

Escobar, G., Clark, R., & Greene, J. (2006). Short-term outcomes of infants born at 35 and 36 weeks' gestation: We need to ask more questions. *Seminars in Perinatology, 30,* 28–33.

Gardner, S. L. (2008). How will I know if my newborn is sick? *Nurse Currents, 2*(2), 1–8.

Gardner, S. L. (2009). Sepsis in the neonate. *Critical Care Clinics of North America, 21*(1), 121–141.

Gardner, S. L., Enzman, M., & Agarwal, R. (2016). Pain and pain relief. In S. L. Gardner, B. S. Carter, M. Enzman Hines, & J. A. Hernandez (Eds.), *Merenstein and Gardner's handbook of neonatal intensive care* (8th ed., pp. 218–261). St. Louis, MO: Mosby-Elsevier.

Gardner, S. L., Enzman, M., & Nyp, M. (2016). Respiratory diseases. In S. L. Gardner, B. S. Carter, M. Enzman Hines, & J. A. Hernandez (Eds.), *Merenstein and Gardner's handbook of neonatal intensive care* (8th ed., pp. 565–643). St. Louis, MO: Mosby-Elsevier.

Gardner, S. L., Goldson, M., & Hernandez, J. A. (2016). The neonate and the environment: Impact on development. In S. L. Gardner, B. S. Carter, M. Enzman Hines, & J. A. Hernandez (Eds.), *Merenstein and Gardner's handbook of neonatal intensive care* (8th ed., pp. 262–314). St. Louis, MO: Mosby-Elsevier.

Gardner, S. L., & Hernandez, J. A. (2016a). Heat balance. In S. L. Gardner, B. S. Carter, M. Enzman Hines, & J. A. Hernandez (Eds.), *Merenstein and Gardner's handbook of neonatal intensive care* (8th ed., pp. 105–125). St. Louis, MO: Mosby-Elsevier.

Gardner, S. L., & Lawrence, R. A. (2016). Breastfeeding the neonate with special needs. In S. L. Gardner, B. S. Carter, M. Enzman Hines, & J. A. Hernandez (Eds.), *Merenstein and Gardner's handbook of neonatal intensive care* (8th ed., pp. 419–463). St. Louis, MO: Mosby-Elsevier.

Hansen, A. K., Wisborg, K., Uldbjerg, N., & Henriksen, T. B. (2007). Elective C-section and respiratory morbidity in the term and near-term neonate. *Acta Obstetricia et Gynecologica Scandinavica, 86*(4), 389–394.

Haroon, A., Ali, S. R., Ahmed, S., & Maheen, H. (2014). Short-term neonatal outcome in late preterm vs. term infants. *Journal of the College of Physicians and Surgeons Pakistan, 24*(1), 34–38.

Hegar, B., Dewanti, N. R., Kadim, M., Alatas, S., Firmansyah, A., & Vandenplas, Y. (2009). Natural evolution of regurgitation in healthy infants. *Acta Paediatrica, 98*, 1189–1193.

Horgan, M. J. (2015). Management of the late preterm infant: Not quite ready for prime time. *Pediatric Clinics of North America, 62*(2), 439–451.

Hyman, P. E., Milla, P. J., Benninga, M. A., Davidson, G. P., Fleisher, D. F., & Taminiau, J. (2006). Childhood functional gastrointestinal disorders: Neonate/toddler. *Gastroenterology, 130*, 1519–1526.

Kamath-Rayne, B. D., Thilo, E. H., Deacon, J., & Hernandez, J. A. (2016). Neonatal hyperbilirubinemia. In S. L. Gardner, B. S. Carter, M. Enzman Hines, & J. A. Hernandez (Eds.), *Merenstein and Gardner's handbook of neonatal intensive care* (8th ed., pp. 511–536). St. Louis, MO: Mosby-Elsevier.

Kattan, J. D., Cocco, R. R., & Jarvinen, K. M. (2011). Milk and soy allergy. *Pediatric Clinics of North America, 58*(2), 407–426.

Kattwinkel, J. (Ed.). (2011). *Textbook of neonatal resuscitation* (6th ed.). Elk Grove Village, IL: American Academy of Pediatrics & American Heart Association.

Khashu, M., Narayanan, M., Bhargava, S., & Osiovich, H. (2009). Perinatal outcomes associated with preterm birth at 33 to 36 weeks' gestation: A population-based cohort study. *Pediatrics, 123*(1), 109–113.

Klemola, T., Vanto, T., Juntunen-Backman, K., Kalimo, K., Korpela, R., & Varjonen, E. (2002). Allergy to soy formula and to extensively hydrolyzed whey formula in infants with cow's milk allergy: A prospective, randomized study with a follow-up to the age of 2 years. *Journal of Pediatrics, 140*(2), 219–224.

Madar, J., Richmond, S., & Hey, E. (1999). Surfactant-deficient respiratory distress syndrome after elective delivery at "term." *Acta Paediatrica, 88*(11), 1244–1248.

Mahoney, A. D., & Jain, L. (2013). Respiratory disorders in moderately preterm, late preterm, and early term infants. *Clinics in Perinatology, 40*(4), 665–678.

Maisels, M. J., Bhutani, V. K., Bogen, D., Newman, T. B., Stark, A. R., & Watchko, J. F. (2009). Hyperbilirubinemia in the newborn infant 35 or more weeks' gestation. *Pediatrics, 124*, 1193–1198.

Mally, P. V., Hendricks-Munoz, K. D., & Bailey, S. (2013). Incidence and etiology of late preterm admissions to the neonatal intensive care unit and its associated respiratory morbidities when compared to term infants. *American Journal of Perinatology, 30*(5), 425–431.

Martinez, J. A., & Ballew, M. P. (2011). Infant formulas. *Pediatrics in Review, 32*, 179–189.

Mathews, T. J., MacDorman, M. F., & Thoma, M. E. (2015). Infant mortality statistics from the 2013 period linked birth/infant death data set. *National Vital Statistics Reports, 64*(9), 1–28.

Meissner-Cutler, S., & Gardner, S. L. (1997). Maternal–child nursing and the law. In S. L. Gardner & M. Enzman Hagedorn (Eds.), *Legal aspects of maternal–child nursing practice.* Menlo Park, CA: Addison-Wesley.

Minkoff, H., & Chervenak, F. (2003). Elective primary cesarean delivery. *New England Journal of Medicine, 348*(10), 946–950.

Morrison, J., Rennie, J., & Milton, P. (1995). Neonatal respiratory morbidity and mode of delivery at term: Influence of timing of elective cesarean section. *British Journal of Obstetrics & Gynaecology, 102*(2), 101–106.

National Association of Pediatric Nurse Practitioners. (2010). *PNPs role in supporting infant and family well-being in the first year of life.* New York, NY: Author.

National Association of Neonatal Nurses. (2010). Position statement #3049: *Prevention of acute bilirubin encephalopathy and kernicterus in newborns.* Glenview, IL: Author.

National Association of Pediatric Nurse Practitioners. (2012). *Breastfeeding.* New York, NY: Author.

National Organization of Nurse Practitioner Faculty (NONPF). (2014). *Population-focused nurse practitioner competencies: Family/across the lifespan, neonatal, acute care pediatric, primary care pediatric, psychiatric–mental health, & women's health/gender-related.* Washington, DC: Author.

Neu, M., Corwin, E., Lareau, S. C., & Marcheggiani, H. C. (2012). A review of non-surgical treatment for the symptom of irritability in infants with GERD. *Journal for Specialists in Pediatric Nursing, 17,* 177–192.

Olsen v. St. Croix Valley Memorial Hospital, 55 Wisc. 2d 628, 201 N.W. 63 (1972).

Pantoja, A. F., & Enzman Hines, M. (2016). Evidence-based clinical practice. In S. L. Gardner, B. S. Carter, M. Enzman Hines, & J. A. Hernandez (Eds.), *Merenstein and Gardner's handbook of neonatal intensive care* (8th ed., pp. 1–10). St. Louis, MO: Mosby-Elsevier.

Parsons, J. A., Seay, A. R., & Jacobson, M. (2016). Neurologic disorders. In S. L. Gardner, B. S. Carter, M. Enzman Hines, & J. A. Hernandez (Eds.), *Merenstein and Gardner's handbook of neonatal intensive care* (8th ed., pp. 262–314). St. Louis, MO: Mosby-Elsevier.

Pike v. Honsinger, 49 N.E. 760 (N.Y. 1898).

Prosser, W. (1984). *The law of torts* (5th ed.). St. Paul, MN: West.

Renslow v. Mennonite Hospital, 67 IL. 2d 348, 367 N.E. 2d 1250 (1977).

Rozance, P. J., McGowan, J. E., Price-Douglas, W., & Hay, W. W. (2016). Glucose homeostasis. In S. L. Gardner, B. S. Carter, M. Enzman Hines, & J. A. Hernandez (Eds.), *Merenstein and Gardner's handbook of neonatal intensive care* (8th ed., pp. 337–359). St. Louis, MO: Mosby-Elsevier.

Rubaltelli, F. F., Bonafe, L., Tangucci, M., Spagnolo, A., & Dani, C. (1998). Epidemiology of acute respiratory disorders: A multicenter study on incidence and fatality rates of neonatal acute respiratory disorders according to gestational age, maternal age, pregnancy complications and type of delivery. Italian Group of Neonatal Pneumology. *Biology of the Neonate, 1,* 7–15.

Sinclair, J. C., & Bracken, M. B. (1992). *Effective care of the newborn infant.* New York, NY: Oxford University Press.

Straus, S. E., Glasziou, P., Richardson, W. S., & Haynes, R. B. (2011). *Evidence-based medicine: How to practice and teach it* (4th ed.). London, UK: Harcourt.

Teeters v. Currey, 518 S.W. 2d 512 (Tenn. 1974).

The Joint Commission (TJC). (2011). Perinatal care core measures. Retrieved from https://tjc.org/releases/TJC2013A/PerinatalCarehtm

Tita, A., Landon, M., Spong, C., Lai, Y., Leveno, K. J., & Varner, M. W. (2009). Timing of elective cesarean delivery at term and neonatal outcomes. *New England Journal of Medicine, 360,* 111–120.

Van Den Berg, A., Van Elburg, R. M., Van Geijn, H. P., & Fetter, W. P. (2001). Neonatal respiratory morbidity following elective caesarean section in term infants: A five year retrospective study and a review of the literature. *European Journal of Obstetrics, Gynecology, and Reproductive Biology, 89*(1), 9–13.

Vandenplas, Y., & Alarcon, P. (2015). Updated algorithms for managing frequent gastro-intestinal symptoms in infants. *Beneficial Microbes, 6,* 199–208.

Volpe, J. J. (2008). *Neurology of the newborn* (5th ed.). Philadelphia, PA: Saunders/Elsevier.

Walden, M., & Gibbins, S. (2013). *Newborn pain assessment and management guideline for practice* (3rd ed.). Glenview, IL: National Association of Neonatal Nurses.

Zanardo, V., Simbi, A., Franzoi, M., Solda, G., Salvadori, A., & Trevisanuto, D. (2004). Neonatal respiratory morbidity risk and mode of delivery at term: Influence of timing of elective caesarean delivery. *Acta Paediatrica, 93*(5), 643–647.

CHAPTER 2

PERINATAL HISTORY: INFLUENCES ON NEWBORN OUTCOME

Pamela J. Reis and Amy Jnah

Care of all patients, including newborns and neonates, begins with a thorough history. For the newborn, a thorough review of maternal prenatal care records coupled with interviewing the mother to verify and clarify history is critical. During prenatal care, family history of importance focuses mostly on maternal history. For prenatal assessment, genetic screening of both mother and father is accomplished. However, prenatal assessment may not be as thorough for other family conditions, such as cancer risk, neurologic disorders, and other conditions.

A composite perinatal history provides for newborn risk assessment and anticipatory care planning—processes that are especially important when there is a poor or slow transition to extrauterine life. Identification of risk factors from the perinatal history enables newborn care providers to target specific assessment strategies, initiate appropriate screening tests and interventions, and improve outcomes by decreasing morbidity and mortality (Gardner & Hernandez, 2016). As an example, consider the identification of perinatal risk factors that result in preterm birth and adverse neonatal outcomes. Several published accounts describe incidents of prematurity or severe cardiorespiratory depression at birth among well-known historical figures. Sir Isaac Newton (1642–1727) was noted to be "as good as dead" at birth and tiny enough to fit inside a quart mug (Raju, 2015). Pablo Picasso (1881–1973) was labeled a stillbirth until resuscitated by a family member (Raju, 2015). Franklin D. Roosevelt (1882–1945) was described as weighing 10 pounds at delivery, and being blue, limp, and apneic (Raju, 2015). A complete physical examination follows the history and is reviewed elsewhere in this text.

Currently, neonatal deaths—defined as those occurring within the first 28 days of life—account for more than 45% of all deaths worldwide (World Health Organization [WHO], 2015). Prematurity and low birth weight are the leading causes of neonatal mortality, especially among black infants. Infants born at less than 32 weeks' gestation are at greatest risk for death and long-term disability (Bettegowda, Lackritz, & Petrini, 2011).

The in utero environment of the developing fetus not only critically affects immediate birth outcomes, but also has implications for long-term health and well-being. Neonatal surveillance is intimately linked to maternal preconception and perinatal history, as well as to family history. This chapter seeks to identify aspects of family, maternal, and intrapartum history that contribute to newborn outcomes at birth and beyond. In doing so, it emphasizes conditions commonly encountered in care of the late-preterm and term newborn.

Components of the Perinatal Health Record

The majority of perinatal risk factors resulting in adverse newborn outcomes are identified prior to birth. The perinatal health record provides essential information for anticipatory guidance and care of the neonate. A thorough exploration of conditions and circumstances that may affect the health of women during their childbearing years can lead to timely identification and management of perinatal factors that may influence maternal, infant, and family outcomes.

Family History

The prenatal record should contain detailed information on all known factors that might affect the newborn's health. Family history encompasses shared medical and genetic factors, environmental influences, and behavioral practices that occur within families (Dolan & Moore, 2007). A thorough and comprehensive family history requires collection of data on the complete medical history of nuclear family members as well as extended family members. If information is missing from the prenatal record, the neonatal provider *must* get the detailed history from the mother for the newborn's record.

Since 2004, the Surgeon General's Family Health Initiative has declared Thanksgiving to be National Family History Day, in an effort to highlight the importance of family history to individual health. This initiative encourages Americans to spend time during family gatherings to discuss and document health conditions that appear in their family. A web-based "My Family Health Portrait" tool and other helpful instructions are available at the Surgeon General's Family Health History Initiative website (U.S. Department of Health and Human Services [USDHHS], 2015).

Table 2-1: Family History and Risk of Selected Diseases and Chronic Health Conditions

Autism	Incidence of familial autism is 36–95% in identical twins, 0–31% in nonidentical twins, and 2–18% for siblings.
Breast and ovarian cancer	Approximately 3 of every 100 women who develop breast cancer will have a *BRCA1* or *BRCA2* mutation. Approximately 10% of women who develop ovarian cancer will have a *BRCA1* or *BRCA2* mutation. Women who have a *BRCA1/2* mutation are at high risk for early breast and ovarian cancer. In some families, inherited mutations in genes other than *BRCA1/2* result in breast cancer or ovarian cancer (uncommon).
Colorectal cancer	Risk is higher for individuals with first-degree relatives (parent, sibling, or child) who developed cancer at a younger age, or for those with multiple affected first-degree relatives.
Heart disease	Can cluster in families. The risk is higher with familial hypercholesterolemia.
Primary hemochromatosis	One of the most common inherited disorders. It is more common among U.S. non-Hispanic whites, and less common among African Americans, Asian Americans, Hispanics/Latinos, and American Indians.
Mental health	Studies of identical twins have provided evidence of genetic contributions to depression, bipolar disorder, schizophrenia, autism, and other mental disorders. Even if genetic risk is present, environmental factors can play a role in determining whether an individual actually develops the disorder and in the severity of the illness.
Obesity	Patterns of inherited obesity within a family caused by a single gene mutation are rare. Obesity is most likely the result of interactions among multiple genes and environmental factors.
Stroke	Stroke can occur as a complication of several genetic disorders. Increased familial risk may be due to common behavioral factors.

Data from Genetic Alliance. (2008). *Understanding genetics: A New York, Mid-Atlantic guide for patients and health professionals.* Washington, DC: Author; National Cancer Institute. (2015). *BRCA1* and *BRCA2*: Cancer risk and genetic testing. Retrieved from http://www.cancer.gov/about-cancer/causes-prevention/genetics/brca-fact-sheet#q1; National Library of Medicine. (2015). *Genetics home reference* [Internet]. Bethesda, MD: Author. Retrieved from http://ghr.nlm.nih.gov/.

Table 2-1 lists selected chronic health conditions, the incidence of their genetic predisposition, and familial inheritance patterns. Common disease states such as cardiovascular diseases, diabetes, and many cancers result from a combined influence of genetic susceptibility, shared environmental exposures, and common behaviors among relatives (Reid & Emery, 2006). The incidence of familial, chronic illnesses may increase anywhere from twofold to fivefold among affected families, depending on the age of onset of the disease and the number of affected relatives.

Genetic Conditions

Genetic disorders are classified into three broad categories: monogenetic, multifactorial, and chromosomal (**Table 2-2**). Of the thousands of known genetic disorders, most do not occur according to classic Mendelian patterns. Providers must be aware of "red flags" that signal risk for potential inherited disorders, such as recurrent pregnancy loss, one or more family members who died at a young age from unknown causes, and known or suspected consanguinity (Genetic Alliance, 2008).

A comprehensive family history includes a three-generation account of the health status of all biological members, and should be regularly updated with each death and new diagnosis of all family members. The degree to which family members share common genes depends on how closely they are related. First-degree relatives (children, parents, and siblings) share 50% of their genes; second-degree relatives (aunts, uncles, grandparents, half-siblings, nieces, and nephews) share 25% of their genes; and third-degree relatives (cousins and great-grandparents) share 12.5% of their genes (Wattendorf & Hadley, 2005).

Genomics—that is, the identification of genetic risk profiles for specific medical conditions—is a growing field in terms of both research and therapy. A primary goal of personalized genomics is modification of treatments or therapies based on genotype. In addition to identifying susceptibility for disease, personalized genomics may predict response to treatment. Even though personalized genomics is an important adjunct to traditional screening measures, longitudinal data to determine the efficacy of personalized genomic technology in ameliorating disease are generally unavailable (Schaefer & Thompson, 2014). **Table 2-3** describes 12 genetically influenced conditions with significant health consequences that advanced practice providers should routinely screen for in the family history.

Table 2-2: Classification of Genetic Disorders

Type of Disorder	Definition
Monogenetic	Caused by a single gene mutation
Multifactorial	Combination of gene variations that may be environmentally influenced
Chromosomal	Excess or deficiency of genes located on chromosomes, or by structural changes within chromosomes

Data from National Institutes of Health, National Human Genome Institute. (2012). What are genetic disorders? Retrieved from http://www.genome.gov/19016930.

Table 2-3: Genetic Conditions in the Newborn

Condition	Incidence	Means of Acquisition	Highest Risk	Clinical Presentation
Beta-thalassemia	1:100,000	Autosomal recessive	Individuals of Italian, Greek, Middle Eastern, Southern Asian, and African descent. The most common inherited single-gene disorder in the world; highest prevalence is in areas where malaria is endemic.	Confirmed with hemoglobin electrophoresis. Individuals may be asymptomatic or present with severe anemia. Signs and symptoms usually occur within the first 2 years of life (American College of Obstetricians and Gynecologists [ACOG], 2013; National Library of Medicine [NLM], 2015).
Cystic fibrosis (CF)	1:2500–3500	Autosomal recessive	Individuals of European Ashkenazi Jewish descent and Mormon faith. Most common autosomal recessive trait of live-born infants.	Identified through newborn screening at 2–3 days of life. Early identification leads to improved pulmonary status, adequate weight gain, reduced hospital stay, and longevity (Comeau et al., 2007; Cystic Fibrosis Foundation, 2015; NLM, 2015).
Fragile X syndrome	1:4000 males and 1:8000 females	X chromosome–linked dominant	Males are more severely affected than females.	Intellectual disability, autism, dysmorphic facial features, prominent ears, soft skin, flat feet, hyperextensible finger

(Continued)

Table 2-3: Genetic Conditions in the Newborn (*Continued*)

Condition	Incidence	Means of Acquisition	Highest Risk	Clinical Presentation
				joints, strabismus, seizures, otitis media (McLennan, Polussa, Tassone, & Hagerman, 2011; NLM, 2015).
Hemophilia A and B	Hemophilia A is most common, occurring in 1:4000–5000 males	X chromosome–linked recessive	Males are at higher risk than females.	Neonatal diagnoses involve persistent bleeding from the umbilical stump or circumcision. Typically diagnosed between 4 and 8 years of age (NLM, 2015).
Huntington disease	3–7:100,000	Autosomal dominant	Individuals of European descent.	Progressive brain disorder causing uncontrolled movements, emotional lability, and loss of cognition. Adult onset is most common; juvenile form begins in childhood or adolescence (NLM, 2015).
Neurofibromatosis I	1:3000–4000	Autosomal dominant	Individuals with a family history are at highest risk.	Multiple café-au-lait spots; growth of tumors in the nervous system, skin, brain, and other parts of the body. Optic tumors may cause vision loss; otic tumors cause deafness.

Condition	Incidence	Means of Acquisition	Highest Risk	Clinical Presentation
				At increased risk for developing leukemia (NLM, 2015).
X-linked severe combined immunodeficiency disorder (SCID)	Estimated at 1:50,000	X chromosome–linked recessive is the most common type	Occurs almost exclusively in males.	Severe immunodeficiency due to a defect in T-cell production/function and defects in β-lymphocytes. Recurrent opportunistic infections. If untreated, death occurs in infancy (NLM, 2015).
Sickle cell disease	1:500 African Americans and 1:1000–1400 Hispanic Americans	Autosomal recessive	Individuals of African, Asian Indian, Middle East, and Mediterranean descent.	Positive newborn metabolic screening test is confirmed with hemoglobin electrophoresis. Symptoms associated with sickle cell anemia present in infancy or early childhood (NLM, 2015).
Tay-Sachs disease	1:250	Autosomal recessive	Jewish individuals of Eastern European ancestry and French Canadians.	Irritability and hypersensitivity to auditory stimuli, red spot on retina, seizures, motor deterioration, and blindness. Symptoms typically present after 12 weeks of age and death usually occurs by age 5. There is no cure (NLM, 2015).

(Continued)

Table 2-3: Genetic Conditions in the Newborn (*Continued*)

Condition	Incidence	Means of Acquisition	Highest Risk	Clinical Presentation
Trisomy 13 (Patau syndrome)	1:16,000	Nondisjunction results in aneuploidy (3 copies of chromosome 13)	Risk increases with advanced maternal age. Most cases are not inherited and result from nondisjunction during gametogenesis. Translocation trisomy 13 can be inherited.	Intrauterine growth restriction, brain anomalies (microcephaly, holoprosencephaly), cardiac defects, cleft lip or palate, low-set ears, anomalies of the extremities (rocker-bottom feet), and renal and gastrointestinal anomalies. Many infants die within the first days or weeks of life; only 5–10% live beyond the first year (NLM, 2015).
Trisomy 18 (Edwards syndrome)	1:5000	Nondisjunction results in aneuploidy (3 copies of chromosome 18)	Risk increases with advanced maternal age. Most cases are not inherited and result from nondisjunction during gametogenesis. Translocation trisomy 18 can be inherited.	Intrauterine growth restriction, brain anomalies (microcephaly, ventriculomegaly), cardiac defects, cleft lip or palate, low-set ears, micrognathia, extremity anomalies (rocker-bottom feet, short long bones), pleural effusion, diaphragmatic hernia, renal anomalies, omphalocele, and small or absent stomach (NLM, 2015).

Condition	Incidence	Means of Acquisition	Highest Risk	Clinical Presentation
Trisomy 21 (Down syndrome)	1:800	Nondisjunction results in aneuploidy (3 copies of chromosome 21)	Risk increased with advanced maternal age. Approximately 95% of cases occur sporadically, due to nondisjunction during gametogenesis. Translocation trisomy 21 can be inherited.	Failure to thrive, intellectual disability, low-set ears, short neck, overlapping fingers, congenital heart defect(s), renal malformations, micrognathia, prominent occiput, and duodenal atresia (NLM, 2015).

Maternal Medical History

More than half of all women of childbearing age have at least one risk factor for developing a chronic illness (Centers for Disease Control and Prevention [CDC], 2015a). Common maternal conditions that affect newborn outcomes include diabetes mellitus, thyroid disorders, and hypertensive disorders.

Diabetes Mellitus Diabetes prior to pregnancy may result in adverse maternal, fetal, and neonatal outcomes. Approximately 50% of neonatal deaths among the children of women with diabetes occur due to congenital anomalies (Lee-Parritz & Cloherty, 2012). The risk for congenital anomalies is increased in women with poor glycemic control. Women with type 1 and type 2 diabetes are at high risk for hypertensive disorders, including preeclampsia. Maternal ketoacidosis carries a 50% risk of fetal death, especially before the third trimester. Stillbirth, while uncommon in women with diabetes, is more often associated with poor glycemic control, fetal anomalies, severe vascular disease, and intrauterine growth restriction (IUGR). Preeclampsia is often present in women with diabetes who experience intrauterine fetal demise. Polyhydramnios is common in diabetic pregnancies, and should be evaluated in the newborn within the context of both maternal diabetes mellitus and potential fetal anomalies.

Neonatal hypoglycemia (blood glucose level < 40 mg/dL) may occur in the presence of neonatal macrosomia due to hyperinsulinemia, and in small-for-gestational-age infants due to inadequate glycogen stores. Infants of mothers with diabetes who are less than 35 weeks' gestation are at greater risk for respiratory distress syndrome than infants born to mothers without diabetes because hyperinsulinemia blocks cortisol, which is necessary for lung maturation. Infants of mothers with diabetes may also have hypocalcemia, hypomagnesemia, polycythemia, jaundice, poor feeding, myocardial dysfunction due to transient hypertrophic subaortic stenosis, renal vein and other thromboses, and small left colon syndrome.

Thyroid Disorders   The thyroid undergoes multiple changes during pregnancy. Hyperthyroidism is present in as many as 1% of pregnancies, and the presence of goiter, ophthalmopathy, or myxedema suggests Graves's disease (Lee-Parritz & Cloherty, 2012). Maternal Graves's disease may result in fetal and neonatal goiter. Maternal hypothyroidism is present in as many as 3% of pregnancies and may be subclinical. During pregnancy, the most common cause of hypothyroidism is chronic autoimmune response. Chronic immune thyroiditis is common in patients with type 1 diabetes mellitus. Fetal goiter is treated with maternal L-thyroxine administration.

Congenital hypothyroidism—one of the most common, preventable causes of developmental disability—is prevalent among Hispanic (1:1600) and Asian Indian (1:1757) infants (Lee-Parritz & Cloherty, 2012). Females are twice as likely as males to have this disorder. Transient congenital hypothyroidism is caused by intrauterine exposure to antithyroid drugs or large amounts of iodine, and generally resolves within a week after birth. Newborn screening for congenital hypothyroidism is routine in most developed countries. Because minimal amounts of antithyroid drugs and L-thyroxine are excreted in breastmilk, breastfeeding is considered to be safe for women who are prescribed these medications (Hale & Rowe, 2014).

Hypertensive Disorders   Hypertensive disorders are among the leading causes of maternal mortality in the United States, responsible for approximately 9.4% of all pregnancy-related mortality (Creanga et al., 2015). Chronic hypertension is defined as hypertension that occurs prior to pregnancy, or is first diagnosed before 20 weeks' gestation.

Approximately 7% of women of childbearing age have been diagnosed with chronic hypertension. Although chronic hypertension usually improves during early pregnancy, the disease is much less predictable later in pregnancy. The development of superimposed preeclampsia in a woman with chronic hypertension increases the risk for maternal and perinatal morbidity and mortality. In the presence of chronic hypertension, the risk for placental abruption is 2 to 3 times higher, and is further exacerbated if the woman smokes. Intrauterine fetal growth restriction may occur in women with chronic hypertension (Cunningham et al., 2014).

Guidelines for the management of hypertension were established by the Eighth Joint National Committee (JNC-8) based on evidence from randomized controlled trials. For most populations, the therapeutic goal for blood pressure maintenance is less than 140/90 mm Hg (James et al., 2014).

Obstetric History

Table 2-4 presents selected components of the perinatal history that have the potential to influence neonatal outcomes. Two of the most common pregnancy complications—gestational diabetes mellitus and hypertensive disorders—are discussed here.

Table 2-4: Perinatal History and Related Neonatal Outcomes

Maternal Medical/ Obstetric History	Neonatal Outcomes
Age: • Less than 18 years • Greater than 35 years	Adolescents are at risk for poor nutrition, emotional instability, and sexually transmitted infections. Infants born to older mothers are at risk for chromosomal abnormalities. Men aged 55 and older are at risk for fathering an infant with a genetic defect (Bettegowda et al., 2011).
Prior pregnancy outcome	A history of a previous neonatal death, stillbirth, or preterm birth increases the risk for the same adverse outcomes in the current pregnancy (American Academy of Pediatrics [AAP] & ACOG, 2012b; Johnson & Cochran, 2012).
Bariatric surgery	Increased risk for preterm birth and small-for-gestational-age infant. Increased risk for altered breastfeeding success related to nutritional deficiencies and/or unstable maternal weight and caloric consumption after delivery (AAP & ACOG, 2012c).
Infertility treatment/assisted reproductive technology	Increased risk of multiple gestation. Use of in vitro fertilization or intracytoplasmic sperm injection increases the risk for congenital anomalies (AAP & ACOG, 2012b).
Gestational age	Ultrasound measurement of crown–rump length between 6 and 14 weeks' gestation enables the most accurate assessment of gestational age (AAP & ACOG, 2012b).
Gravidity and parity	Increased risk of significant growth disparity in multiple-gestation pregnancies. Vascular anastomoses that connect monochorionic/diamniotic gestations can result in twin-to-twin transfusion and discordant growth (Johnson, 2012).
Prenatal laboratory tests	Blood type: Identifies risk for Rh or ABO isoimmunization. Antibody screen: If positive, may indicate isoimmunization.

(Continued)

Table 2-4: Perinatal History and Related Neonatal Outcomes (*Continued*)

Maternal Medical/ Obstetric History	Neonatal Outcomes
	Complete blood count (CBC): Identifies anemia or potential hemoglobinopathies.
	Venereal Disease Research Laboratory (VDRL)/rapid plasma reagin (RPR) (nontreponemal tests): Test for syphilis. If untreated, can result in perinatal transmission from mother to infant.
	Urine culture: Tests for asymptomatic bacteriuria and group B *Streptococcus*.
	Urinalysis (U/A): Screens for proteinuria and hematuria.
	Hepatitis B surface antigen (HBsAg): If positive, infant will need prophylaxis and vaccination at birth.
	Human immunodeficiency virus (HIV): If positive, maternal antiretroviral therapy is indicated to prevent maternal-to-child transmission of HIV, and neonatal prophylaxis after birth is recommended.
	Gonorrhea/chlamydia: If untreated can cause ophthalmia neonatorum and/or chlamydial pneumonia.
	Mantoux tuberculin skin test or interferon gamma release assay: If positive, mother may need treatment and should be tested for HIV (AAP & ACOG, 2012b).
Perinatal-acquired infectious conditions	See Table 2-5.
Chronic maternal illness	Depending on the condition, can lead to intrauterine growth restriction, fetal anomalies, macrosomia, congenital thyroid disease, and other conditions (AAP & ACOG, 2012b).
Depressive disorder	Some studies suggest that untreated gestational depression may have untoward effects on the developing fetus and newborn, and the negative effects can extend into childhood (Lancaster et al., 2010).
Tobacco, alcohol, and illegal substance use	Strong association between smoking during pregnancy and sudden infant death syndrome (CDC 2015c; Task Force on Sudden Infant Death Syndrome & Moon, 2011).
	Alcohol use during pregnancy increases the risk for fetal alcohol spectrum disorder (Williams, Smith, & Committee on Substance Abuse, 2015).

Maternal Medical/ Obstetric History	Neonatal Outcomes
	Substance abuse results in neonatal abstinence syndrome and neurodevelopmental delays. See the section on opioid exposure during pregnancy (AAP & ACOG, 2012a).
Intimate partner violence	Associated with stillbirth, placental abruption, fetal injury, preterm birth, and low birth weight (ACOG, 2012a).
Exposure to occupational and environmental toxins	The mother should avoid exposure to known teratogens, such as drugs (anticonvulsants, lithium, angiotensin-converting enzyme [ACE] inhibitors, retinoic acids, megadoses of vitamin A, selective serotonin reuptake inhibitors [SSRIs], and nonsteroidal anti-inflammatory drugs [NSAIDs]) (Swanson & Erickson, 2016) and lead (CDC, 2010). Prenatal and lactational lead exposure increases the risk for neurodevelopmental abnormalities (CDC, 2010). Prenatal exposure to the drugs listed previously increases the risk of congenital heart defect (Swanson & Erickson, 2016).
Uterine anomaly/diethylstilbesterol (DES)	DES (prescribed 1938–1971) increases the risk of vaginal, uterine, and breast cancer in human and animal models. Animal studies have demonstrated adverse effects in unexposed generations (Schrager & Potter, 2004).

Gestational Diabetes Diabetes mellitus is present in approximately 6% to 7% of pregnancies; the majority of women with diabetes in pregnancy (90%) meet the criteria for having gestational diabetes mellitus (GDM). Hispanic, African American, Native American, Asian, and Pacific Islander women are at greatest risk for GDM. The increasing incidence of obesity and sedentary lifestyle is a factor contributing to the rising incidence of GDM. Gestational hypertension, preeclampsia, and cesarean birth are common complications of GDM, and women with GDM are at increased risk for developing type 2 diabetes later in life.

Newborns of mothers with GDM are at risk for macrosomia, neonatal hypoglycemia, hyperbilirubinemia, shoulder dystocia, birth trauma, and operative delivery. Poor maternal glycemic control during pregnancy is strongly correlated with macrosomia, neonatal hypoglycemia, and cesarean birth (Metzger et al., 2008). Maternal and newborn outcomes are graver for women with advanced stages of the disease as described by White's classification of gestational diabetes (Hare & White, 1980).

Screening for GDM usually occurs at 24 to 28 weeks' gestation, or sooner if risk factors are identified in the maternal history. A two-step approach to screening is most commonly used in the United States: 50 g of an oral glucose solution is administered, followed by a 1-hour venous blood glucose test. Women who meet or exceed the threshold of 130–140 mg/dL should undergo further screening with a 100 g, 3-hour diagnostic oral glucose tolerance test (American College of Obstetricians and Gynecologists [ACOG], Committee on Practice Bulletins—Obstetrics, 2013).

Surveillance of blood glucose levels in women with GDM is critical to monitor glycemic control. The glycemic targets recommended by both the American Diabetes Association and the American College of Obstetricians and Gynecologists to reduce the risk of macrosomia are 140 mg/dL at 1 hour postprandial or 120 mg/dL at 2 hours postprandial (ACOG, Committee on Practice Bulletins—Obstetrics, 2013).

Hypertensive Disorders of Pregnancy   Hypertensive disorders of pregnancy include chronic hypertension, gestational hypertension, preeclampsia, preeclampsia superimposed on chronic hypertension, and eclampsia. Each of these conditions is a serious threat to maternal and newborn health. Gestational hypertension is defined as hypertension without proteinuria that develops after 20 weeks' gestation (ACOG & Task Force on Hypertension in Pregnancy, 2013). Preeclampsia alone, or superimposed on existing chronic hypertension, is a serious consequence of gestational hypertension. The greatest risk for adverse newborn outcome occurs when preterm birth becomes necessary to resolve acute maternal illness from preeclampsia.

The diagnostic criteria for preeclampsia are hypertension (blood pressure equal to or greater than 140/90 mm Hg) and proteinuria (more than 300 mg/24 hours) after 20 weeks' gestation. If proteinuria is absent, then the diagnosis requires at least one of the following: thrombocytopenia (fewer than 100,000 platelets/µL), impaired liver function, new renal insufficiency, pulmonary edema, or new-onset cerebral or visual disturbances. Severe preeclampsia is diagnosed if systolic blood pressure is equal to or greater than 160 mm Hg or diastolic blood pressure is equal to or greater than 110 mm Hg on 2 occasions at least 4 hours apart during bed rest, and there is evidence of significant and progressive hematologic, renal, liver, pulmonary, or cerebrovascular disease. Eclampsia is defined as new-onset grand mal seizures in women with preeclampsia (ACOG & Task Force on Hypertension in Pregnancy, 2013).

In cases of severe preeclampsia at gestation less than 33 weeks and 6 days, if preterm delivery is indicated, corticosteroids should be administered to the mother and delivery should be deferred for 48 hours (ACOG & Task Force on Hypertension in Pregnancy, 2013). Fetal growth restriction (less than the 5th percentile), oligohydramnios (amniotic fluid index less than 5 cm), and reversed end-diastolic flow on umbilical artery Doppler studies indicate significant fetal compromise. If delivery cannot be deferred due to severe maternal illness, placental abruption, or neonatal compromise, corticosteroids should be administered for a fetus less than 34 weeks' gestation, and delivery should proceed after maternal stabilization (ACOG & Task Force on Hypertension in Pregnancy, 2013). Research is ongoing to predict antecedents of preeclampsia and to test the efficacy of a number of antepartum prophylactic measures that are posited to prevent the disease (ACOG & Task Force on Hypertension in Pregnancy, 2013).

Perinatally Acquired Infections

Perinatally acquired infectious diseases may have devastating and debilitating neonatal outcomes. During the perinatal period, screening for common infectious agents is recommended because of the potential for adverse neonatal outcomes (**Table 2-5**).

Table 2-5: Perinatal Infectious Diseases

Infectious Agent	Newborn/Neonatal Sequelae
Hepatitis B virus (HBV)	Approximately 40% of infants born to HBV-infected women who do not receive immunoprophylaxis at birth will develop chronic hepatitis B infection.
	About 25% of infants who develop chronic infection will not survive.
Hepatitis C virus (HCV)	Approximately 6% of infants born to HCV-infected mothers will be infected with the virus. There is an increased risk of transmission with maternal HCV viremia at birth and coinfection with HIV. Prophylaxis to prevent transmission is currently not available.
	At birth, most infants infected are asymptomatic.
	Long-term effects of perinatal HCV infection are not well known.
Tuberculosis (TB)	Infants and children younger than 4 years of age are at high risk for developing disseminated tuberculosis.
Herpes simplex (HSV)	Incidence of perinatal transmission is highest during a maternal primary outbreak.
	Disseminated infection is the most severe form of neonatal herpes, with an 85% mortality rate for untreated neonates.
Rubella	The risk of congenital infection and anomalies is increased during the first 12 weeks of gestation.
Human immunodeficiency virus (HIV)	A 6-week neonatal zidovudine prophylaxis regimen is generally recommended for all HIV-exposed neonates to reduce perinatal transmission of HIV. A 4-week neonatal zidovudine prophylaxis

(Continued)

Table 2-5: Perinatal Infectious Diseases (*Continued*)

Infectious Agent	Newborn/Neonatal Sequelae
	regimen can be considered for full-term infants when the mother has received standard combination antiretroviral therapy during pregnancy with consistent viral suppression, and there are no concerns related to maternal adherence.
Sexually transmitted infections (gonorrhea, chlamydia, human papillomavirus)	Gonorrhea: gonococcal ophthalmia neonatorum Chlamydia: *Chlamydia trachomatis* ophthalmia neonatorum and/or pneumonia Human papillomavirus: can cause laryngeal papillomatosis (rare)
Group B *Streptococcus* (GBS)	Early-onset disease occurs during the first week of life; late-onset disease occurs from the first week through 3 months of life. Can cause sepsis, pneumonia, and meningitis.
Congenital syphilis	Neonatal treatment decisions are based on the diagnosis of syphilis in the mother, adequacy of maternal treatment, clinical evidence of syphilis in the neonate, and comparison of maternal titers at delivery and neonatal nontreponemal serologic titers of same test (by the same laboratory). Newborns suspected of having syphilis should be evaluated and tested for HIV.

Data from Centers for Disease Control and Prevention. (2003). Treatment of tuberculosis: American Thoracic Society, CDC, and Infectious Diseases Society of America. *Morbidity and Mortality Weekly Report, 52*(No. RR-11), 1–77; Centers for Disease Control and Prevention. (2010). 2010 guidelines for the prevention of perinatal group B streptococcal disease. *Morbidity and Mortality Weekly Report, 59*(RR-10), 1–32; Centers for Disease Control and Prevention. (2012). Congenital rubella infection. In *Manual for the surveillance of vaccine-preventable diseases*. Atlanta, GA: Author; Centers for Disease Control and Prevention. (2015). Viral hepatitis: hepatitis B information: Perinatal transmission. Retrieved from http://www.cdc.gov/hepatitis/HBV/PerinatalXmtn.htm; Centers for Disease Control and Prevention. (2015). Viral hepatitis: hepatitis C information: Hepatitis C FAQs for health professionals. Retrieved from http://www.cdc.gov/hepatitis/hcv/hcvfaq.htm#section4; Centers for Disease Control and Prevention. (2015). 2015 sexually transmitted diseases guidelines: Congenital syphilis. Retrieved from http://www.cdc.gov/std/tg2015/congenital.htm; Knezevic, A., Martic, J., Stanojevic, M., Jankovic, S., Nedeljkovic, J., Nikolic, L. (2007). Disseminated neonatal herpes caused by herpes simplex virus types 1 and 2. *Emerging Infectious Diseases, 13*(2), 302–304; Panel on Antiretroviral Therapy and Medical Management of HIV-Infected Children. (2015). Guidelines for the use of antiretroviral agents in pediatric HIV infection. Retrieved from http://aidsinfo.nih.gov/contentfiles/lvguidelines/pediatricguidelines.pdf.

Perinatal Substance Abuse

Internationally, perinatal substance abuse is a significant problem, posing a number of health risks for the pregnant woman, fetus, and newborn. During the embryonic period of gestation (the first trimester), maternal substance abuse may result in significant teratogenic effects. After the first trimester, abnormal growth patterns, alterations in neurotransmitters and their receptors, and disturbances in brain development and organization may occur with such abuse (Behnke, Smith, Committee on Substance Abuse, & Committee on Fetus and Newborn, 2013). Maternal substance abuse may be the result of or trigger intimate partner violence; places the pregnant woman at risk for sexually transmitted infections, including HIV and viral hepatitis; and may impair parenting behaviors (WHO, 2014).

Alcohol consumption during pregnancy is common. In the 2011–2013 Behavioral Risk Factor Surveillance System survey, 1 in 10 pregnant women reported consuming alcohol in the past 30 days, and 1 in 33 reported binge drinking (Tan, Denny, Cheal, Sniezek, & Kanny, 2015). Fetal alcohol spectrum disorder (FASD) is among the most common identifiable causes of developmental delay and intellectual disability. In 2015, the American Academy of Pediatrics' Committee on Substance Abuse strongly affirmed that *no* amount of alcohol intake at any time during pregnancy should be considered safe. Furthermore, the AAP warned of the dose-related risk of FASD from binge drinking (Williams et al., 2015).

The National Survey on Drug Use and Health (NSDUH) (Substance Abuse and Mental Health Services Administration [SAMHSA], 2014) is an annual survey that provides national and state-level information about the use of alcohol, tobacco, and illicit drugs, and nonmedical use of prescription drugs. Approximately 70,000 individuals older than the age of 12, including pregnant women, are represented in the survey. From the NSDUH data, inferences about the prevalence, incidence, and effects of perinatal substance abuse can be surmised. **Table 2-6** summarizes the short- and long-term effects of perinatal substance exposure on the infant/child.

Opioid Use During Pregnancy

The United States is currently experiencing an epidemic of abuse of *prescribed* controlled substances, often originally administered for the management of chronic pain. More than 116 million Americans report chronic pain and receive pharmacologic treatment for this condition (CDC, 2012, 2015b; Manchikanti et al., 2012). The abuse of prescription analgesics, including the misuse of opioids prescribed for chronic pain, increased sevenfold from 1999 to 2010. Opioid addiction often begins with a prescription for a controlled substance to manage chronic pain (CDC, 2012, 2013). According to a CDC (2013) report, opioids prescribed by providers currently account for more unintended overdose deaths than heroin and cocaine

Table 2-6: Effects of Perinatal Substance Exposure on the Infant

Effects	Nicotine	Alcohol	Marijuana	Opiates	Cocaine	Methamphetamine
Short-Term/Birth						
Fetal growth	Effect	Strong effect	No effect	Effect	Effect	Effect
Anomalies	No consensus	Strong effect	No effect	No effect	No effect	No effect
Withdrawal	No effect	No effect	No effect	Strong effect	No effect	Limited data
Neuro-behavioral	Effect	Effect	Effect	Effect	Effect	Effect
Long-Term						
Growth	No consensus	Strong effect	No effect	No effect	No consensus	Limited data
Behavior	Effect	Strong effect	Effect	Effect	Effect	Limited data
Cognition	Effect	Strong effect	Effect	No consensus	Effect	Limited data
Language	Effect	Effect	No effect	Limited data	Effect	Limited data
Achievement	Effect	Strong effect	Effect	Limited data	No consensus	Limited data

Reproduced with permission from Behnke, M., and Smith, V. C. (2013). Prenatal substance abuse, long- and short-term effects on the exposed fetus. *Pediatrics, 131*(3), p. e1016. Copyright (c) 2013 by the AAP.

combined. The majority of those who died from opioid overdose were given a prescription for the substance within 60 days of the reported overdose (CDC, 2013).

In addition to prescribed analgesics, the use of illicit opioid drugs by pregnant women is increasing. Opioid use among pregnant women increased sixfold from 2000 to 2009 and continues to rise (Patrick et al., 2012). When stratified by age, women of childbearing age (25 to 34 years) are most likely to abuse prescription painkillers (CDC, 2013). In addition, the 2013 National Survey on Drug Use and Health found that pregnant females, aged 15 to 17, now account for an alarming 14.6% of illicit drug users (SAMHSA, 2014).

Studies are inconclusive regarding the teratogenic effects of opioid use during pregnancy (ACOG, 2012b). While some studies have found an association between first-trimester use of opiates and congenital anomalies, results are inclusive due to small sample sizes and methodological problems in the study designs. The overall rate of birth defects is low, with only a small increase in absolute risk (ACOG, 2012b). Opioid abuse during pregnancy may result in fetal IUGR, placental abruption, preterm labor and birth, fetal death, and in utero passage of meconium (ACOG, 2012b). In addition, women who abuse opioids often engage in behaviors that place them at risk for sexually transmitted infections, becoming victims of violence, and legal prosecution (ACOG, 2012b). Opioids are also clearly associated with an increased potential for psychological and physical dependence for the pregnant woman and newborn infant (SAMHSA, 2014). As a result, from 2004 to 2013, the incidence of neonatal intensive care unit (NICU) admissions for the treatment of neonatal abstinence syndrome (NAS) across the United States rose dramatically, from 7 to 27 cases per 1000 admissions (Tolia et al., 2015).

Transfer of Substances to the Fetus and Newborn

The vast majority of substances, including drugs, cross the placenta by way of passive diffusion (**Table 2-7**). The degree of drug transfer is contingent on the drug's chemical makeup (Concheiro, Jones, Johnson, Choo, & Huestis, 2011). Clinicians are encouraged to consider not "if" a drug crosses the placenta, but rather how much, how quickly, and by which mechanism (Blackburn, 2013). For example, lipid-soluble drugs cross the placenta more readily than water-soluble drugs. Developmental changes in the placenta's surface area, diffusion distance, permeability, and blood flow, as well as advancing gestational age of the fetus may act individually or in aggregate to affect placental transfer. As a result, drugs may be either completely transferred from mother to fetus (equivocal levels between mother and fetus), partially transferred (higher concentrations in the mother than in the fetus), or transferred in excess (higher concentrations in the fetus than the mother) (Blackburn, 2013).

Table 2-7: Mechanisms by Which Substances Cross the Placenta

Mechanism	Substance
Simple (passive) diffusion	Water, electrolytes, oxygen, carbon dioxide, urea, simple amines, creatinine, fatty acids, steroids, fat-soluble vitamins, narcotics, antibiotics, barbiturates, anesthetics
Facilitated diffusion	Glucose, oxygen
Active transport	Amino acids, water-soluble vitamins, calcium, iron, iodine
Pinocytosis and endocytosis	Globulins, phospholipids, lipoproteins, antibodies, viruses
Bulk flow/solid drag	Water, electrolytes

Two commonly encountered opioid-based therapies for pregnant women are buprenorphine and methadone. Rationales for use of either medication include (1) prevention of complications associated with opioid use and narcotic withdrawal, (2) appropriate and close monitoring by obstetric providers, (3) reduction in diversionary drug-seeking activities by pregnant women, and (4) reduction in obstetric complications (ACOG, 2012b). Both buprenorphine and methadone have a low molecular weight, are lipophilic, and passively diffuse across the placenta (Blackburn, 2013). However, their diffusion across the placenta is mitigated by syncytiotrophoblast tissues, which tend to sequester the drugs within these placental tissues (Blackburn, 2013). Several other factors—for example, gestational age, activity of the enzyme that metabolizes methadone, genetics, preexisting maternal/fetal complications, and concurrent use of drugs such as heroin and cocaine—also influence the rate of diffusion of methadone (Hieronymus et al., 2006).

Buprenorphine is a water-soluble, lipophilic drug. Approximately 10% to 50% of maternally ingested buprenorphine diffuses across the placenta, with approximately 5% to 10% of that amount being metabolized to norbuprenorphine (Bartu, Ilett, Hackett, Doherty, & Hamilton, 2012). Norbuprenorphine is the metabolite form of the drug and has 25% of the analgesic activity and 10 times the respiratory depressant effect of buprenorphine (Bartu et al., 2012). Using 1- and 5-minute Apgar scores, no studies have documented statistically significant depressive effects as a result of maternal buprenorphine ingestion in the third trimester. Measured by the modified Finnegan scoring system, NAS occurs with a mean onset of treatable symptoms at 36 to 60 hours of life and average withdrawal period lasting 30 or more days (Kocherlakota, 2014). A dose–response relationship between maternal ingestion of buprenorphine and NAS remains inconclusive. Breastfeeding is recommended, with a relative infant dose of buprenorphine ingested via breastmilk of 0.09% to 1.9% (clinically insignificant) (Hale & Rowe, 2014).

Variation in methadone concentration and diffusion across the placenta in pregnant women is high. Nanovskaya, Nekhayeva, Hankins, and Ahmed (2008) reported transfer of methadone from mother to fetus at rates as high as 31%. Similar to buprenorphine, methadone is reported to become sequestered within placental syncytiotrophoblasts, making the placenta somewhat of a gatekeeper or protective mechanism for the fetus. Measured by the modified Finnegan scoring system, NAS is most often reported with a mean onset of treatable symptoms at 48 to 72 hours of life and average withdrawal lasting 28 or more days (Kocherlakota, 2014). No studies were found that indicated a dose–response relationship with maternal ingestion of methadone and NAS. Breastfeeding is recommended, with a relative infant dose of methadone ingested via the breastmilk of 1.9% to 6.5% (Hale & Rowe, 2014). A reduction in the incidence and severity of NAS has been observed in women who ingest methadone and breastfeed (Dryden, Young, Hepburn, & Mactier, 2009).

Screening for Substance Abuse

Screening pregnant women for substance abuse should be done with a nonjudgmental, information-seeking attitude on the part of the healthcare provider (ACOG, 2012b). At each prenatal visit, each pregnant woman should be screened by using specific terminology to elicit feedback about alcohol, drug, and prescription opioid use (ACOG, 2012b). The two recommended screening tools are presented in **Table 2-8** and **Table 2-9**.

Table 2-8: Ewing's Four P's Screening Tool

Question	Response*
Did any of your *parents* have a problem with alcohol or drug abuse?	Yes/no
Does your *partner* have a problem with alcohol or drug use?	Yes/no
In the *past*, have you had difficulties in your life because of alcohol or drugs, including prescription medications?	Yes/no
In the past month have you *presently* drunk any alcohol or used other drugs?	Yes/no

* Any positive response should elicit further questioning.
Modified from American College of Obstetricians and Gynecologists, Committee on Health Care for Underserved Women & American Society of Addiction Medicine. (2012). Opioid abuse, dependence, and addiction in pregnancy. *Obstetrics & Gynecology, 119,* 1071. Copyright 2012 by the American College of Obstetrics & Gynecologists.

Table 2-9: CRAFFT Substance Abuse Screen for Adolescents and Young Adults

Question	Response*
Have you ever ridden in a *car* driven by someone (including yourself) who was high or had been using alcohol or drugs?	Yes/no
Do you ever use alcohol or drugs to *relax*, feel better about yourself, or fit in?	Yes/no
Do you ever use alcohol or drugs while you are by yourself or *alone*?	Yes/no
Do you ever *forget* things you did while using alcohol or drugs?	Yes/no
Do your *family* or friends ever tell you that you should cut down on your drinking or drug use?	Yes/no
Have you ever gotten in *trouble* while you were using alcohol or drugs?	Yes/no

* Two or more positive responses should elicit further questioning.
Modified from American College of Obstetricians and Gynecologists, Committee on Health Care for Underserved Women & American Society of Addiction Medicine. (2012). Opioid abuse, dependence, and addiction in pregnancy. *Obstetrics & Gynecology, 119,* 1071. From Center for Adolescent Substance Abuse Research, Children's Hospital Boston. (2009). The CRAFFT screening interview.

Intrapartum History

After reviewing the prenatal history to identify any pregnancy-related issues, the provider should review the intrapartum history. Reviewing the conduct of labor and birth is important in identifying influences on the newborn's health after birth and during the first few weeks of life. In addition to the method of birth (i.e., spontaneous vaginal birth, assisted vaginal birth, or cesarean section), the initial transition and treatment may be affected by the conditions identified in **Box 2-1**.

Normal Physiologic Childbirth

Normal physiologic childbirth is characterized by the spontaneous onset and progression of labor, within a process that utilizes biologic and physiologic conditions to promote effective labor ("Supporting Healthy and Normal Physiologic Childbirth," 2013). Maternal and neonatal benefits of physiologic birth include (1) the reduction of perinatal morbidity and mortality from complications of invasive procedures, (2) reduced iatrogenic causes of harm to the newborn, and (3) the promotion of breastfeeding and maternal attachment.

Box 2-1: Conditions Affecting the Care of the Newborn

- Premature rupture of membranes
- Length of rupture of membranes
- Meconium staining
- GBS status and treatment if done
- Total length of labor
- Presentation of newborn
- Maternal medications, pain management, tocolysis, Pitocin, antibiotics
- Complications during labor and delivery
- Birth trauma
- Apgar scores
- Resuscitation
- Cord gas, if completed

Data from American Academy of Pediatrics (AAP), Committee on Fetus and Newborn, & American College of Obstetricians and Gynecologists (ACOG), Committee on Obstetric Practice (2012a). Intrapartum and postpartum care of the mother. In AAP, Committee on Fetus and Newborn, & ACOG, Committee on Obstetric Practice (Eds.), *Guidelines for perinatal care* (7th ed., pp. 169–210). Elk Grove Village, IL: AAP; Smith, V. C. (2012). The high-risk newborn: Anticipation, evaluation, management, and outcome. In J. P. Cloherty, E. C. Eichenwald, A. R. Hansen, & A. R. Stark (Eds.), *Manual of neonatal care* (7th ed., pp. 74–90). Philadelphia, PA: Wolters Kluwer.

Cesarean Birth

Although 1 in 3 women in the United States gives birth by cesarean section, the rapid rise in the number of cesarean births (from 1996 to 2011) did not decrease maternal or neonatal morbidity and mortality (ACOG, 2015b). Cesarean birth occurs when the mother/fetus pair experience labor dystocia, abnormal or indeterminate fetal heart rate tracing, fetal malpresentation, multiple gestation, or suspected fetal macrosomia. Significant variations in the rates of cesarean birth for primiparous and multiparous women occur from state to state, from hospital to hospital, and from provider to provider. Cesarean birth is associated with a higher incidence of complications, such as amniotic fluid embolism, abnormal placentation with each subsequent pregnancy, and neonatal laceration and respiratory distress. Efforts to reduce cesarean birth include (1) an evidence-based approach to defining labor dystocia, (2) standardization of fetal heart rate interpretation, (3) external cephalic version for breech presentation, and (4) supporting women with twin gestations who desire a trial of labor when the first twin is in cephalic presentation (ACOG, 2015b).

While rates of cesarean birth have been rising, rates of vaginal operative deliveries (forceps or vacuum extraction) have declined significantly in the last 15 years. In 2015, ACOG affirmed support for the safe and effective use of operative vaginal delivery to avoid cesarean birth. ACOG (2015b) identifies the indications for operative vaginal delivery as prolonged second stage of labor, immediate or potential fetal compromise, and shortening the second stage of labor for maternal benefit.

The overall risk of injury to newborns from operative vaginal delivery is estimated to be low, although large studies are necessary to reliably establish the extent of risk and complications. The type of neonatal injury experienced usually depends on the type and frequency of the instrument used. **Table 2-10** lists potential neonatal injuries based on the instrument used for operative delivery. In a review of 13 randomized trials that compared forceps with vacuum

Table 2-10: Potential Neonatal Injuries from Operative Delivery

Forceps	Vacuum Extractor
• Laceration	• Facial lacerations
• Cephalohematoma	• Facial nerve palsy
• Subgaleal or intracranial hemorrhage	• Corneal abrasions
• Retinal hemorrhages	• External ocular trauma
• Hyperbilirubinemia	• Skull fracture
	• Intracranial hemorrhage

Data from American College of Obstetricians and Gynecologists (ACOG). (2015). Practice bulletin no. 154: Operative vaginal delivery. *Obstetrics & Gynecology, 126*(5), e56–65. doi: 10.1097/AOG.0000000000001147

extraction, no significant differences were found in umbilical arterial pH, morbidity, or death with these techniques (ACOG, 2015b).

Neonatal Resuscitation

In 2015, the International Consensus on Cardiopulmonary Resuscitation and Emergency Cardiovascular Care Science with Treatment Recommendations Task Force published updates to the 2010 Neonatal Resuscitation Program guidelines (Perlman, Wyllie, & Kattwinkel, 2015). These recommendations and conclusions were reached by consensus after a comprehensive systematic review. Key differences from the 2010 guidelines are summarized in **Box 2-2**.

Box 2-2: 2015 Updated Neonatal Resuscitation Recommendations

- Delayed cord clamping for greater than 30 seconds is reasonable for both term and preterm infants who do not require resuscitation at birth, but there is insufficient evidence to recommend a specific approach to cord clamping for infants who require resuscitation at birth.
- The routine use of cord milking for infants born at less than 29 weeks' gestation should be avoided until more is known about the benefits and complications of this procedure.
- The neonate's temperature should be maintained between 36.5°C and 37.5°C after birth and recorded as a predictor of outcomes and quality indicator. Use of radiant warmers, plastic wrap with a cap, thermal mattress, warmed and humidified gases, and increased room temperature with a cap and thermal mattress are strategies to establish and maintain euthermia.
- Hyperthermia (temperature greater than 38°C) should be avoided.
- If an infant is born through meconium-stained amniotic fluid and presents with poor muscle tone and inadequate breathing efforts, positive-pressure ventilation should be initiated, after suctioning the oro-nasopharynx, if needed. Routine intubation for tracheal suction is no longer suggested due to insufficient evidence to support this practice.
- Assessment of heart rate remains critical during the first minute of resuscitation, and the use of a 3-lead ECG may be reasonable. Use of the ECG does not replace the need for pulse oximetry.
- Resuscitation of preterm newborns born at less than 35 weeks' gestation should be initiated with 21% to 30% oxygen, and titrated to achieve preductal oxygen saturation in the range of healthy term infants.
- There are insufficient data about the safety and method of application of sustained inflation for the transitioning newborn.

Data from Perlman, J. M., Wyllie, J., Kattwinkel, J., Wyckoff, M. H., Aziz, K., Guinsburg, R., . . . Velaphi, S. (2015). Part 7: Neonatal resuscitation: 2015 International Consensus on Cardiopulmonary Resuscitation and Emergency Cardiovascular Care Science with treatment recommendations. *Circulation, 132*(suppl 1), S204–S241.

The majority of infants who require resuscitation at birth are identified before birth. **Table 2-11** lists risks for resuscitation at birth based on perinatal history and the maternal and fetal status during labor. The need for resuscitation at birth is rapidly assessed by answering these three questions:

- Is the newborn at term gestation?
- Is the tone good?
- Is the baby breathing or crying?

The "Golden Minute" is the first minute of life, when initial steps to resuscitate the newborn should result in stabilization of the infant. Although the 60-second time limit to implement successful resuscitation is not based on data from randomized clinical trials, it is a reasonable window within which the effectiveness of resuscitation efforts can be evaluated, and additional measures can be implemented to prevent hypoxia and asphyxia (Perlman et al., 2015).

Table 2-11: Risk Factors Identifying the Need for Resuscitation at Birth

Perinatal History	Maternal Status in Labor	Fetal Status in Labor
• Intrauterine growth restriction • Decreased fetal movement • Congenital anomalies • Prematurity • Multiple gestation • Hydrops fetalis • Suspicion of macrosomia and concern about possible shoulder dystocia • Known sexually transmitted infection • Maternal diabetes, hypertension, or renal, pulmonary, or cardiac disease	• Acute event (abruption, cord prolapse) • Significant vaginal bleeding • Fever • Membranes ruptured for more than 24 hours • Chorioamnionitis	• Abnormal or indeterminate fetal heart rate tracing • Abnormal fetal presentation • Meconium-stained amniotic fluid • Administration of maternal narcotics shortly prior to delivery

Data from American Academy of Pediatrics (AAP), Committee on Fetus and Newborn, & American College of Obstetricians and Gynecologists (ACOG), Committee on Obstetric Practice (2012a). Intrapartum and postpartum care of the mother. In AAP, Committee on Fetus and Newborn, & ACOG, Committee on Obstetric Practice (Eds.), *Guidelines for perinatal care* (7th ed., pp. 169–210). Elk Grove Village, IL: AAP; Smith, V. C. (2012). The high-risk newborn: Anticipation, evaluation, management, and outcome. In J. P. Cloherty, E. C. Eichenwald, A. R. Hansen, & A. R. Stark (Eds.), *Manual of neonatal care* (7th ed., pp. 74–90). Philadelphia, PA: Wolters Kluwer.

The Apgar Score

In 1953, Virginia Apgar, MD, proposed a system for evaluation of the newborn at birth based on heart rate, respiratory effort, reflex irritability, muscle tone, and color at 1 and 5 minutes of age. The Apgar score is still accepted as a convenient method for determining the newborn's status immediately after birth. This score is not predictive of neonatal mortality or neurologic outcome, however, and it should not be considered as evidence of birth asphyxia. Both the AAP and the ACOG encourage use of an expanded Apgar score. Extending newborn Apgar scoring up to 20 minutes after birth reflects resuscitation efforts, cardiorespiratory status, and neurologic conditions (ACOG, 2015a).

Cultural Considerations During Childbirth

The culture in which a mother gives birth, as well as the culture she identifies with, will likely influence her experience of childbirth (Greene, 2007; National Perinatal Association & Shah, 2004). On both individual and community levels, a person's culture influences her or his perceptions and beliefs about healthcare practices (Dreachslin, Gilbert, & Malone, 2013). Even within a given culture, however, wide variations in nationality, language, religion, and customs may exist.

More than 40% of the U.S. population reports their race or ethnicity as non-white (U.S. Census Bureau, 2015). In the United States, non-white race and ethnicity are associated with inequities in access to health care and poorer outcomes.

Acculturation is the process by which individuals adopt the beliefs and behaviors of another group, usually the dominant culture in a society (O'Brien, Alos, Davey, Bueno, & Whitaker, 2014). Newly arrived immigrants tend to closely adhere to the beliefs and practices of their native culture regarding care of mothers and newborns. When immigrants live for longer periods within the dominant culture, however, more acculturation occurs, which may negatively impact maternal child health and birth outcomes (O'Brien et al., 2014; Pak-Gorstein, Haq, & Graham, 2009).

While newborn care varies widely across and among cultures, care at birth focuses on six common themes: naming rituals, feeding practices, bathing and hygiene, caregiver roles, beliefs about the placenta, and beliefs about circumcision. Discussing newborn care prior to birth can prevent conflict and misunderstanding between healthcare providers, the mother, and her family. Open discussion may also identify practices that may be potentially harmful to the neonate. Many people of other cultures mistrust Western traditional healthcare practices and prefer indigenous practices that are familiar to them and supported within their communities. Principles of culturally sensitive communication to enhance respect and understanding between providers and patients of different cultures are listed in **Box 2-3**.

Box 2-3: Principles of Culturally Sensitive Communication Data

- Personalize interactions with first and last name introductions, addressing patients and their significant others by name.
- Be prepared for patient encounters by investigating healthcare practices that are specific to the mother's and family's culture.
- Understand personal fears and biases when interacting with individuals from different cultures.
- Don't assume one size fits all because significant differences in beliefs and practices among individuals of the same culture or ethnicity do exist.
- Be mindful of body language and aware of specific gestures and behaviors that can be interpreted as disrespectful.
- Use language that is clearly understood and be aware that words may not have the same meaning in other cultures.
- Be a good listener—ask for clarification of points that are not well understood, and follow-up after conversations to confirm understanding.
- Provide positive reinforcement, reassurance, and encouragement to the patient and her family to ask questions and express concerns.
- Promote a family-centered team approach to health promotion and disease prevention.
- Be a conduit for the reciprocal sharing of information.

Data from Dreachslin, J. L., Gilbert, M. J., & Malone, B. (2013). *Diversity and cultural competence in healthcare: A systems approach*. San Francisco, CA: Jossey-Bass; National Perinatal Association & Shah, M. A. (Ed.) (2004). *Transcultural aspects of perinatal health care: A resource guide*. Tampa, FL: National Perinatal Association; Pak-Gorstein, S., Haq, A., & Graham, E. A. (2009). Cultural influences on infant feeding practices. *Pediatrics in Review/American Academy of Pediatrics, 30*(3), e11–e21. doi: 10.1542/pir.30-3-e11.

Conclusion

The newborn's clinical course after birth is intimately linked to fetal and maternal history, as well as intrapartum events. A risk-oriented assessment of the perinatal record facilitates the proactive and timely management of newborns who are at risk for adverse birth outcomes. Because shared chronic illness and genetically acquired conditions among family members are common, a careful review of the family history is essential in care of the neonate. A careful review of the intrapartum history should identify any events that might negatively impact the health of the neonate at and after birth.

An ongoing challenge for healthcare providers is the widespread use of electronic health records that often fail to connect maternal and family health information with the newborn's medical record. Providers of newborn care must know which perinatal risk factors might potentially affect birth outcomes, whether or not they are captured in the newborn electronic health record.

Student Practice Activities

Baby Boy M. is a 38-week-gestational-age infant who is now 12 hours old. His mother is a 24-year-old G1P0 who gave birth within an hour of admission. The newborn weighed 2850 g and had Apgar scores of 3 and 8 at 1 and 5 minutes, respectively. He required a brief period of positive-pressure ventilation for respiratory depression. The perinatal history is significant for inadequate prenatal care. The mother had one prenatal visit at 15 weeks' gestation, for confirmatory ultrasound. At this prenatal visit, she denied alcohol or drug use, although her urine toxicology screen was positive for opiates. Her history is significant for a back injury suffered during a car accident 1 year ago. She stated that she takes over-the-counter analgesics to control her pain. You review her record and note that she was seen in four different emergency departments within the past 6 months for her back pain, including a visit 3 months ago. At each of these visits, opioids were prescribed. Concerns for maternal drug abuse are reported to the pediatric team, and the infant is monitored for signs of neonatal abstinence syndrome.

1. Which components of the perinatal history identify this infant as at risk for neonatal abstinence syndrome?

2. What is neonatal abstinence syndrome?

3. How does NAS affect the newborn?

4. How is NAS diagnosed in newborns?

5. Describe discharge planning for the newborn with NAS.

Multiple Choice

1. Narcotics cross the placenta and enter the fetal circulation through:
   A) active transport.
   B) simple diffusion.
   C) pinocytosis.
   D) independent movement.

2. First-degree relatives share approximately _____ of their genes.
   A) 20%
   B) 25%
   C) 50%
   D) 75%

3. Which of the following disorders has the highest risk for mortality during early childhood?
   A) Tay-Sachs disease
   B) Beta-thalassemia
   C) Huntington disease
   D) Fragile X syndrome

4. Which of the following statements about inherited genetic disorders is false?
   A) The incidence of shared chronic illnesses among family members can be increased by 2 to 5 times.
   B) Most genetic disorders are inherited through classic Mendelian patterns.
   C) Personalized genomics can predict an individual's response to treatment.
   D) Disability from congenital hypothyroidism is preventable.

5. According to the 2015 updated neonatal resuscitation guidelines, which of the following statements is true?
   A) There is strong evidence to support the routine use of cord clamping for infants who require resuscitation.
   B) During resuscitation, the use of a neonatal ECG can be substituted for pulse oximetry.
   C) Routine intubation for tracheal suction is recommended for infants born through meconium-stained fluid.
   D) Preterm infants requiring resuscitation should be initially resuscitated with 21% to 30% oxygen.

6. Baby Girl F. is a 2-day-old infant born to a mother who recently emigrated to the United States from Haiti. The mother is breastfeeding her daughter. Which of the following statements reflect culturally sensitive communication in talking to her about the care of her newborn?
   A) Explain to her that naming her infant is required before discharge and offer her a book of common American names.
   B) Limit the number of visitors to prevent the baby from becoming ill.
   C) Discourage her family from bringing her food from home because you do not know how it will affect breastfeeding.
   D) Talk to her about the significance of the band of cloth she placed around the baby's abdomen.

7. Which of the following set of questions can quickly identify a baby in need of resuscitation?

    A) Did the mother receive narcotics? Is the baby full term? Is the baby breathing?

    B) Is the baby term? Is the tone good? Is the baby breathing or crying?

    C) Is the baby pink? Are there congenital anomalies? What is the cord pH?

    D) Is the baby appropriate for gestational age? Is there acrocyanosis? Are there sternal retractions?

8. What is the most common cause of neonatal death as a result of diabetes mellitus?

    A) Hyperglycemia

    B) Seizures

    C) Congenital anomalies

    D) Hyperbilirubinemia

9. What is the greatest risk for adverse neonatal outcomes for a mother with preeclampsia?

    A) Preterm birth

    B) Eclampsia

    C) Renal disease

    D) Congenital heart disease

10. Baby Boy G. is a 2800 g infant born by an uncomplicated spontaneous vaginal delivery at 39 weeks' gestation to a 21-year-old G1P0 mother. The mother did not begin prenatal care until 20 weeks' gestation. During her pregnancy, she was treated for gonorrhea and chlamydia. She admits to smoking one pack of cigarettes per day and denies alcohol or other substance use. She was treated with ferrous sulfate during her pregnancy for anemia. Which of the following aspects of the perinatal history places the infant at highest risk for sudden infant death syndrome?

    A) Low birth weight

    B) Late onset of prenatal care

    C) Anemia during pregnancy

    D) Cigarette smoking

References

American Academy of Pediatrics (AAP), Committee on Fetus and Newborn, & American College of Obstetricians and Gynecologists (ACOG), Committee on Obstetric Practice. (2012a). Intrapartum and postpartum care of the mother. In AAP, Committee on Fetus and Newborn, & ACOG, Committee on Obstetric Practice (Eds.), *Guidelines for perinatal care* (7th ed., pp. 169–210). Elk Grove Village, IL: AAP.

American Academy of Pediatrics (AAP), Committee on Fetus and Newborn, & American College of Obstetricians and Gynecologists (ACOG), Committee on Obstetric Practice. (2012b). Preconception and antepartum care. In: AAP, Committee on Fetus and Newborn, & ACOG, Committee on Obstetric Practice (Eds.), *Guidelines for perinatal care* (7th ed., pp. 95–167). Elk Grove Village, IL: AAP.

American Academy of Pediatrics (AAP), Committee on Fetus and Newborn, & American College of Obstetricians and Gynecologists (ACOG), Committee on Obstetric Practice. (2012c). Obstetric and medical complications. In AAP, Committee on Fetus and Newborn, & ACOG, Committee on Obstetric Practice (Eds.), *Guidelines for perinatal care* (7th ed., pp. 211–264). Elk Grove Village, IL: AAP.

American College of Obstetricians and Gynecologists (ACOG). (2012). ACOG committee opinion no. 518: Intimate partner violence. *Obstetrics & Gynecology, 119*(2 Pt 1), 412–417. doi: 10.1097/AOG.0b013e318249ff74

American College of Obstetricians and Gynecologists (ACOG). (2013). Practice bulletin no. 138: Inherited thrombophilias in pregnancy. *Obstetrics & Gynecology, 122*(3), 706–717. doi: 10.1097/01.AOG.0000433981.36184.4e

American College of Obstetricians and Gynecologists (ACOG). (2015a). ACOG committee opinion no. 644: The Apgar score. *Obstetrics & Gynecology, 126*(4), e52–e55.

American College of Obstetricians and Gynecologists (ACOG). (2015b). Practice bulletin no. 154: Operative vaginal delivery. *Obstetrics & Gynecology, 126*(5), e56–65. doi: 10.1097/AOG.0000000000001147

American College of Obstetricians and Gynecologists (ACOG), Committee on Practice Bulletins—Obstetrics. (2013). Practice bulletin no. 137: Gestational diabetes mellitus. *Obstetrics & Gynecology, 122*(2 Pt 1), 406–416. doi: 10.1097/01.AOG.0000433006.09219.f1

American College of Obstetricians and Gynecologists (ACOG) & Task Force on Hypertension in Pregnancy. (2013). Hypertension in pregnancy. *Obstetrics & Gynecology, 122*(5), 1122–1131. doi: 10.1097/01.AOG.0000437382.03963.88

Backes, C. H., Backes, C. R., Gardner, G., Nankervis, C. A., & Giannone, P. J. (2012). Neonatal abstinence syndrome: Transitioning methadone-treated infants from an inpatient to outpatient setting. *Journal of Perinatology, 32*(6), 425–430.

Bartu, A. E., Ilett, K. F., Hackett, L. P., Doherty, D. A., & Hamilton, D. (2012). Buprenorphine exposure in infants of opioid-dependent mothers at birth. *Australian & New Zealand Journal of Obstetrics & Gynaecology, 52*(4), 342–347. doi: 10.1111/j.1479-828X.2012.01424.x

Behnke, M., Smith, V. C., Committee on Substance Abuse, & Committee on Fetus and Newborn. (2013). Prenatal substance abuse: Short- and long-term effects on the exposed fetus. *Pediatrics, 131*(3), e1009–e1024. doi: 10.1542/peds.2012-3931

Bettegowda, V., Lackritz, E., & Petrini, J. (2011). Epidemiologic trends in perinatal data. In S. D. Berns (Ed.), *Toward improving the outcome of pregnancy III: Enhancing perinatal health through quality, safety and performance initiatives* (pp. 20–32). White Plains, NY: March of Dimes Foundation.

Blackburn, S. T. (2013). *Maternal, fetal, and neonatal physiology: A clinical perspective* (4th ed.). Maryland Heights, MO: Elsevier Saunders.

Centers for Disease Control and Prevention (CDC). (2010). *Guidelines for the identification and management of lead exposure in pregnant and lactating women.* Atlanta, GA: Author.

Centers for Disease Control and Prevention (CDC). (2012). Prescription drug overdose: State laws. [Data file]. pp.1–25. Retrieved from http://www.cdc.gov/homeandrecreationalsafety/pubs/RXReport_web-a.pdf

Centers for Disease Control and Prevention (CDC). (2013). Prescription painkillers. Retrieved from http://www.cdc.gov/vitalsigns/PrescriptionPainkillerOverdoses/index.html

Centers for Disease Control and Prevention (CDC). (2015a). Chronic diseases: The leading causes of death and disability in the United States. Retrieved from http://www.cdc.gov/chronicdisease/overview/

Centers for Disease Control and Prevention (CDC). (2015b). Injury prevention and control: Prescription drug overdose. Retrieved from http://www.cdc.gov/drugoverdose/index.html

Centers for Disease Control and Prevention (CDC). (2015c). Sudden infant death syndrome. Retrieved from http://www.cdc.gov/Features/SidsAwarenessMonth/index.html

Comeau, A. M., Accurso, F. J., White, T. B., Campbell, P. W. 3rd, Hoffman, G., Parad, R. B.,. . . & the Cystic Fibrosis Foundation. (2007). Guidelines for implementation of cystic fibrosis newborn screening programs: Cystic fibrosis foundation workshop report. *Pediatrics, 119*(2), e495–e518. doi: 119/2/e495

Concheiro, M., Jones, H. E., Johnson, R. E., Choo, R., & Huestis, M. A. (2011). Preliminary buprenorphine sublingual tablet pharmacokinetic data in plasma, oral fluid, and sweat during treatment of opioid-dependent pregnant women. *Therapeutic Drug Monitoring, 33*(5), 619–626. doi: 10.1097/FTD.0b013e318228bb2a

Creanga, A. A., Berg, C. J., Syverson, C., Seed, K., Bruce, F. C., & Callaghan, W. M. (2015). Pregnancy-related mortality in the United States, 2006–2010. *Obstetrics & Gynecology, 125*(1), 5–12. doi: 10.1097/AOG.0000000000000564

Cunningham, F. G., Leveno, K. J., Bloom, S. L., Spong, C. Y., Dashe, J. S., Hoffman, B. L.,. . . Sheffield, J. C. (Eds.). (2014). Chronic hypertension. In *Williams Obstetrics* (pp. 1000–1010). New York, NY: McGraw-Hill Education.

Cystic Fibrosis Foundation. (2015). Newborn screening for CF. Retrieved from https://www.cff.org/What-is-CF/Testing/Newborn-Screening-for-CF/

Dolan, S. M., & Moore, C. (2007). Linking family history in obstetric and pediatric care: Assessing risk for genetic disease and birth defects. *Pediatrics, 120*(suppl 2), S66–S67. doi: 120/SUPPLEMENT_2/S66

Dreachslin, J. L., Gilbert, M. J., & Malone, B. (2013). *Diversity and cultural competence in healthcare: A systems approach.* San Francisco, CA: Jossey-Bass.

Dryden, C., Young, D., Hepburn, M., & Mactier, H. (2009). Maternal methadone use in pregnancy: Factors associated with the development of neonatal abstinence syndrome and implications for healthcare resources. *BJOG: An International Journal of Obstetrics & Gynaecology, 116*(5), 665–671. doi: 10.1111/j.1471-0528.2008.02073.x

Gardner, S. L., & Hernandez, J. A. (2016). Heat balance. In S. L. Gardner, B. S. Carter, M. Enzman-Hines, & J. A. Hernandez (Eds.), *Merenstein and Gardner's handbook of neonatal intensive care* (8th ed., pp. 105–125). St. Louis, MO: Elsevier-Mosby.

Genetic Alliance. (2008). *Understanding genetics: A New York, Mid-Atlantic guide for patients and health professionals.* Washington, DC: Author.

Greene, M. J. (2007). Strategies for incorporating cultural competence into childbirth education curriculum. *Journal of Perinatal Education, 16*(2), 33–37. doi: 10.1624/105812407X191489

Hale, T. W., & Rowe, H. E. (2014). *Medications and mother's milk* (16th ed.). Plano, TX: Hale Publishing.

Hare, J. W., & White, P. (1980). Gestational diabetes and the white classification. *Diabetes Care, 3*(2), 394.

Hayes, M. J., & Brown, M. S. (2012). Epidemic of prescription opiate abuse and neonatal abstinence. *Journal of the American Medical Association, 307,* 1974–1975.

Hieronymus, T. L., Nanovskaya, T. N., Deshmukh, S. V., Vargas, R., Hankins, G. D., & Ahmed, M. S. (2006). Methadone metabolism by early gestational age placentas. *American Journal of Perinatology, 23*(5), 287–294. doi: 10.1055/s-2006-947160

James, P. A., Oparil, S., Carter, B. L., Cushman, W. C., Dennison-Himmelfarb, C., Handler, J.,. . . Ortiz, E. (2014). 2014 evidence-based guideline for the management of high blood pressure in adults: Report from the panel members appointed to the eighth Joint National Committee (JNC 8). *Journal of the American Medical Association, 311*(5), 507–520. doi: 10.1001/jama.2013.284427

Johnson, L., & Cochran, W. D. (2012). Assessment of the newborn history and physical examination of the newborn. In J. P. Cloherty, E. C. Eichenwald, A. R. Hansen, & A. R. Stark (Eds.), *Manual of neonatal care* (7th ed., pp. 91–102). Philadelphia, PA: Wolters Kluwer.

Johnson, Y. R. (2012). Multiple births. In J. P. Cloherty, E. C. Eichenwald, A. R. Hansen, & A. R. Stark (Eds.), *Manual of neonatal care* (7th ed., pp. 124–133). Philadelphia, PA: Wolters Kluwer.

Kelly, L. E., Knoppert, D., Roukema, H., Rieder, M. J., & Koren, G. (2015). Oral morphine weaning for neonatal abstinence syndrome at home compared with in-hospital: An observational cohort study. *Pediatric Drugs, 17*(2), 151–157. doi: 10.1007/s40272-014-0096-y

Kocherlakota, P. (2014). Neonatal abstinence syndrome. *Pediatrics, 134*(2), e547–e561. doi: 10.1542/peds.2013-3524

Lancaster, C. A., Gold, K. J., Flynn, H. A., Yoo, H., Marcus, S. M., & Davis, M. M. (2010). Risk factors for depressive symptoms during pregnancy: A systematic review. *American Journal of Obstetrics & Gynecology, 202*(1), 5–14. doi: 10.1016/j.ajog.2009.09.007

Lee-Parritz, A., & Cloherty, J. P. (2012). Diabetes mellitus. In J. P. Cloherty, E. C. Eichenwald, A. R. Hansen, & A. R. Stark (Eds.), *Manual of neonatal care* (pp. 11–23). Philadelphia, PA: Wolters Kluwer.

Manchikanti, L., Helm, S. 2nd, Fellows, B., Janata, J. W., Pampati, V., Grider, J. S., & Boswell M. V. (2012). Opioid epidemic in the United States. *Pain Physician, 15*(3 suppl), ES9–ES38.

McLennan, Y., Polussa, J., Tassone, F., & Hagerman, R. (2011). Fragile X syndrome. *Current Genomics, 12*(3), 216–224. doi:1 0.2174/138920211795677886

Metzger, B. E., Lowe, L. P., Dyer, A. R., Trimble, E. R., Chaovarindr, U., Coustan, D. R., . . . Sacks, D. A. (2008). Hyperglycemia and adverse pregnancy outcomes. HAPO Study Cooperative Research Group. *New England Journal of Medicine, 358*, 1991–2002.

Nanovskaya, T. N., Nekhayeva, I. A., Hankins, G. D., & Ahmed, M. S. (2008). Transfer of methadone across the dually perfused preterm human placental lobule. *American Journal of Obstetrics & Gynecology, 198*(1), 126.e1–126.e4. doi: 10.1016/j.ajog.2007.06.073

National Library of Medicine. (2015). *Genetics home reference* [Internet]. Bethesda, MD: Author. Retrieved from http://ghr.nlm.nih.gov/

National Perinatal Association & Shah, M. A. (Ed.) (2004). *Transcultural aspects of perinatal health care: A resource guide*. Tampa, FL: National Perinatal Association.

O'Brien, M. J., Alos, V. A., Davey, A., Bueno, A., & Whitaker, R. C. (2014). Acculturation and the prevalence of diabetes in US Latino adults: National Health and Nutrition Examination Survey 2007–2010. *Prevention of Chronic Disease, 11*, 140–142. doi: http://dx.doi.org/10.5888/pcd11.140142

Pak-Gorstein, S., Haq, A., & Graham, E. A. (2009). Cultural influences on infant feeding practices. *Pediatrics in Review/American Academy of Pediatrics, 30*(3), e11–e21. doi: 10.1542/pir.30-3-e11

Patrick, S. W., Schumacher, R. E., Benneyworth, B. D., Krans, E. E., McAllister, J. M., & Davis, M. M. (2012). Neonatal abstinence syndrome and associated health care expenditures: United States, 2000–2009. *Journal of the American Medical Association, 307*(18), 1934–1940. doi: 10.1001/jama.2012.3951

Perlman, J. M., Wyllie, J., Kattwinkel, J., Wyckoff, M. H., Aziz, K., Guinsburg, R., . . . Velaphi, S. (2015). Part 7: Neonatal resuscitation: 2015 International Consensus on Cardiopulmonary Resuscitation and Emergency Cardiovascular Care Science with treatment recommendations. *Circulation, 132*(suppl 1), S204–S241.

Raju, T. N. (2015). Growth of neonatal–perinatal medicine: A historical perspective. In R. Martin, A. Fanaroff, & M. Walsh (Eds.), *Fanaroff & Martin's neonatal–perinatal medicine: Diseases of the fetus and infant* (10th ed., pp. 1–15). Philadelphia, PA: Elsevier Saunders.

Ramsey, K. (2015, October). *Examination of an outpatient approach to the treatment of neonatal abstinence syndrome*. Poster session presented at the meeting of the Vermont Oxford Network, Chicago, IL.

Reid, G., & Emery, J. (2006). Chronic disease prevention in general practice: Applying the family history. *Australian Family Physician, 35*(11), 879–882, 884–885.

Schaefer, G. B., & Thompson, J. N. (2014). Population genetics and genetic diversity. In *Medical genetics* (pp. 309–323). New York, NY: McGraw-Hill.

Schrager, S., & Potter, B. E. (2004). Diethylstilbestrol exposure. *American Family Physician, 69*(10), 2395–2400.

Substance Abuse and Mental Health Services Administration (SAMHSA). (2014). *Results from the 2013 National Survey on Drug Use and Health: Summary of national findings*. NSDUH Series H-48, HHS Publication No. (SMA) 14-4863. Rockville, MD: Author.

Supporting healthy and normal physiologic childbirth: A consensus statement by ACNM, MANA, and NACPM. (2013). *Journal of Perinatal Education, 22*(1), 14–18. doi: 10.1891/1058-1243.22.1.14

Swanson, T., & Erickson, L. (2016). Cardiovascular diseases and surgical interventions. In S. L. Gardner, B. S. Carter, M. Enzman-Hines, & J. A. Hernandez (Eds.), *Merenstein and Gardner's handbook of neonatal intensive care* (8th ed., pp. 644–688). St. Louis, MO: Elsevier-Mosby.

Tan, C. H., Denny, C. H., Cheal, N. E., Sniezek, J. E., & Kanny, D. (2015). Alcohol use and binge drinking among women of childbearing age—United States, 2011-2013. *Morbidity and Mortality Weekly Report, 64*(37), 1042–1046. doi: 10.15585/mmwr.mm6437a3

Task Force on Sudden Infant Death Syndrome & Moon, R. Y. (2011). Technical report: SIDS and other sleep-related infant deaths: Expansion of recommendations for a safe infant sleeping environment. *Pediatrics, 128*(5), e1341–e1367. doi: 10.1542/peds.2011-2285

Tolia, V. N., Patrick, S. W., Bennett, M. M., Murthy, K., Sousa, J., Smith, P. B.,. . .Spitser, A. R. (2015). Increasing incidence of the neonatal abstinence syndrome in U.S. neonatal ICUs. *New England Journal of Medicine, 372*(22), 2118–2126. doi: 10.1056/NEJMsa1500439

U.S. Census Bureau. (2015). Annual estimates of the resident population by sex, race alone or in combination, and Hispanic origin for the United States, states, and counties: April 1, 2010 to July 1, 2014. Retrieved from http://factfinder.census.gov/bkmk/table/1.0/en/PEP/2014PEPSR5H

U.S. Department of Health and Human Services (USDHHS). (2015). My family health portrait. Retrieved from https://familyhistory.hhs.gov/FHH/html/index.html

Wattendorf, D. J., & Hadley, D. W. (2005). Family history: The three-generation pedigree. *American Family Physician, 72*(3), 441–448.

Williams, J. F., Smith, V. C., & Committee on Substance Abuse. (2015). Fetal alcohol spectrum disorders. *Pediatrics*. doi: peds.2015-3113

World Health Organization (WHO). (2014). *Guidelines for the identification and management of substance use and substance use disorders in pregnancy*. Geneva, Switzerland: Author.

World Health Organization (WHO). (2015). Neonatal mortality. Retrieved from http://www.who.int/gho/child_health/mortality/neonatal/en/

CHAPTER 3

NEWBORN TRANSITION: THE JOURNEY FROM FETAL TO EXTRAUTERINE LIFE

Jenna Shaw-Battista and Sandra L. Gardner

A newborn's birth is a unique and meaningful time for both the infant and his or her family. Most infants transition uneventfully from fetal to extrauterine life. This transition is remarkable given the complex and profound changes in anatomy and physiology that occur in the first minutes and hours of life. Many factors in the fetal, maternal, and perinatal history may complicate or facilitate a successful newborn transition and should be assessed to inform birth preparations and newborn care. Sensitivity and awareness of families' social, cultural, and religious beliefs and preferences are also important parts of the quality of newborn care. Caring for essentially healthy newborns undergoing a physiologic process versus a pathophysiologic process at birth, however, requires a different skill set than caring for sick infants. Expectant management of the well newborn, or watchful waiting, and support for family participation and bonding are emphasized rather than diagnostic and treatment skills. When a newborn's transition is compromised, clinical skill is paramount, along with skills in educating and counseling parents that may include management of unmet expectations, grief, and loss.

Regardless of the child's health status, the newborn's transition from fetal to extrauterine life is critically important, and events during birth and the newborn transition are linked to a range of both immediate and lifelong health conditions. Emerging data demonstrate the probable intergenerational and whole-family effects of newborn birth method and early life experiences including postnatal care.

This chapter presents up-to-date recommendations for family-centered care during the normal newborn transition, evidence-based strategies to promote newborn health, and risk assessment strategies for compromised and failed transition, along with a review of potential adverse sequelae.

Epigenetics

A helpful new framework for assessing the newborn transition is the epigenetic impact of childbirth hypothesis, which includes the concept of evolutionary eustress resulting from normal physiological labor and birth. Eustress is defined as a health-promoting form of fetal–neonatal stress. A growing body of research suggests that eustress has an "epigenomic effect on particular genes, particularly those that program immune responses, genes responsible for weight regulation, and specific tumor-suppressor genes. Reduced or elevated levels of cortisol, adrenalin, and oxytocin produced during labor may lead to fetal epigenomic remodeling anomalies which exert influence on abnormal gene expression" (Dahlen et al., 2013, p. 3). This reprogramming is theorized to be the etiology for a range of non-contagious diseases and neonatal biobehavioral differences observed in newborns through adulthood following specific intrapartum and early life events (e.g., mode of delivery, circumcision, neonatal intensive care experience). To date, there has been very little research about the possible epigenetic consequences of most obstetric interventions, intrapartum events, and environmental factors (Dahlen et al., 2013).

Research on the relationships among many maternity care practices and perinatal outcomes is limited, primarily observational versus experimental, and often restricted to neonatal and maternal morbidity and mortality, which are rare in healthy populations. A promising area of research to address these limitations is grounded in the *optimality principle* first described by Dutch pediatric neurologists, who assessed the healthiest newborns following physiologically normal labors and births, without complications or obstetric interventions (Prechtl, 1967, 1980). These observations gave rise to optimality indices, which have since been adapted and validated for use in multiple settings, including healthy women and newborns in the United States (Fullerton, Low, Shaw-Battista, & Murphy, 2011). These instruments measure perinatal optimality, defined as the balance of risk factors and care practices appropriate to achieve ideal maternal and newborn outcomes (Kennedy, 2006). The optimality concept and measurement tools assign values to health-promoting activities (e.g., delayed cord clamping, skin-to-skin contact, and breastfeeding), the absence of adverse outcomes, and evidence-based restricted use of obstetric interventions.

The concept that "nature knows best" (in most cases) is not new. Indeed, a growing body of evidence supports the contention that physiologic birth is biologically ideal for most women and newborns. Normal childbirth is increasingly being studied as an antidote to the high levels of obstetric intervention employed during most births in the United States, often without supportive data, and frequently leading to maternal, newborn, and public health sequelae. For example, researchers are exploring oxytocin dosing regimens that mimic physiological hormonal release patterns and promote cervical ripening during induction of labor to increase the likelihood of success, fetal tolerance, and the spontaneous vaginal birth rate. Similarly, a national initiative to reduce iatrogenic prematurity has decreased the rate of elective induction of labor at less than 39 weeks' gestation with significant positive public health ramifications (Chescheir & Menard, 2012).

Research on the support and promotion of physiological birth is growing exponentially. Prevention of primary and repeat cesarean sections has become an interprofessional public health goal worldwide. Significant potential health benefits are associated with evidence-based restriction of cesarean section during normal labors among healthy women and babies. Recent research has also documented positive outcomes of family-centered, "natural" cesarean sections, which may include delayed cord clamping or cord milking, skin-to-skin contact, and other practices that support the newborn's physiologic transition to extrauterine life despite surgical delivery (Smith, Plaat, & Fisk, 2008; Stevens, Schmied, Burns, & Dahlen, 2014).

Going forward, perinatal epigenetics and new areas of research, such as the newborn microbiome, hold great promise to inform care practices and promote optimal health in infancy, across the life span, and intergenerationally. In light of emerging research in this area, it is prudent to provide newborn care with evolutionary biology and normal physiology in mind—for example, to assist with maternal closeness, skin-to-skin contact, and breastfeeding, whenever possible.

Newborn care has implications beyond the infant, including support of the mother's postpartum health and parenting abilities, along with assessment and health education for the whole family. Newborn care practices often have both infant and maternal health-promoting effects. For example, skin-to-skin contact after birth helps with infant thermoregulation, promotes maternal oxytocin release to control postpartum bleeding, and facilitates breastfeeding. Successful breastfeeding provides optimal newborn nutrition, reduces immediate and lifelong health risks for both mother and child, and engenders hormonal reinforcement of bonding and family integration.

Historically, there has been cross-cultural recognition of the vulnerability and interdependence of mothers and their newborns, with modern references to the "motherbaby" that reflect the symbiotic relationship of this dyad and their existence as a conceptual unified organism (Davis-Floyd, Pascali-Bonaro, Sagady Leslie, & Ponce de León, 2011). Physical and emotional closeness and interdependence persist throughout breastfeeding or bottle-feeding, with the first few months postpartum sometimes referred to as the "fourth trimester." This "exterogestational period" (Montagu, 1961) is roughly equivalent to the length of pregnancy and encompasses significant maternal and neonatal growth and development milestones.

The First Hour of Life

A 2011 study demonstrated universal and common activities among newborns in the first 70 minutes after delivery onto their mother's abdomens, where they were left undisturbed (Widström et al., 2011). Nine sequential behavioral phases were identified, as outlined in **Table 3-1**.

Table 3-1: Behavioral Phases of Term Newborns in the First Hour of Life

Behavior	Significance
Crying at birth	Robust crying at birth helps dissipate remaining lung fluid and facilitate extrauterine pulmonary transition.
Relaxation (within a few minutes after birth)	Stops crying; relaxed, quiet, and still behavior—may be an evolutionary mechanism to avoid detection by predators.
Awakening (2–5 minutes of life; median = 2.5 minutes)	Opening of eyes; beginning to move the head and open the mouths.
Activity (4–12 minutes of life; median = 8 minutes)	Activity increases; keeps eyes open for longer than 5 minutes. Becomes interested in the mother's face and breast. Looks at both the mother's face and breasts while rooting, moving the hands to the mouth, and making soliciting noises that signal hunger. Other hunger cues include head turning from side to side, and opening and closing the mouth with lips in the position to breastfeed.
Resting (13–27 minutes of life; median = 18 minutes)	Rest; becomes quiet and sleeps.
Crawling (18–54 minutes of life; median = 36 minutes)	Renewed and more vigorous efforts to breastfeed. Uses smell to locate the maternal breast. Instinctual behaviors such as the stepping reflex and head bobbing assist the newborn to physically move toward the breast in a crawling fashion.
Familiarization (29–62 minutes of life; median = 43 minutes)	Licks the areola and touches the maternal nipple in a pattern of hand–breast–mouth movements.
Sucking (44–90 minutes of life; median = 62 minutes)	Nursing and suckling without assistance.
Sleeping (by 70 minutes of life)	Rests/naps by 70 minutes of age, so it is optimal to initiate breastfeeding prior to this time.

Reproduced from Widström, A.-M., Lilja, G., Aaltomaa-Michalias, P., Dahllöf, A., Lintula, M., & Nissen, E. (2011). Newborn behaviour to locate the breast when skin-to-skin: A possible method for enabling early self-regulation. *Acta Paediatrica, 100*, 79–85.

Neonatal Transition Period

After birth, healthy newborns progress through a fairly predictable sequence of events, recovering from the stress of birth and adapting to extrauterine life (Gardner & Hernandez, 2016). **Figure 3-1** shows the classic description of neonatal transition, which includes the three stages of transition described in **Box 3-1**.

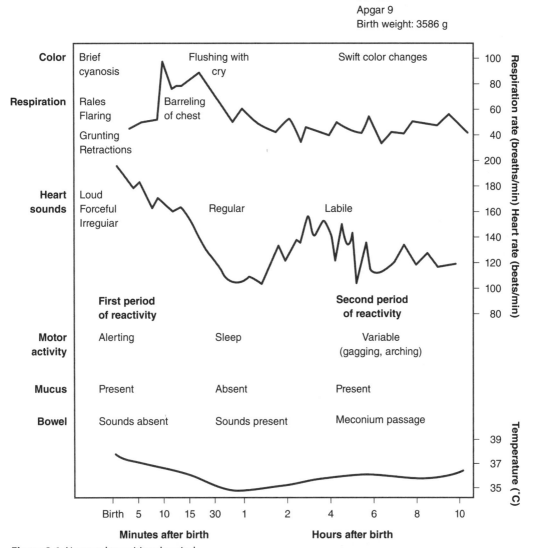

Figure 3-1: Neonatal transitional period.
Reproduced from Desmond, M. M., Rudolph, A. J., Phitaksphraiwan, P., et al. (1966). The transitional care nursery: a mechanism for preventive medicine in the newborn. *Pediatr Clin North Am, 13*, 651–68, Copyright Elsevier 1966.

...ional Period

...30 minutes): First Period of Reactivity

...se in heart rate to a range of 160–180 beats/min (0–15 min).
...rease in heart rate over 30 minutes to baseline rate of 100–120 beats/min.
- ❑ Irregular respirations (first 15 minutes), peak respiratory rate of 60–80 breaths/min.
- ❑ Rales present on auscultation.
- ❑ Grunting, flaring, and retractions may be noted, as well as brief periods of apnea (less than 10 seconds in duration).
- ❑ Plethora.
- ❑ Alert with spontaneous startle reactions, gustatory movements, tremors, crying, and side-to-side head movements.
- ❑ Decrease in body temperature.
- ❑ Generalized increase in motor activity, with increased muscle tone.
- ❑ Bowel sounds absent, and abdomen distended.
- ❑ Minimal production of saliva.

Second Stage (30 minutes to 2 hours): Period of Decreased Responsiveness
- ❑ Newborn either sleeps or has a marked decrease in motor activity.
- ❑ Muscle tone returns to normal, but responsiveness is diminished.
- ❑ Fast, shallow, synchronous breathing (60 breaths/min) without dyspnea occurs.
- ❑ Newborn's color is pale but pink with excellent perfusion and capillary refill.
- ❑ Increase in anterior–posterior diameter (barreling) of the chest is usually present.
- ❑ Heart rate decreases to 100–120 beats/min or less; the newborn is relatively less responsive to external stimuli.
- ❑ Abdomen is rounded, and bowel sounds are audible; peristaltic waves may be visible, and meconium may be passed.
- ❑ Oral mucus is absent.
- ❑ Spontaneous jerks and twitches are common, but the newborn quickly returns to rest.

Third Stage (2–8 hours): Second Period of Reactivity
- ❑ Return of and possible exaggeration of responsiveness.
- ❑ Labile heart rate: periods of tachycardia.
- ❑ Brief periods of rapid respirations.
- ❑ Abrupt changes in tone, color, and bowel sounds.
- ❑ Possible prominence of oral mucus; gagging and vomiting not unusual.
- ❑ Possible clearing of meconium from the bowel.
- ❑ Increased responsiveness to endogenous and exogenous stimuli.
- ❑ Newborn hunger cues; quiet, alert periods when maternal bonding is established.

Modified from Hernandez, J. A., & Thilo, E. (2005). Routine care of the full-term newborn. In L. C. Osborn, T. G. DeWitt, L. R. First, & J. Zenel (Eds.), (2004). Pediatrics. St. Louis, MO: Mosby. Copyright 2005, with permission from Elsevier.

Physiology and Pathophysiology of the Neonatal Transition

Pulmonary and Cardiac Newborns are dependent on others for care, but in utero they were completely reliant on their mothers for survival. The placenta delivers oxygen and nutrients to the fetus and removes accumulated wastes via exchange at the uterine implantation site. Uterine venous blood enters the placental intervillous space, where gas exchange occurs. The umbilical vein carries relatively oxygenated blood from the placenta to the fetus. The placenta has low circulatory resistance and utilizes much of the glucose and oxygen it receives for its own metabolic needs (McNanley & Woods, 2008).

The fetal pulmonary system, though physiologically functional close to term, is incapable of directly participating in oxygenation before birth. Less than 10% of cardiac output circulates to the fetal lungs in utero, due to pressure and resistance in the fetal pulmonary circuit. Anatomic shunts favor right-to-left shunting of blood, and optimize delivery of oxygen and other nutrients to the tissues (Fraser, 2014) (**Figure 3-2**):

- The *ductus venosus* directs oxygenated blood from the umbilical vein to the infant's inferior vena cava.

- The *foramen ovale* directs intra-arterial blood flow from right to left in the fetal heart.

- The *ductus arteriosus* directs blood from the pulmonary artery to the descending aorta.

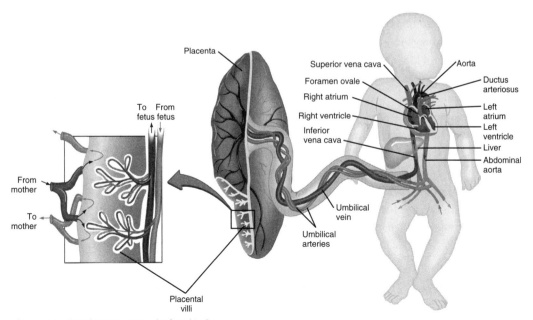

Figure 3-2: Circulatory pattern before birth.

Physiological responsibility for gas exchange is transferred from the placenta to the newborn's lungs and pulmonary system at birth. The fetal alveoli are filled with lung fluid, which is necessary for development in utero but creates a diffusion barrier that must be overcome during the first postnatal breaths. Ventilation of the lungs dramatically decreases pulmonary vascular resistance and creates a 10-fold increase in pulmonary blood flow. This enhanced pulmonary blood flow increases the infant's left atrial volume and pressure; as left atrial pressure exceeds that in the right atrium, the foramen ovale closes and the contribution of the placenta to the infant's circulation ceases (Fraser, 2014; Hillman, Kallapur, & Jobe, 2012).

With the termination of the placental contribution (including via cord clamping), the newborn's circulation redistributes the infant's blood flow, increases systemic vascular resistance, and decreases right atrial pressure. When systemic vascular resistance exceeds that in the pulmonary bed, right-to-left shunting through the ductus arteriosus ceases, and a left-to-right flow pattern is generated instead. Functional closure of the ductus arteriosus occurs due to a progressive increase in oxygenation (increased pO_2) and elimination of prostaglandin as a ductal relaxant by the lung; permanent closure and remodeling occurs within weeks after birth (Fraser, 2014).

Paralleling the circulatory changes, spontaneous infant ventilation mobilizes lung fluid into the pulmonary lymphatic system and recruits alveoli to generate functional residual capacity (FRC). FRC requires sustained pressure, functionally adequate surfactant to overcome resistance forces, and normal chest wall/lung compliance. The initiation and maintenance of respirations are triggered by a drop in ambient temperatures as the newborn enters the extrauterine environment, along with potent chemical (hypoxia, hypercarbia, and acidosis), mechanical (vaginal squeeze, infant crying), and sensory (tactile, visual, auditory, and olfactory) stimuli. Fetal lung fluid must be cleared from alveoli, and two-thirds of fetal lung fluid is typically cleared during vaginal birth. The clearance of fetal lung fluid is enhanced by passive forces (e.g., bulk movement created by vaginal squeeze and evaporation), epithelial reabsorption, and decreased fetal lung fluid secretion due to hormonal influences in late pregnancy and in labor—for example, intrapartum eustress is characterized by a surge in cortisol and catecholamine levels (Fraser, 2014; Hillman et al., 2012).

Complications of the Pulmonary Transition Approximately 10% of newborns will require assistance following delivery to initiate or sustain effective respiratory effort (Fernandes, 2015; Pramanik, Rangaswamy, & Gates, 2015). Respiratory distress is a common complication seen in the early neonatal period, and is a major cause of mortality and morbidity. The cause of newborn respiratory distress varies, but the result is impaired oxygenation to vital organs and inadequate ventilation, accompanied by retention of carbon dioxide and alteration of acid–base status. Respiratory distress can be an isolated condition or associated with other problems, and may be due to structural or functional abnormality or acquired injury

Box 3-2: Symptoms of Respiratory Distress in the Neonate

❑ Tachypnea (more than 60 breaths/min at more than 60 minutes of life): The earliest symptom of respiratory, cardiac, and metabolic conditions.

❑ Grunting (forced expiration through a partially closed glottis): Grunting increases trans-pulmonary pressure to stabilize the alveoli and increases gaseous exchange by delaying expiration.

❑ Retractions (inward pull of the pliable chest wall of a newborn on inspiration): Observed and reported in relation to the sternum (substernal/suprasternal) and the ribs (intercostal, supracostal, or subcostal).

❑ Nasal flaring (increasing the size of the nares with inspiration): An attempt to take in more oxygen by increasing the size of the nares and decreasing the resistance (by as much as 40%) of the narrow airways.

❑ Hypoxemia/hypoxia (low concentration of oxygen in the blood and in the tissues): Can be assessed noninvasively by pulse oximetry (PO) that gives the saturation of oxygen (normal saturation = 92–94%).

❑ Color changes:
   ❑ Pink (within 10–15 minutes of birth): Skin color should be pink.
   ❑ Pallor: Pale skin color with poor peripheral circulation may indicate systemic hypotension.
   ❑ Cyanosis: Blue discoloration.
      ○ Acrocyanosis (peripheral cyanosis of hands/feet): Occurs in the first 24 hours of life and is normal; also occurs with cold stress.
      ○ Central cyanosis of the skin, nailbeds, and mucous membranes: A late and serious sign because with the presence of fetal hemoglobin, the newborn must be at least 60% to 65% desaturated (PO = 60–65%) before cyanosis becomes visible.

Data from Gardner, S. L., Enzman-Hines, M., & Nyp, M. (2016). Respiratory diseases. In S. L. Gardner, B. S. Carter, M. Enzman-Hines, & J. A. Hernandez (Eds.), *Merenstein and Gardner's handbook of neonatal intensive care* (8th ed., pp. 565–643). St. Louis, MO: Elsevier-Mosby; Pramanik, A. K., Rangaswamy, N., & Gates, T. (2015). Neonatal respiratory distress: A practical approach to its diagnosis and management. *Pediatric Clinics of North America, 62*(2), 453–469. doi: 10.1016/j.pcl.2014.11.008

of the pulmonary system. **Box 3-2** lists the clinical findings of respiratory distress and their significance; **Table 3-2** identifies five common causes of respiratory distress.

Thermoregulation and Newborn Heat Loss Newborns must be supported to maintain their temperature while transitioning from the warm intrauterine environment to external ambient temperatures. The typical term infant has accumulated fat stores that provide insulation as well as metabolic fuel to sustain body temperature while the infant transitions to

Table 3-2: Common Causes of Respiratory Distress in Newborns

Medical Diagnosis	Etiology	Incidence	Signs/Symptoms	Mortality	Management
Transient tachypnea of the newborn (TTN)	Failure to clear lung fluid by usual mechanisms (i.e., absence of labor, cesarean section) and inadequate sodium transport at the cellular level (Hillman et al., 2012).	0.3–0.5% of term and late-preterm infants. Onset immediately after birth.	Self-limiting condition presenting with tachypnea and no other abnormalities. Tachypnea lasting 12–72 hours, until the excess lung fluid is reabsorbed.	Low	Supportive care—NPO due to tachypnea; IVs for fluids and calories until respirations slow and the newborn is able to take PO feeds; oxygen supplementation; warmth. Support with CPAP or mechanical ventilation is rarely needed and warrants a diagnostic workup for other pathology (e.g., pneumonia; PPHN).
Meconium aspiration syndrome (MAS)	Aspiration of meconium, an irritant that produces inflammation, creates obstruction (ball-valve effect), and interferes with surfactant activity (Pramanik et al., 2015).	2–10% of term and post-term infants exposed to MSAF; 5–30% of term and post-term births occur with MSAF (Edwards, Kotecha, & Kotecha, 2013).	Progressive disorder with symptoms increasing from inflammation to inability to oxygenate/ventilate. Tachypnea, grunting, flaring, retracting, hypoxemia, acidosis. Increased risk for pneumothorax and PPHN.	4–40%	Supplemental oxygen and CPAP to improve oxygenation. Mechanical ventilation for persistent respiratory acidosis and hypoxemia, iNO, surfactant, and ECMO at a tertiary center (Edwards et al., 2013; Pramanik et al., 2015).
Respiratory distress syndrome (RDS)	Insufficient surfactant, a phospholipid that lowers alveolar surface tension, prevents alveolar collapse at expiration, and maintains FRC.	Inversely related to gestational age: <28 weeks: 60%; <34 weeks: 5%. Occurs in preterm and late-preterm infants (<39 weeks).	Tachypnea, grunting, flaring, retracting, hypoxemia, hypercarbia/respiratory acidosis that begins soon after birth.	10%	Supportive care: warmth, fluids/calories; oxygen supplementation with oxygen hood, nasal cannula, CPAP, or mechanical ventilation. Surfactant replacement therapy.

Persistent pulmonary hypertension of the newborn (PPHN)	Failure to relax the pulmonary vasculature after breathing oxygen at birth; pulmonary vasoconstriction due to hypoxia after birth, resulting in elevated PVR and decreased SVR.	1:500 to 1:1500 live births. Affects term and post-term newborns due to pulmonary or nonpulmonary conditions.	Tachypnea, grunting, flaring, retracting, hypoxemia, hypercarbia/respiratory acidosis. Hypoxemia and acidosis are severe and intractable.	High. PPHN is generally reversible when diagnosed early and treated aggressively.	Supportive care: warmth, fluids/calories; oxygen supplementation with oxygen hood, nasal cannula, CPAP, mechanical ventilation, iNO, or ECMO (Jain & McNamara, 2015).
Pneumonia	Acquired as early onset (first week of life) or late onset (after first week of life). Early onset due to pathogens in utero (i.e., chorioamnionitis, congenital, or aspiration) or from infected personnel, equipment, or cohorts.	<1% of term neonates (Speer, 2015).	Tachypnea, grunting, flaring, retracting, hypoxemia, hypercarbia/respiratory acidosis.	Varies with organism virulence, hypoxemia, acidosis, and secondary PPHN.	Supportive care: warmth, fluids/calories; oxygen supplementation with oxygen hood, nasal cannula, CPAP, mechanical ventilation, iNO, or ECMO. Empiric and/or therapeutic antibiotic/antiviral therapy.

Abbreviations: CPAP, continuous positive airway pressure; ECMO, extracorporeal membrane oxygenation; FRC, functional residual capacity; iNO, inhaled nitric oxide; IV, intravenous; MSAF, meconium-stained amniotic fluid; NPO, non per os; PO, per os; PVR, peripheral vascular resistance; SVR, systemic vascular resistance.

Data from Gardner, S. L., Enzman-Hines, M., & Nyp, M. (2016). Respiratory diseases. In S. L. Gardner, B. S. Carter, M. Enzman-Hines, & J. A. Hernandez (Eds.), *Merenstein and Gardner's handbook of neonatal intensive care* (8th ed., pp. 565–643). St. Louis, MO: Elsevier-Mosby; Smith, J. R., & Carley, A. (2014). Common neonatal complications. In K. R. Simpson & P. A. Creehan (Eds.), *Perinatal nursing* (4th ed., pp. 662–698). Philadelphia, PA: Wolters Kluwer.

breastfeeding and lactation becomes well established. Oxidative glucose, fat and protein metabolism, nonshivering thermogenesis of brown fat, and muscle activity are all mechanisms to generate heat in the term newborn. Peripheral vasoconstriction helps prevent heat loss, as does normal newborn flexion (decreased body surface area exposed to air) (Fraser, 2014; Hillman et al., 2012; Interprofessional Education & Research Committee, Champlain Maternal Newborn Regional Program [IPERC], 2013). However, even healthy term newborns are at risk for heat loss due to their relatively large body surface area, immature permeable skin, limited subcutaneous fat stores, poorly developed shivering thermogenesis, and emergence from the birth canal wet with amniotic fluid (IPERC, 2013). Preterm infants, including late-preterm infants (Gardner, 2007), are often deficient in stored fat, have an immature hypothalamus that regulates temperature, and have more heat and energy challenges; hence, they are at higher risk of heat loss than term infants.

Four mechanisms of heat transfer affect the newborn: conduction, convection, evaporation, and radiation. *Conductive* heat loss refers to the ability to transfer heat to cooler contiguous surfaces, such as from the infant's warm body to a cold table or cold blankets. *Convective* heat loss refers to heat transfer through air currents, such as from the infant's warm body when subjected to cooler airflow from drafts. *Evaporative* heat loss occurs with evaporation of moisture, as when a newborn wet with amniotic fluid is subjected to dry and cooler surrounding air. *Radiant* heat loss occurs from the transfer of heat via thermal waves from the infant's warm body to cooler surrounding objects through air (IPERC, 2013).

Minimizing heat loss and maintaining the newborn in a thermally neutral environment are important in facilitating a normal neonatal transition. Effective strategies will be directed toward limiting any negative consequences of conduction, convection, evaporation, and radiation. In 1997, the World Health Organization (WHO) advocated a 10-step "warm chain" approach to supporting thermal stability in the newborn that included the following elements: environmental modifications such as warming the delivery room and examination or transport areas; skin-to-skin holding, mother–baby care, and breastfeeding; delayed bathing and weighing; immediate drying and clothing/blanketing; and adequate staff training in recognition and management of cold stress (IPERC, 2013).

A highly effective strategy for supporting newborn temperature is the use of skin-to-skin holding, also known as kangaroo care, in which infants are unclothed and placed against the bare skin of the mother or caregiver before being covered with a blanket (Moore, Anderson, & Berman, 2012; Phillips, 2013). Skin-to-skin contact conserves infant heat through tucked positioning and covering, and positively contributes to thermal gain from contiguous adult body heat. In some studies, skin-to-skin contact has been shown to be more effective for the prevention (Ludington-Hoe et al., 2004) and treatment of newborn hypothermia than either an incubator or radiant warmer (Christensson, Bhat, Amadi, Eriksson, & Hojer, 1998; Erlandsson, Dsilna, Fagerberg, & Christensson, 2007).

When heat loss is greater than the infant's ability to conserve and produce heat, the newborn is no longer in thermal neutrality: in such a case, the body temperature drops, and the newborn is cold stressed and becomes hypothermic (IPERC, 2013). Hypothermia in a newborn is defined as body temperature below 36.3–36.5°C (97.3–97.7°F) measured as an axillary temperature. Consequences of cold stress include increased oxygen and glucose consumption, depletion of glycogen, pulmonary vasoconstriction, hypoglycemia, hypoxia, anaerobic metabolism, and metabolic acidosis (IPERC, 2013). Thermal gain can be effectively achieved through heat application, such as via incubators and radiant warmers.

In all birth sites, thermoregulatory principles must be addressed adequately, with creative use of available materials if necessary. Skin-to-skin contact should be universally promoted as an effective and low-cost intervention. Warming options may also include low-tech equipment such as heating pads, hot water bottles, or temporary chemical warmers, but *only* if temperatures can be sufficiently controlled to avoid iatrogenic burns.

Labor and Birth in Water

Intrapartum hydrotherapy and waterbirth are nonpharmacologic labor pain relief methods that may not be available in all facilities and are best restricted to healthy childbearing women with the expectation of a healthy newborn without challenges to extrauterine transition. All women in labor at term may be encouraged to labor in water for pain relief, provided that standard assessments are feasible and hygienic practices are employed. Warm-water immersion hydrotherapy should be recommended to women who desire a normal physiologic birth without analgesia. More than 11 randomized trials of labor in water have demonstrated excellent perinatal outcomes with this approach and shown that routine fetal and newborn care can be safely provided. There is less consensus about the quality of data supporting waterbirth safety, although evidence-based guidelines have been developed to reduce the possible risk of harm and optimize outcomes (Nutter, Shaw Battista, & Marowitz, 2014).

During labor, bathwater should be regulated to normal body temperature and never exceed 37.8°C (100°F), so as to reduce the risk of hypoxic injury to the fetus that could result from excessively warm water. The fetus experiences higher temperatures than the mother and is unable to use normal extrauterine compensatory cooling mechanisms. Cooler water temperatures can be used for hydrotherapy during labor according to the mother's preference. Prior to waterbirth, water temperature should be raised to 36.1–37.8°C (97–100°F) to reduce the risk of premature initiation of newborn respiration during underwater birth (Nutter et al., 2014).

Infants born into water should have their face gently and directly brought to the surface immediately after birth, and the face and head should never be re-submerged (Nutter et al., 2014). Following birth into water, a newborn can remain skin-to-skin with the mother in the tub, with legs and trunk submerged and face and head above water. Do not place wet wash-cloths or linen over the infant's head or shoulders, as this will contribute to heat loss rather than heat gain. The use of warm bathwater to promote newborn thermoregulation permits beneficial delayed cord clamping for vigorous infants, and avoids separation from the mother. Alternatively, the newborn can be dried and held skin-to-skin while covered with warm, dry linens, if the mother chooses to exit the tub soon after birth.

Waterbirth is a key element of the newborn's health history, which should be documented in the birth record and shared with newborn care providers. Isolated case studies report that failure to include a history of waterbirth has delayed the diagnosis and treatment of newborns infected by contaminated bathwater. Overall infection does not appear to be more common among babies born in water compared to standard birthing practices. Research (primarily observational studies) has shown that maternal and neonatal outcomes after waterbirth are excellent, in part because waterbirth is restricted to healthy, low-risk populations.

Data Collection

History

Newborn care providers require information about the mother's health and pregnancy history, complications or interventions in labor or birth, and other known risks for compromised post-natal transition and extrauterine life. **Table 3-3** lists some maternal, obstetric, and neonatal factors that are known to increase the risk of an abnormal neonatal transition.

Signs And Symptoms

"Knowledge of the normal changes occurring during transition enables early recognition of a newborn who is not making a normal extrauterine adaptation" (Gardner & Hernandez, 2016, p. 83). After the first hour of life, if the newborn's respirations, pulse, color, and activity have not stabilized within the normal ranges, a problem should be suspected and investigated (Gardner & Hernandez, 2016). Clinical manifestations of an abnormal transition are listed in **Box 3-3**.

"Initial newborn assessment includes the following:

- Assessments of gestational age and fetal growth
- Newborn classification and neonatal mortality and morbidity risk
- Physical and neurologic examination
- Assessment of neurobiological development" (Gardner & Hernandez, 2016, p. 77)

Tachypnea after the first hour of life is one of the most common deviations from a normal transition. Tachypnea must be investigated with a "minimum" workup of a physical

Table 3-3: Maternal, Obstetric, Neonatal Conditions that Increase the Risk of Abnormal Transition

Maternal factors	Chronic hypertension
	Pregnancy-induced hypertension
	Diabetes mellitus
	Renal disease
	Infection
	Abuse of tobacco, alcohol, or illicit drugs
	Collagen vascular diseases
	Hemizygous hemoglobinopathies
	Certain maternal medications
Obstetric factors	Rh or other isoimmunization
	Fetal growth restriction
	Decreased fetal movements
	Multiple gestation
	Oligohydramnios or polyhydramnios
	Premature rupture of membranes
	Third-trimester bleeding
	Delivery by cesarean section
Neonatal factors	Prematurity ($<$ 37 weeks)
	Postmaturity ($>$ 42 weeks)
	Small for gestational age
	Large for gestational age
	Infection
	Metabolic abnormalities
	Birth trauma
	Major malformations
	Anemia
	Apgar 0–4 at 1 minute or need for resuscitation at delivery

Reproduced from Hernandez, J. A., & Thilo, E. (2005). Routine care of the full-term newborn. In L. C. Osborn, T. G. DeWitt, L. R. First, & J. Zenel (Eds.), *Pediatrics*. St. Louis, MO: Mosby.

examination, chest x-ray, arterial blood gas, and if there is suspicion of infection, complete blood count with differential and platelets, blood culture, and C-reactive protein measurement.

To conserve energy, provide developmentally supportive care, and stabilize a tachypneic late-preterm or term infant, use of evidence-based nursing strategies to assist transition includes the following measures (Gardner, Enzman-Hines, & Nyp, 2016; Gardner, Goldson, & Hernandez, 2016; Gardner & Hernandez, 2016):

- Place the infant prone (in skin-to-skin care on the mother's or father's chest).

    - Prone positioning improves oxygenation by 15% to 25% (Balaguer, Escribano, & Rogue, 2003; Bhat et al., 2003; Dimaguila, DiFore, Martin, & Miller, 1997; Martin, Herrell, Rubin, & Fanaroff, 1979; McEvoy et al., 1997; Schwartz, 1993; Wagaman et al., 1979).

    - Prone positioning improves lung mechanics and lung volumes (i.e., lung compliance and tidal volumes) (Dimaguila et al., 1997; Hutchison, Ross, & Russell, 1979; Wagaman et al., 1979).

    - Prone positioning enhances respiratory control (Bolton & Herman, 1974; Martin, DiFiore, Korenke, Randal, & Miller, 1995; Martin et al., 1979).

    - Prone positioning decreases the infant's energy expenditure (Goto et al., 1999; Kahn et al., 1993; Lawson, Anday, & Guillet,1987; Masterson, Zucker, & Schulze, 1987;

Box 3-3: Neonatal Clinical Manifestations Signaling an Abnormal Transition

❑ Persistent tachypnea, flaring, grunting, and retractions (respiratory score > 4; duration lasting past the first hour of life); fixed bradycardia

❑ Diffuse and persistent rales, retractions, flaring, and grunting (respiratory score > 4; duration lasting past the first hour of life)

❑ Persistent cyanosis (persistent oxygen saturation < 90% in room air) and prolonged requirements for supplemental oxygen (after 2–3 hours of age)

❑ Episodes of prolonged apnea (>20 seconds) and bradycardia (< 80 beats/min)

❑ Marked pallor or ruddiness

❑ Temperature instability, persistently (after 2–3 hours of age) low temperature (< 36.5°C [97.7°F])

❑ Poor capillary filling (>3 seconds) and blood pressure instability

❑ Unusual neurologic behavior (lethargy, decreased activity with marked and persistent hypotonia, irritability, excessive tremors and jitteriness)

❑ Excessive oral secretions, drooling, and choking/coughing spells, cyanosis

Modified from Hernandez, J. A., & Thilo, E. (2005). Routine care of the full-term newborn. In L. C. Osborn, T. G. DeWitt, L. R. First, & J. Zenel (Eds.), *Pediatrics*. St. Louis, MO: Mosby; Gardner, S. L., & Hernandez, J. A. (2016). Initial nursery care. In S. L. Gardner, B. S. Carter, M. Enzman-Hines, & J. A. Hernandez (Eds.), *Merenstein and Gardner's handbook of neonatal intensive care* (8th ed., p. 84). St. Louis, MO: Elsevier-Mosby.

Schwartz, 1993), as evidenced by less crying (Brackbill, Douthitt, & West, 1973; Chang, Anderson, & Lin, 2002), lower levels of activity (Casaer, O'Brien, & Prechtl, 1973; Chang et al., 2002; Hashimoto, Hirua, & Endo,1983), and less awake time and more sleep time (Chang et al., 2002).

- Elevate the head of the bed; the gravity-assisted downward position of the diaphragm will facilitate the infant's chest excursion.

- Place a pulse oximeter and titrate supplemental oxygen (FiO_2) to maintain PO saturations between 92% and 94% or higher (a normal oxygen saturation value) (Barry, Deacon, Hernandez, & Jones, 2016). For late-preterm and term newborns, there is less concern about the effect of supplemental oxygen on their eyes and much more concern about the effects of hypoxemia and acidosis on their pulmonary vasculature (i.e., vasoconstriction of pulmonary vessels in the presence of hypoxemia and acidosis).

- Ensure minimal handling of the infant, so as to avoid iatrogenic hypoxemia and reflexive pulmonary vasoconstriction with the onset of persistent pulmonary hypertension of the newborn (PPHN).

  Maintaining adequate oxygenation is a prime goal to prevent (and care for) infants with PPHN, so that alterations in routine care and handling are essential. Because handling a sick newborn for any reason causes a fall in PaO_2, the benefits of handling for routine care such as changing linens, weighing, suctioning, and taking vital signs must be balanced against the risk of iatrogenic hypoxia. PaO_2 variations in the newborn are as follows (Dangeman et al., 1976; Evans, 1991):

  - At rest $\pm$ 15 mm Hg variation
  - While crying: decrease of PaO_2 by as much as 50 mm Hg
  - With routine care: decrease of PaO_2 by as much as 30 mm Hg

  Maintaining organized, coordinated care and minimizing disturbances are therefore very important. Keeping the infant calm is important because severe hypoxia accompanies crying. Using pacifiers and decreasing noxious stimuli (e.g., invasive procedures) keeps struggling and crying to a minimum. Continuously monitoring vital signs, blood pressure, and pulse oximetry decreases the need for physical manipulation and disturbance. (Gardner et al., 2016)

- Maintain thermal neutrality. Axillary temperatures should be maintained at 36.5–37.5°C (97.7–99.5°F) in term infants. Thermal neutrality is the temperature at which oxygen consumption is minimal and basal metabolic rate is minimal (Gardner & Hernandez, 2016).

- Relieve pain. Pain from invasive procedures is a physiologic stress that results in an increase in heart and respiratory rates, blood pressure, carbon dioxide retention, pulmonary vascular tone, and oxygen consumption. Pain also decreases the depth of respirations, oxygenation (PaO_2, PO_2 saturation) (Gardner, Enzman-Hines, & Agarwal, 2016).

- Maintain blood sugar in the normal range. Hypoglycemia may cause respiratory depression/apnea, alterations in the level of consciousness, hypothermia, hypotonia, limpness, and inactivity (Rozance, McGowan, Price-Douglas, &Hay, 2016).

With adequate support and a minimum of stress, these newborns may be able to slow their respirations and make a successful transition to extrauterine life. If the transition remains abnormal, these supportive strategies will prevent worsening of their condition by maintaining adequate oxygenation and ventilation (and thereby reducing hypoxemia and acidosis) and avoiding pulmonary hypertension, pulmonary hypoperfusion, opening of the ductus arteriosus, and the development of PPHN with subsequent mechanical ventilation, pneumothorax inhaled nitric oxide and/or and extracorporeal membrane oxygenation (ECMO) treatment.

Physical Examination

The normal newborn assessment includes a brief initial evaluation immediately following birth, and a complete physical exam with gestational age assessment on the day of delivery. Newborn care includes ongoing support and observation of the physiological transition to extrauterine life and adaptive infant behaviors including feeding. These assessments occur with simultaneous evaluations of maternal health and mothering, family dynamics, the safety of the care and home environments and anticipatory discharge planning, and health education. Examination of the newborn with the parents present is also a teaching opportunity.

Newborn Competencies and Behaviors

Both the fetus and the newborn have well-developed sensory pathways with which to experience and interact with the environment. Newborns have a well-developed ability to hear, recognize their parents' voices, and turn their heads toward sounds (DeCasper & Fifer, 1980; DeCasper & Spence, 1986; Widström et al., 2011). They also have a preference for their mother's face and her unique scent. Newborns are able to localize smells (e.g., amniotic fluid), turn toward the familiar smell of their own mother's breastmilk, and withdraw from unpleasant smells (Association of Women's Health, Obstetric, and Neonatal Nurses [AWHONN], 2006; Sullivan & Toubas, 1998). Newborns have visual acuity of approximately 8 to 12 inches, can fix their gaze and follow a moving object, and are visually attracted to items with contrasts (e.g., the human face, and black-and-white patterns) (AHWONN, 2006). The newborn's tongue has more taste buds than that of an adult, keen detection of sour tastes, and a preference for sweet breastmilk (AWHONN, 2006).

The normal newborn experiences cyclical sleep and alert states with six identified levels of consciousness (outlined in **Table 3-4**). Neonatal reflexes are discussed elsewhere in this text.

Table 3-4 : Newborn States and Considerations for Caregiving

Newborn State	Comments
Sleep States	
Deep sleep (non-rapid-eye-movement [non-REM] or quiet sleep): • Slow state changes • Regular breathing • Eyes closed; no eye movements • No spontaneous activity except startles and jerky movements • Startles with some delay and suppresses rapidly • Lowest oxygen consumption	Infant is very difficult if not impossible to arouse. Infant will not breastfeed or bottle-feed in this state, even after vigorous stimulation. Infant is unable to respond to environment, which is frustrating for caregivers. Term infants may exhibit a "slow" heart rate (80–90 beats/min). At birth, preterm infants, including late-preterm infants, have altered states of consciousness. Early dominant states are light sleep, quiet, and active alert. "Protective apathy" enables the preterm infant to remain inactive, unresponsive, and in a sleep state to conserve energy, grow, and maintain physiologic homeostasis (Tronick, Scanlon, & Scanlon, 1990). As maturation occurs, there is an increase in quiet alert.
Light sleep (REM or active sleep): • Low activity level • Random movements and startles • Respirations irregular and abdominal • Intermittent sucking movements • Eyes closed; REM • Higher oxygen consumption	Full-term infants begin and end sleep in active sleep; preterm infants are more responsive (than term infants) to stimuli in active sleep. Infants may cry or fuss briefly in this state and be awakened to feed before truly awake and ready to eat. Lower and more variable oxygenation states.
Awake States	
Drowsy or semi-dozing: • Eyelids fluttering • Eyes open or closed (dazed) • Mild startles (intermittent) • Delayed response to sensory stimuli • Smooth state change after stimulation • Fussing may or may not be present • Respirations are more rapid and shallow	Infants may awaken further or return to sleep (if left alone). Quietly talking and looking at the infant or offering a pacifier or an inanimate object to see and listen to may arouse the infant to the quiet, alert state. Less mature infants (30 weeks) demonstrate a more drowsy than quiet alert state than more mature infants (36 weeks).

(Continued)

Table 3-4: Newborn States and Considerations for Caregiving (*Continued*)

Awake States	
Quiet alert, with bright look: • Focuses attention on source of stimulation • Impinging stimuli may break through; may have some delay in response • Minimal motor activity	Immediately after birth, term newborns exhibit a period of quiet alert, which is their first opportunity to "take in" their parents and the extrauterine environment. Dimmed lights, quiet talking, and stroking optimize this time for parents. This is the best state for learning to occur, because the infant focuses all of his or her attention on visual, auditory, tactile, and sucking stimuli; this is also the best state for interaction with parents—the infant is maximally able to attend and reciprocally respond to parents.
Active alert—eyes open: • Considerable motor activity—thrusting movements of extremities; spontaneous startles • Reacts to external stimuli with increase in movements and startles (discrete reactions difficult to differentiate because of general higher activity level) • Respirations irregular • May or may not be fussy	Infant has decreased threshold (increased sensitivity) to internal (hunger, fatigue) and external (wet, noise, handling) stimuli. Infant may quiet self, may escalate to crying, or with consolation by caregiver, may become quiet alert or go to sleep. Infant is unable to maximally attend to the caregiver or environment because of increased motor activity and increased sensitivity to stimuli.
Crying—intense and difficult to disrupt with external stimuli Respirations rapid, shallow, and irregular	Crying is the infant's response to unpleasant internal or external stimulation—the infant's tolerance limits have been reached (and exceeded). Infant may be able to quiet self with hand-to-mouth behaviors; talking may quiet a crying infant; holding, rocking, or putting the infant upright on the caregiver's shoulder may quiet the infant.

Reproduced from Gardner, S. L., Goldson, E. & Hernandez, J. A. (2016). The neonate and the environment: Impact on development. In Gardner, S. L., Carter, B. S., Enzman-Hines, M., & Hernandez, J. A., (Eds.), *Merenstein and Gardner's handbook of neonatal intensive care* (8th ed., pp. 262–315). St Louis, MO, Elsevier- Mosby.

Routine Care During Transition

Glucose Screening

The assessment of the newborn's glucose level is complicated by the lack of universally accepted definitions of normal and abnormal glucose levels. What is known is that blood glucose in the newborn at birth is approximately 70% of the maternal value. Within the first postnatal hour, the newborn's glucose level may drop to as low as 25 mg/dL. The significance of these transient, asymptomatic glucose levels is less clear, however. It has been postulated that postnatal decreases in glucose are necessary to appropriately induce physiologic processes such as gluconeogenesis or oxidative metabolism of fat that are necessary for ultimate stabilization of glucose supply. Due to the lack of sufficiently clear data, the American Academy of Pediatrics (AAP) has proposed age-based "operational thresholds" for use in the management of suspected neonatal hypoglycemia. Within the first 4 hours after birth, for example, an operational threshold of 25–35 mg/dL serum glucose concentration is an indication for consideration of glucose support (**Figure 3-3**). For the subsequent 20 hours, the AAP has proposed

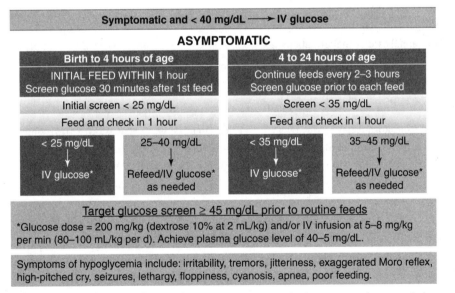

Figure 3-3: American Academy of Pediatrics algorithm: Screening and management of postnatal glucose homeostasis in late preterm and term small-for-gestational age (SGA) infants, infants of diabetic mothers (IDM), and large-for-gestational-age (LGA) infants.

Reproduced with permission from Adamkin, D. H., and the Committee on Fetus and Newborn of the American Academy of Pediatrics. (2011). Clinical report–postnatal glucose homeostasis in late-preterm and term infants. *Pediatrics, 127*(3), 575–9. Copyright (c) 2011 by AAP.

Box 3-4: Indications for Routine Monitoring of Blood Glucose for Prevention of Neonatal Hypoglycemia

Maternal Conditions

- ❏ Presence of diabetes or abnormal result of glucose tolerance test
- ❏ Preeclampsia and pregnancy-induced or essential hypertension
- ❏ Previous macrosomic infants
- ❏ Substance abuse
- ❏ Treatment with beta-agonist tocolytics
- ❏ Treatment with oral hypoglycemic agents
- ❏ Late antepartum to intrapartum administration of intravenous glucose

Neonatal Conditions

- ❏ Prematurity
- ❏ Intrauterine growth restriction
- ❏ Perinatal hypoxia–ischemia
- ❏ Sepsis
- ❏ Hypothermia
- ❏ Polycythemia–hyperviscosity
- ❏ Erythroblastosis fetalis
- ❏ Iatrogenic administration of insulin
- ❏ Congenital cardiac malformations
- ❏ Persistent hyperinsulinemia
- ❏ Endocrine disorders
- ❏ Inborn errors of metabolism

Reproduced from Rozance, P. J., McGowan, J. E., Price-Douglas, W., & Hay, W. W. (2016). Glucose homeostasis. In S. L. Gardner, B. S. Carter, M. Enzman-Hines, & J. A. Hernandez (Eds.), *Merenstein and Gardner's handbook of neonatal intensive care* (8th ed., p. 352). St. Louis, MO: Elsevier-Mosby.

35–45 mg/dL as an operational glucose threshold. Values below these thresholds are an indication for increasing serum glucose levels (Adamkin, 2015).

Indications for routine monitoring of blood glucose for the prevention of neonatal hypoglycemia are listed in **Box 3-4**. Signs and symptoms of neonatal hypoglycemia are nonspecific and extremely variable; clinical signs of this condition are listed in **Box 3-5**. Most asymptomatic newborns with hypoglycemia can be treated with early and frequent feedings (breastfeeding, expressed breastmilk, donor human milk, or formula) (Rozance et al., 2016). All symptomatic newborns should receive treatment with intravenous dextrose solution. Guidelines for management of newborns with hypoglycemia are shown in **Figure 3-4**.

Box 3-5: Clinical Signs of Hypoglycemia

- ❏ Mild to moderate changes in level of consciousness*
- ❏ Stupor or lethargy*
- ❏ Tremulousness*
- ❏ Irritability*
- ❏ Coma
- ❏ Seizures (depend on duration, repetitive occurrence, and severity of hypoglycemia)

- ❏ Respiratory depression or apnea, leading to cyanosis
- ❏ Hypotonia, limpness, inactivity
- ❏ High-pitched cry
- ❏ Poor feeding (after previously feeding well)
- ❏ Hypothermia

*Most frequent, and should be alleviated with correction of low glucose concentrations.
Reproduced from Rozance, P. J., McGowan, J. E., Price-Douglas, W., & Hay, W. W. (2016). Glucose homeostasis. In S. L. Gardner, B. S. Carter, M. Enzman-Hines, & J. A. Hernandez (Eds.), *Merenstein and Gardner's handbook of neonatal intensive care* (8th ed., p. 351). St. Louis, MO: Elsevier-Mosby.

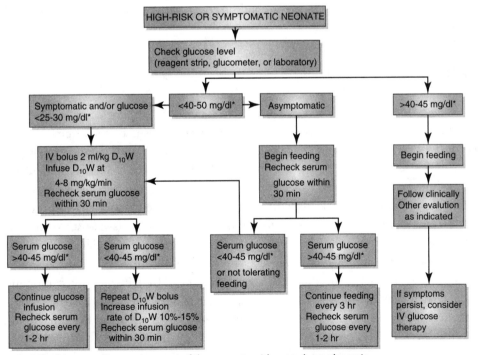

Figure 3-4: Decision tree for management of the neonate with acute hypoglycemia.
Reproduced from Rozance, P. J., McGowan, J. E., Price-Douglas, W., & Hay, W., W. (2016). Glucose homeostasis. In S. L. Gardner, B. S. Carter, M. Enzman Hines, & J. A. Hernandez (Eds.), *Merenstein and Gardner's handbook of neonatal intensive care* (8th ed., p. 352). St Louis, MO: Elsevier-Mosby.

Vitamin K Administration

Newborns are at risk for bleeding complications due to their immature hepatic system and their inability to produce several key coagulation factors dependent on vitamin K. Specifically, vitamin K is necessary for the synthesis of coagulation factors II, VII, IX, and X. Administration of a single intramuscular dose of vitamin K (1 mg for infants weighing more than 1.5 kg at birth) is recommended within the first postnatal hour (Fraser, 2014). Oral dosing with vitamin K_1 (2 mg PO) requires repeated dosing (e.g., first feed, 1 week, 4 weeks, 8 weeks). There is an increased risk for late-onset hemorrhagic disease when an infant receives only one dose (Gardner & Hernandez, 2016).

Eye Prophylaxis

Universal newborn ophthalmologic prophylaxis against gonococcal and chlamydia infections has been recommended in most U.S. states. A single application of ointment into the conjunctival sac is recommended within the first postnatal hour (Fraser, 2014). Either erythromycin (0.5%) or tetracycline (1%) is applied as a ribbon of ointment into the conjunctival sac. The bacteriocidal effects depend on the tissue concentrations of microorganisms and the drug (Gardner & Hernandez, 2016).

Standards of Care

Routine newborn care is provided by an interprofessional workforce including registered nurses, nurse practitioners, midwives, physicians, physician assistants, and respiratory therapists. The specific newborn care providers in attendance at an infant's birth vary by risk assessment and site, and necessarily take into consideration the availability of staff and other resources, unit census, and proximity to newborn intensive care services. Regardless of the birth setting, standards established by the Neonatal Resuscitation Program (NRP) can reduce morbidity and mortality if universally applied. NRP recommends at least two birth attendants capable of performing initial neonatal resuscitation be present, along with at least one attendant capable of providing advanced support, such as intubation and vascular access (AAP & American Heart Association, 2011; Smith & Carley, 2014). Providers in community and home birth settings require both NRP certification and routine practice "drills" to maintain these skills, as the use of resuscitation techniques is infrequent in healthy populations. The American Association of Birth Centers (AABC) standards require routine maternal and newborn emergency drills on a quarterly or more-frequent basis to maintain and demonstrate current knowledge and skill (AABC, 2013).

Guidelines for Perinatal Care (AAP & ACOG, 2012) sets the standard of care for maternal and neonatal care. The current standards require skilled healthcare providers to be available 24 hours/day to care for newborns during and after birth (AAP & ACOG, 2012; Gardner & Hernandez, 2016; Hernandez & Thilo, 2005). "All newborns are to be cared for, regarded and observed as recovering patients until they have successfully completed a smooth transition" (Gardner & Hernandez, 2016, p. 73). Meeting this criterion requires care providers who are familiar with normal transition and deviations from normal transition. "After birth, at 15 minute intervals, *every* newborn must be assessed for general condition, respiratory effort, color, muscle tone, and temperature; all assessments must be documented" (Gardner & Hernandez, 2016, p. 74). "By 30 minutes of age, every newborn, regardless of where the baby is being cared for, must be examined by a neonatal–perinatal nurse. During the first 6 hours after birth, heart rate, respirations, blood pressure, degree of alertness, and color of skin and mucous membranes should be assessed frequently and the findings recorded" (Gardner & Hernandez, 2016, p. 74).

"During the transitional period, vital signs should be recorded frequently enough to monitor the infant's condition and provide appropriate care:

- If the newborn is distressed . . . , vital signs may be required every 10 minutes.

- If the baby's vital signs are normal after birth . . . , vital signs may be required every 30 to 45 minutes until the infant's condition has remained stable for 2 to 4 hours.

- Vital signs should be recorded at least once every 8 hours.

- Measuring the temperature rectally is contraindicated in newborns because of the risk of perforation." (Gardner & Hernandez, 2016, p. 98)

Skin-to-skin (kangaroo) care is recommended for the term newborn at birth by the World Health Organization, the AAP (2012), the Academy of Breastfeeding Medicine (2008), NRP (AAP & AHA, 2011), and the Centers for Disease Control and Prevention (CDC). The AAP and the ABM recommend that full-term newborns should be immediately placed into skin-to-skin (kangaroo care) after birth and remain there until after the first breastfeeding. The International Network on Kangaroo Mother Care (Nyqvist et al., 2010) and the CDC recommend that term babies remain in skin-to-skin care throughout the postpartum period as a strategy to facilitate breastfeeding.

Cultural Considerations

Cross-culturally, families frequently mark the arrival of a newborn with celebrations and formal welcomes into their community. The timing and number of social, spiritual, and religious ceremonies for newborns vary but do not usually occur for several weeks or months after birth. This may be an adaptation to historically high perinatal death rates with inadvertent or intentional delayed bonding, infection prevention considerations, and recognition of mothers' need for postpartum recovery. A rest period of 20 to 40 days is commonly prescribed for new mothers and infants in Asia and Latin America, often with partial or complete seclusion, and with support by family or community members who perform the cooking, cleaning, and cultural rituals. The timing of earlier rituals may have similarly evolved to be protective— for example, Jewish circumcision occurs at 8 days of life, when the infant gut is sufficiently colonized to ensure endogenous vitamin K production and blood clotting. Regardless of theoretical or demonstrable benefit, the absence of evidence of harm supports providers in encouraging families' cultural practices for welcoming the newborn along with support for bonding and parenting skill development.

Families may describe welcoming their newborns "earthside" at birth, either in recognition of the approximately 10 months of pregnancy or in acknowledgment of a longer relationship history (e.g., if the baby resulted from eggs carried by the mother since her birth, intergenerational gene transmission). Some families' spiritual or religious beliefs include infant souls that accompanied humans in spirit form beforehand (e.g., angels) or previously inhabited one or more bodies (i.e., past lives of ancestors or others). It is recommended that you take the lead from families in terms of language selection, ask questions if their beliefs are unfamiliar to you, verify that you understand their cultural preferences, and refrain from making assumptions based on race or ethnicity.

Health Education

Ongoing infant care and feeding may present challenges, especially for the inexperienced family. Parenting requires cognitive, motor, social, and behavioral skills development amidst significant and often stressful family transitions and sleep challenges (AWHONN, 2006). The healthcare provider should offer encouragement and support for the development of competence, and confidence should be emphasized due to its correlation with long-term parenting satisfaction and behaviors as well as positive parent–child interactions (AWHONN, 2006; Hudson, Elek, & Fleck, 2001).

The assessment and resolution of parent and caregiver knowledge deficits are also key to newborn care. A recent review of non-acute emergency care visits for neonates revealed the most common reasons for care seeking included jaundice, irritability, and emesis. These researchers concluded that improved caretaker education and postnatal supports would moderate the frequency of these care-seeking encounters (Batu, Yeni, & Teksam, 2015). In addition to common infant health conditions and concerns, providers should ensure that parents and other infant caregivers are aware of danger signs and symptoms requiring immediate evaluation, and know how and when to access emergency versus routine care.

Conclusion

The newborn transition period is an important time to provide careful assessment, early recognition of difficulty, and proper management. Assessment at birth that demonstrates initial adjustment to the extrauterine environment provides a foundation for continued normal transition. Keeping the newborn in the mother's arms allows for the normal transition but does not relieve the providers from the responsibility of performing a careful assessment. This chapter has outlined the parameters for the normal transition and the systems and signs that are critical to appraise. Recognizing normal changes that occur in the newborn provides a foundation for initial, ongoing, and supportive care. It is critical to perform frequent observations and assessments to have early recognition of deviations from normal. Specifically focusing on the respiratory and cardiovascular systems provides initial assurance that the newborn is adjusting appropriately. Supportive care that maintains a thermoneutral environment and pays attention to glycemic regulation allows the newborn to transition from fetal to neonatal life. Generally within 4 hours of age, a newborn either will have successfully transitioned or will be recognized to need additional support and observation. The thorough provider will support the normal transition by keeping a watchful eye and presence while the mother–baby dyad adjust to their new environment.

Student Practice Activities

Baby Boy N.T. is the product of a full-term pregnancy from a 27-year-old G2P1. The pregnancy was uncomplicated, and the mother was induced because she was 40 weeks, 6 days. Her labor was a total of 3.5 hours from the initiation of the Pitocin. Near the end of the labor, significant variable decelerations were noted during the 4-minute second stage. The variable decelerations were noted to coincide with a finding of complete dilation. Artificial rupture of membranes (AROM) was done with crowning, with clear fluid being noted. The fetus had a tight nuchal cord × 2 that needed to be clamped and cut to allow for the release of the shoulders and birth of baby. Initially the baby was moderately floppy without initial cry, responding to vigorous stimulation and blow-by oxygen within the first minute of life. The baby "perked up" quickly and continues to be in skin-to-skin contact with his mother. While heart rate never fell below 100 beats/min, the initial respiratory evaluation found a rate of 60 beats/min at 5 minutes of age, and noted crackles in the upper lung fields. The Apgar score at 5 minutes is 9.

1. What should be a consideration at this point to evaluate the neonate?
    You find the temperature to be 97.8°F axillary, and suctioning produced a moderate amount of clear mucus and seemed to improve with episodes of crying and good tone. With suctioning, you notice that there is mild bruising of the neck and face. At 30 minutes of age, the baby continues to need stimulation to cry and begins to have some nasal flaring.

2. Which other signs might you need to evaluate?
    With closer evaluation, you find poor suck or rooting and the baby is "not interested" in nursing at 40 minutes of life. You find that the baby has some "wimpy" crying during the weight and length measurements. Respiratory rate is 58, and lung fields are not clear. The baby is found to weigh 8 lb, 8 oz and be 19 inches long.

3. What would be your next steps?

4. Which information should you provide for the parents about what is going on with the baby?

Multiple Choice

1. Transient tachypnea of the newborn develops more often in the infant who is born:
    A) by cesarean section.
    B) after a prolonged first stage of labor.
    C) with intrauterine growth restriction.

2. The physiologic effect of pulmonary surfactant is to:
    A) increase alveolar surface tension.
    B) decrease alveolar surface tension.
    C) improve chest wall compliance.

3. A consequence of hypothermia in the newborn is:
    A) decreased metabolic demand.
    B) hypoglycemia.
    C) metabolic alkalosis.

4. In which of the following cases is it most appropriate to screen for hypoglycemia?
    A) The second of twins, who weighs 3 kg at birth
    B) A male born at 38 weeks' gestation
    C) A small-for-gestational-age female infant

5. Physiologic hyperbilirubinemia in the newborn is characterized by serum bilirubin that peaks at:
   A) 24 hours of age.
   B) 48 hours of age.
   C) 72 hours of age.

6. A potential association of hypoglycemia in the newborn infant due to impaired production of glucose is:
   A) cold stress.
   B) infant of a diabetic mother.
   C) infant small for gestational age.

References

Academy of Breastfeeding Medicine Protocol Committee. (2008, June). ABM clinical protocol #5: Peripartum breastfeeding management for the healthy mother and infant at term. *Breastfeeding Medicine, 30,* 129. Retrieved from http://www.bfmed.org

Adamkin, D. H. (2015). Metabolic screening and postnatal glucose homeostasis in the newborn. *Pediatric Clinics of North America, 62,* 385–409.

American Academy of Pediatrics (AAP), Section on Breastfeeding. (2012). Breastfeeding and the use of human milk. *Pediatrics, 129,* e827–e841.

American Academy of Pediatrics (AAP) & American College of Obstetricians and Gynecologists (ACOG). (2012). *Guidelines for perinatal care* (7th ed.). Elk Grove Village, IL: Authors.

American Academy of Pediatrics (AAP) & American Heart Association (AHA). (2011). *Textbook of neonatal resuscitation* (6th ed.). Elk Grove Village, IL: Authors.

American Association of Birth Centers (AABC). (2013). Standards for Birth Centers. Available at: http://aabc.site-ym .com/?page=standards

Association of Women's Health, Obstetric, and Neonatal Nurses (AWHONN). (2006). *The compendium of postpartum care.* Washington, DC: Author.

Balaguer, A., Escribano, J., & Rogue, M. (2003). Infant position in neonates receiving mechanical ventilation. *Cochrane Database of Systematic Reviews, 2,* CD 003668.

Barry, J. S., Deacon, J., Hernandez, C., & Jones, M. D. (2016). Acid–base homeostasis and oxygenation. In S. L. Gardner, B. S. Carter, M. Enzman-Hines, & J. A. Hernandez (Eds.), *Merenstein and Gardner's handbook of neonatal intensive care* (8th ed., pp. 145–157). St. Louis, MO: Elsevier-Mosby.

Batu, E. D., Yeni, S., & Teksam, O. (2015). The factors affecting neonatal presentations to the pediatric emergency department. *Journal of Emergency Medicine, 48*(5), 542–547.

Bhat, R., Leipala, J., Singh, N., Rafferty, G. F., Hannam, S., & Greenough, A. (2003). Effect of posture on oxygenation, lung volume, and respiratory mechanics in premature infants studied before discharge. *Pediatrics, 112,* 29–32.

Bolton, D., & Herman, S. (1974). Ventilation and sleep state in the newborn. *Journal of Physiology, 24*(1), 67–77.

Brackbill, Y., Douthitt, T., & West, H. (1973). Neonatal posture: Psychophysiological effects. *Neuropadiatrie, 4*(2), 145–150.

Casaer, P., O'Brien, M., & Prechtl, H. (1973). Postural behavior in human newborns. *Agressologie, 14B*, 49–57.

Chang, Y., Anderson, G., & Lin, C. (2002). Effects of prone and supine positions on sleep state and stress responses in mechanically ventilated preterm infants during the first postnatal week. *Journal of Advanced Nursing, 40*, 161–169.

Chescheir, N., & Menard, M. (2012). Scheduled deliveries: Avoiding iatrogenic prematurity. *American Journal of Perinatology, 9*(1), 27–34.

Christensson, K., Bhat, G. J., Amadi, B. C., Eriksson, B., & Hojer, B. (1998). Randomized study of skin-to-skin versus incubator care for rewarming low-risk hypothermic neonates. *Lancet, 352*, 1115.

Dahlen, H. G., Kennedy, H. P., Anderson, C. M., Bell, A. F., Clark, A., Foureur, M., & Downe, S. (2013). The EPIIC hypothesis: Intrapartum effects on the neonatal epigenome and consequent health outcomes. *Medical Hypotheses, 80*(5), 656–662.

Dangeman, B. C. (1976). The variability of PaO$_2$ in newborn infants. *Pediatric Research, 10*, 149.

Davis-Floyd, R., Pascali-Bonaro, D., Sagady Leslie, M., & Ponce de León, R. G. (2011). The International MotherBaby Childbirth Initiative: Working to create optimal maternity care worldwide. *International Journal of Childbirth, 1*(3), 126–212.

DeCasper, A. J., & Fifer, W. P. (1980). Of human bonding: Newborns prefer their mother's voices. *Science, 208*, 1174–1176.

DeCasper, A. J., & Spence, M. J. (1986). Prenatal maternal speech influences newborns' perception of speech sounds. *Infant Behavior and Development, 9*, 133.

Dimaguila, M., DiFore, J., Martin, R., & Miller, M. (1997). Characteristics of hypoxemia episodes in VLBW infants on ventilator support. *Journal of Pediatrics, 130*, 577–583.

Edwards, M. O., Kotecha, S. J., & Kotecha, S. (2013). Respiratory distress of the term newborn infant. *Paediatric Respiratory Reviews, 14*(1), 29–36.

Erlandsson, K., Dsilna, A., Fagerberg, I., & Christensson, K. (2007). Skin-to-skin care with the father after cesarean birth and its effect on newborn crying and prefeeding behavior. *Birth, 34*(2), 105–114.

Evans, J. (1991). Incidence if hypoxia associated with caregiving in premature infants. *Neonatal Network, 10*, 17–24.

Fernandes, C. J. (2015). Neonatal resuscitation in the delivery room. *UpToDate.* Retrieved from http://www.uptodate.com/contents/neonatal-resuscitation-in-the-delivery-room

Fraser, D. (2014). Newborn adaptation to extrauterine life. In K. R. Simpson & P. A. Creehan (Eds.), *Perinatal nursing* (4th ed., pp. 581–596). Philadelphia, PA: Wolters Kluwer.

Fullerton, J. T., Low, L. K., Shaw-Battista, J., & Murphy, P. A. (2011). Measurement of perinatal outcomes: A decade of experience and future vision for the Optimality Index—US. *International Journal of Childbirth, 1*(3), 171–178.

Gardner, S. L. (2007). Late-preterm ("near-term") newborns: A neonatal nursing challenge. *Nurse Currents, 1*, 1–8.

Gardner, S. L., Enzman-Hines, M., & Agarwal, R. A. (2016). Pain and pain relief in the neonate. In S. L. Gardner, B. S. Carter, M. Enzman-Hines, & J. A. Hernandez (Eds.), *Merenstein and Gardner's handbook of neonatal intensive care* (8th ed., p. 261). St. Louis, MO: Elsevier-Mosby.

Gardner, S. L., Enzman-Hines, M., & Nyp, M. (2016). Respiratory diseases. In S. L. Gardner, B. S. Carter, M. Enzman-Hines, & J. A. Hernandez (Eds.), *Merenstein and Gardner's handbook of neonatal intensive care* (8th ed., pp. 565–643). St. Louis, MO: Elsevier-Mosby.

Gardner, S. L., Goldson, E., & Hernandez, J. A. (2016). The neonate and the environment: Impact on development. In S. L. Gardner, B. S. Carter, M. Enzman-Hines, & J. A. Hernandez (Eds.), *Merenstein and Gardner's handbook of neonatal intensive care* (8th ed., pp. 262–314). St. Louis, MO: Elsevier-Mosby.

Gardner, S. L., & Hernandez, J. A. (2016). Heat balance. In S. L. Gardner, B. S. Carter, M. Enzman-Hines, & J. A. Hernandez (Eds.), *Merenstein and Gardner's handbook of neonatal intensive care* (8th ed., pp. 105–125). St. Louis, MO: Elsevier-Mosby.

Goto, K., Mirmiran, M., Adams, M., Longford, R. V., Baldwin, R. B., Boeddiker, M. A., & Ariagno, R. L. (1999). Effects of prone and supine sleeping position on heart rate variability in preterm infants. *Pediatric Research, 45,* 199A.

Hashimoto, T., Hirua, K., & Endo, S. (1983). Postural effects on behavioral states of newborn infants: A sleep polygraphic study. *Brain Development, 5,* 286–291.

Hernandez, J. A., & Thilo, E. (2005). Routine care of the full-term newborn. In L. C. Osborn, T. G. DeWitt, L. R. First, & J. Zenel (Eds.), *Pediatrics.* St. Louis, MO: Mosby.

Hillman, N. H., Kallapur, S. G., & Jobe, A. H. (2012). Physiology of transition from intrauterine to extrauterine life. *Clinics in Perinatology, 39*(4), 769–783. doi: 10.1016/j.clp.2012.09.009

Hudson, D., Elek, S., & Fleck, M. (2001). First-time mothers' and fathers' transition to parenthood: Infant care self-efficacy, parenting satisfaction, and infant sex. *Issues in Comprehensive Pediatric Nursing, 24,* 31–43.

Hutchison, A., Ross, K., & Russell, G. (1979). Effect of posture on ventilation and lung mechanisms in preterm and light-for-date infants. *Pediatrics, 64,* 429–432.

Interprofessional Education & Research Committee, Champlain Maternal Newborn Regional Program [IPERC]. (2013). Newborn thermoregulation. Retrieved from http://www.cmnrp.ca/uploads/documents//Thermoregulation_Self_Learning_Module_FINAL_2013_06.pdf

Jain, A., & McNamara, P. J. (2015). Persistent pulmonary hypertension of the newborn: Advances in diagnosis and treatment. *Seminars in Fetal & Neonatal Medicine.* doi: 10.1016/j.siny.2015.03.001

Kahn, A., Grosswater, J., Sottiaux, M., Rebuffat, E., Franco, P., & Dramaix, M. (1993). Prone or supine body position and sleep characteristics in infants. *Pediatrics, 91,* 1112–1115.

Kennedy, H. P. (2006). A concept analysis of optimality in perinatal health. *Journal of Obstetrical, Gynecological and Neonatal Nursing, 35*(6), 763–769.

Lawson, B., Anday, E., & Guillet, R. (1987). Brain oxidative phosphorylation following alteration in head positioning in preterm and term infants. *Pediatric Research, 22,* 302–305.

Ludington-Hoe, S., Anderson, G., Swinth, J., Thompson, C., Hadeed, A. J., & Brooks, L. J. (2004). Randomized controlled trial of kangaroo care: Cardiorespiratory and thermal effects on healthy preterm infants. *Neonatal Network, 23,* 39–48.

Martin, R., DiFiore, J. M., Korenke, C. B., Randal, H., & Miller, M. J., (1995).Vulnerability of respiratory control in healthy preterm infants placed supine. *Journal of Pediatrics, 127,* 609–614.

Martin, R. J., Herrell, N., Rubin, D., & Fanaroff, A. (1979). Effect of supine and prone positions on arterial oxygen tensions in the preterm infant. *Pediatrics, 63,* 528–531.

Masterson, J., Zucker, C., & Schulze, K. (1987). Prone and supine positioning effects on energy expenditure and behavior of low birth weight neonates. *Pediatrics, 80,* 689–692.

McEvoy, C., Mendoza, M., Bowling, S., Hewlett, V., Sardesai, S., & Durand, M. (1997). Prone positioning decreases episodes of hypoxemia in ELBW infants (1000 grams or less) with chronic lung disease. *Journal of Pediatrics, 130,* 305–309.

McNanley, T., & Woods, J. (2008). Placental physiology. In T. McNanley & J. Woods, *Global library of women's medicine.* Retrieved from http://www.glowm.com/section_view//heading/Placental%20Physiology/item/195

Montagu, A. (1961). Neonatal and infant immaturity in man. *Journal of the American Medical Association, 178*(1), 56–57.

Moore, E. R., Anderson, G. C., & Berman, N. (2012). Early skin-to-skin contact for mothers and their healthy infants. *Cochrane Database of Systematic Reviews, 5,* CD003519.

Nutter, E., Shaw Battista, J., & Marowitz, A. (2014). Waterbirth fundamentals for clinicians. *Journal of Midwifery & Women's Health, 59*(3), 350–354.

Nyqvist, K. H., Anderson, G. C., Bergman, N., Cattaneo, A., Charpak, N., Davanzo, R., & Widstrom, A. (2010). Towards universal Kangaroo Mother Care: Recommendations and report from the First European conference and Seventh International Workshop on Kangaroo Mother Care. *Acta Paediatrica, 99,* 820–826.

Phillips, R. (2013). Uninterrupted skin-to-skin contact immediately after birth. *Newborn and Infant Nursing Reviews, 13,* 67–72.

Pramanik, A. K., Rangaswamy, N., & Gates, T. (2015). Neonatal respiratory distress: A practical approach to its diagnosis and management. *Pediatric Clinics of North America, 62*(2), 453–469. doi: 10.1016/j.pcl.2014.11.008

Prechtl, H. F. (1967). Neurological sequelae of prenatal and perinatal complications. *British Medical Journal, 4*(5582), 763–767.

Prechtl, H. F. (1980). The optimality principle. *Early Human Development, 4*(3) 201–205.

Rozance, P. J., McGowan, J. E., Price-Douglas, W., & Hay, W. W. (2016). Glucose homeostasis. In S. L. Gardner, B. S. Carter, M. Enzman-Hines, & J. A. Hernandez (Eds.), *Merenstein and Gardner's handbook of neonatal intensive care* (8th ed., p. 351). St. Louis, MO: Elsevier-Mosby.

Schwartz, R. (1993). Effect of position on oxygenation, heart rate, and behavioral state in the transitional newborn infant. *Neonatal Network, 12,* 73–77.

Smith, J. R., & Carley, A. (2014). Common neonatal complications. In K. R. Simpson & P. A. Creehan (Eds.), *Perinatal nursing* (4th ed., pp. 662–698). Philadelphia, PA: Wolters Kluwer.

Smith, J., Plaat, F., &Fisk, N. M. (2008). The anrural caesarean: A woman-centered technique. *BJOG: An International Journal of Obstetrics & Gynaecology, 115*(8), 1037–1042, discussion 1042.

Speer, M. E. (2015). Neonatal pneumonia. *UpToDate.* Retrieved from http://www.uptodate.com/contents/neonatal-pneumonia

Stevens, J., Schmeid, V., Burns, E., & Dahlen, H. (2014). Immediate or early skin-to-skin contact after a caesarean section: A review of the literature. *Maternal & Child Nutrition, 4,* 450–473.

Sullivan, R., & Toubas, P. (1998). Clinical usefulness of maternal odor in newborns: Soothing and feeding preparatory responses. *Biology of the Neonate, 74,* 402–408.

Tronick, E., Scanlon, K. B., & Scanlon, J. W. (1990). Protective apathy, a hypothesis about the behavioral organization and its relation to clinical and physiologic status of the preterm infant during the newborn period. *Clinical Perinatology, 17*(1), 125–154.

Wagaman, M. J., Shutak, J. G., Moomjian, A. S., Schwartz, J. G., Shaffer, T. H., & Fox, W. W. (1979). Improved oxygenation and lung compliance with prone positioning of neonates. *Journal of Pediatrics, 94,* 787–791.

Widström, A.-M., Lilja, G., Aaltomaa-Michalias, P., Dahllöf, A., Lintula, M., & Nissen, E. (2011). Newborn behaviour to locate the breast when skin-to-skin: A possible method for enabling early self-regulation. *Acta Paediatrica, 100,* 79–85.

CHAPTER 4

PHYSICAL EXAMINATION, INTERVENTIONS, AND REFERRALS

Nicole Boucher, Donna Marvicsin, and Sandra L. Gardner

The initial examination of the newly born infant takes place in the delivery/birth room. A brief examination, which includes Apgar scoring and gestational age assessment, is performed immediately after delivery, with a more thorough exam occurring usually 2 to 3 hours after birth.

Apgar Scoring and Gestational Age

A complete assessment of the newborn must take into account risk factors that may have affected fetal intrauterine growth and development. A complete prenatal history, therefore, is vital for the healthcare provider to accurately assess the newborn. For example, factors such as maternal smoking or placental insufficiency may have influenced fetal growth and development.

The physiologic stress of transitioning from the intrauterine environment to the extrauterine environment must also be taken into account when assessing the newborn. The Apgar scoring system (**Figure 4-1**) "provides a comprehensive, objective measure of the infant's condition in the first minutes after birth. The Apgar score does not serve as an indicator of the need for resuscitation; rather, it quantifies an infant's response to the extrauterine environment and resuscitative measures" (Niremeyer, Clarke, & Hernandez, 2016, p. 54). The 1-minute score determines how well the baby tolerated the birthing process. The 5-minute

Sign	0	1	2	1 min	5 min	10 min	15 min	20 min
Color	Blue or pale	Acrocyanotic	Completely pink					
Heart rate	Absent	Less than 100 min	Greater than 100 min					
Reflex irritability	No response	Grimace	Cry or active withdrawal					
Muscle tone	Limp	Some flexion	Active motion					
Respiration	Absent	Weak cry, hypoventilation	Good, crying					
			Total					

Comments:	Resuscitation					
	Min	1	5	10	15	20
	Oxygen					
	PPV/NCPAP					
	ETT					
	Chest compressions					
	Epinephrine					

Figure 4-1: Expanded Apgar score.
Reproduced from American College of Obstetricians and Gynecologists. (2015). The Apgar score. Committee Opinion No. 644. Obstetrics & Gynecology, 126(4): e52–5.

score provides information on how well the baby has completed the neonatal transition. Specifically, the score indicates the extent of the newborn's cardiac and respiratory adjustment.

Gestational age can be calculated based on the date of the last menstrual period, but also by examination of the newborn infant using the Ballard score (Ballard et al., 1991). Newborns are classified as one of the following (Gardner & Hernandez, 2016):

- *Preterm* (PT): less than 37 weeks' gestation (36 6/7 weeks; less than 259 days)
- *Late preterm* (LPT): 34 0/7 to 36 6/7 weeks' gestation; 238 to 259 days
- *Moderate-severe preterm* (MSPT): 28 to 33 6/7 weeks' gestation; 196 to 237 days
- *Extreme preterm* (EPT): 27 6/7 or less weeks' gestation; less than 196 days
- *Full term* (FT): 37 to 41 6/7 weeks' gestation; 239 to 293 days
- *Post-term* (PoT): 42 or more weeks' gestation; 294 or more days

Late preterm infants are at greater risk for short-term morbidities such as hypoglycemia, hypothermia, respiratory distress, sepsis, hyperbilirubinemia, readmission, and feeding difficulties.

The Ballard scale (**Figure 4-2**) is used to determine the gestational age of newborn infants between 20 weeks' and 44 weeks' gestation, based on the assessment of six physical and

Neuromuscular Maturity

Score	−1	0	1	2	3	4	5
Posture							
Square window (wrist)	>90°	90°	60°	45°	30°	0°	
Arm recoil		180°	140°–180°	110°–140°	90°–110°	<90°	
Popliteal angle	180°	160°	140°	120°	100°	90°	<90°
Scarf sign							
Heel to ear							

Physical Maturity

Skin	Sticky, friable, transparent	Gelatinous, red, translucent	Smooth, pink; visible veins	Superficial peeling and/or rash; few veins	Cracking, pale areas; rare veins	Parchment, deep cracking; no vessels	Leathery, cracked wrinkled		
Lanugo	None	Sparse	Abundant	Thinning	Bald areas	Mostly bald	**Maturity Rating**		
Plantar surface	Heel-toe 40–50 mm: −1 <40 mm: −2	>50 mm, no crease	Faint red marks	Anterior transverse crease only	Creases anterior 2/3	Creases over entire sole	Score	Weeks	
							−10	20	
							−5	22	
Breast	Imperceptible	Barely perceptible	Flat areola, no bud	Stippled areola, 1–2 mm bud	Raised areola, 3–4 mm bud	Full areola, 5–10 mm bud	0	24	
							5	26	
Eye/Ear	Lids fused loosely: −1 tightly: −2	Lids open; pinna flat; stays folded	Slightly curved pinna; soft; slow recoil	Well curved pinna; soft but ready recoil	Formed and firm, instant recoil	Thick cartilage, ear stiff	10	28	
							15	30	
							20	32	
Genitals (male)	Scrotum flat, smooth	Scrotum empty, faint rugae	Testes in upper canal, rare rugae	Testes descending, few rugae	Testes down, good rugae	Testes pendulous, deep rugae	25	34	
							30	36	
							35	38	
Genitals (female)	Clitoris prominent, labia flat	Clitoris prominent, small labia minora	Clitoris prominent, enlarging minora	Majora and minora equally prominent	Majora large, minora small	Major cover clitoris and minora	40	40	
							45	42	
							50	44	

Figure 4-2: Clinical estimation of gestational age.

Reprodued from Ballard, J. L., Khoury, J. C., Wedig, K., Wang, L., Eilers-Walsman, B. L., & Lipp, R. (1991). New Ballard score, expanded to include extremely premature infants. *Journal of Pediatrics, 119*(3): 417–423. Copyright 1991, with permission from Elsevier.

six neuromuscular criteria. For most infants, this assessment should occur within 2 hours after birth (American Academy of Pediatrics [AAP] and American College of Obstetricians and Gynecologists [ACOG], 2012). If any complications occurred during the birth process, such as fetal distress or maternal anesthesia, the Ballard scale assessment should be repeated within the first 48 hours of birth.

Additional terms based on the birth weight of the newborn are used to acknowledge intrauterine growth concerns:

- *Appropriate for gestational age* (AGA): Newborn birth weight between the 10th and 90th percentiles for gestational age

- *Small for gestational age* (SGA) or *intrauterine growth restriction* (IUGR): Newborn birth weight less than the 10th percentile for gestational age

- *Large for gestational age* (LGA): Newborn birth weight greater than the 90th percentile for gestational age

Anthropometric Measurements

Head circumference is measured at the largest part of the newborn's head. The head circumference should be measured three times, and the largest measurement should be recorded. The average head circumference for the newborn is 31 to 38 cm (12 to 15 inches). All measurements should be documented and plotted on the correct age-for-gender growth curve.

The newborn should be weighed without clothes or a diaper. Normal birth weight graphs range from 2500 to 4000 g (5 lb 8 oz to 8 lb 13 oz).

For measurement of length, the newborn should be placed on a flat surface, straightened out, and measured from the top of the head to the heel. Normal length for a newborn is 46 to 56 cm (18 to 22 inches).

Physical Examination

Examination of the normal newborn with the parents present enables the healthcare provider to use this encounter as a teaching opportunity for the new parents. The provider is able to show parents and explain the normal variations of newborn anatomy and physiology. This physical examination is an excellent opportunity to provide anticipatory guidance and discuss safety issues in handling and caring for a newborn.

A newborn examination should proceed from the least intrusive to the more intrusive to avoid agitating the newborn and affecting the quality and reliability of data obtained from the exam. Examination proceeds from observation, to the quiet examination, to a head-to-toe examination (**Box 4-1**). The majority of information is obtained by observing the newborn. In addition, the responsiveness of the newborn to the mother and father should be observed.

Vital Signs

Vital signs should be obtained when the infant is quiet and comfortable. Axillary—*never* rectal—temperature should be taken. Normal temperature for a term newborn is 36.5°C to 37.2°C (97.7°F to 99°F). Pain, the fifth vital sign, should be evaluated in all neonates, and adequate nonpharmacologic and pharmacologic pain relief should be given before, during, and after every painful procedure (such as intramuscular injections, heel lance for newborn genetic screening, and circumcision).

Box 4-1: Physical Examination of the Newborn

Observation Examination
- [ ] General condition
  - [ ] Color
  - [ ] Activity and neonatal state
- [ ] Crying
- [ ] Anomalies
- [ ] Resting posture
- [ ] Respirations

Quiet Examination
- [ ] Auscultation
  - [ ] Heart
  - [ ] Lungs
  - [ ] Abdomen
- [ ] Palpation
  - [ ] Fontanels
  - [ ] Abdomen
- [ ] Inspection
  - [ ] Eyes
  - [ ] Blood pressure

Head-to-Toe Examination
- [ ] Skin
- [ ] Head
  - [ ] Ears
  - [ ] Nose
  - [ ] Mouth
- [ ] Thorax
  - [ ] Breast
  - [ ] Clavicles
- [ ] Genitalia
- [ ] Rectum
- [ ] Back
- [ ] Extremities
  - [ ] Upper
  - [ ] Lower

Reproduced from Gardner, S. L., & Hernandez, J. A. (2016). Initial nursery care. In S. L. Gardner, B. S. Carter, M. Enzman Hines, & J. A. Hernandez (Eds.), *Merenstein and Gardner's handbook of neonatal intensive care* (8th ed., pp. 71–104). St. Louis, MO: Mosby-Elsevier.

Respiratory Exam

Without touching the neonate, observe the respiratory rate and rhythm. In newborns, the respiratory rate should be assessed by counting the rise and fall of the chest for one full minute. A normal respiratory rate in the newborn is 30 to 60 breaths per minute. Assess respirations for depth and regularity. Teaching parents about the normal, rapid, and shallow respirations of the newborn can be done here. During the first few hours of life, it is not uncommon to hear crackles when auscultating the lungs of a newborn. **Table 4-1** outlines concerning findings in a neonatal respiratory examination and indicates their clinical significance and the required action.

Cardiac Exam

The heart rate should be auscultated at the point of maximal impulse (PMI) and counted for one full minute. The normal resting heart rate for a newborn is between 120 and 160 beats per minute (BPM). Newborn heart rates vary between a low of 80 to 100 BPM when sleeping to a high of 180 BPM when crying. If the baby is comfortable, move on with the cardiac exam; otherwise, offer a pacifier or rock or quiet a crying newborn before proceeding.

The provider should auscultate in five different areas on the chest (proceeding from the aortic, pulmonic, Erb's point, tricuspid, and mitral areas) for normal S_1 and S_2 heart sounds, as well as for S_3 and S_4. **Table 4-2** outlines concerning findings in a neonatal cardiac examination and indicates their clinical significance and the required action. **Table 4-3** summarizes murmurs commonly auscultated in the first few hours of life in the newborn. Palpate the newborn's chest for heaves, thrills, and the PMI. In the newborn, the PMI should be palpated at the third to fourth intercostal spaces at the left mid-clavicular line.

Screening for Critical Congenital Heart Defects

Newborns with a critical congenital heart defect (CCHD) are at significant risk of disability or death if their condition is not diagnosed soon after birth. Newborn screening using pulse oximetry identifies some infants with CCHD before they become symptomatic. Pulse oximetry of the right hand (preductal) and the right foot (postductal) is performed after the infant reaches 24 hours of age and before hospital discharge. If the baby is born at home or at a birth center, then the screening for CCHD should be done during the first pediatric provider visit. The screening test is normal if oxygen saturation for both hand and foot is greater than 95% and there is less than a 3% difference between the hand and foot saturations. Discrepancy between the preductal and postductal oxygen saturations requires a referral to pediatric cardiology.

Table 4-1: Abnormal Findings in the Respiratory Examination of the Neonate

Red Flags in the Respiratory Assessment	Examination Findings	Clinical Significance	Action Required
Rate	Tachypnea (greater than 60 breaths/min at more than 60 minutes of life) at rest	Earliest sign of a myriad of neonatal conditions: Possible respiratory, metabolic, infectious or congenital cardiac condition or hypothermia	Complete review of perinatal history and respiratory/ cardiac examination. Evaluate oxygenation status with noninvasive PO; evaluate preductally and postductally. POC blood sugar to evaluate for hypoglycemia. Consultation with and referral to neonatology/ pediatrics for diagnosis and intervention based on findings.
Rate	Apnea: Cessation of respirations for 20 seconds or longer, accompanied by physiologic alterations such as color change, bradycardia, and oxygen desaturations as measured on noninvasive PO	Possible metabolic, infectious, respiratory, or neurologic condition or hypothermia	Complete review of perinatal history and respiratory, cardiac, and neurologic examination. POC blood sugar to evaluate for hypoglycemia. Seizures in term newborns due to hypoglycemia, infection, hypoxia–ischemia, and hemorrhage often present as apnea. Consultation with and referral to neonatology or pediatric neurology.
Use of accessory muscles of respiration	Grunting Flaring Retracting	Possible respiratory, metabolic, infectious, or neurologic condition	Same as above.
Chest excursion	Unequal chest excursion	Possible pneumothorax (spontaneous or acquired) Can occur with the first breath of life, after the first cry, or after positive-pressure resuscitation	Consultation with and referral to neonatology/ pediatrics.

Abbreviations: PO, pulse oximetry; POC, point-of-care.

Table 4-2: Abnormal Findings in the Cardiac Examination of the Neonate

Red Flags in the Cardiac Assessment	Examination Findings	Clinical Significance	Action Required
Respiratory rate	Tachypnea (greater than 60 breaths/min at more than 60 minutes of age) at rest	Congenital cardiac disease	Complete cardiac assessment—auscultation, evaluate pulses, blood pressures, and pulse oximetry. Consultation with and referral to neonatology/pediatrics/pediatric cardiology.
Pulses	Unequal pulses: Increased (higher) pulses in the upper extremities and decreased (lower) pulses in the lower extremities	May indicate coarctation of the aorta	Complete cardiac assessment, including pulses (presence, quality, and equality). Evaluate and compare blood pressures and pulse oximetry saturations in upper and lower extremities.
Blood pressure (BP)	Measure in all 4 extremities	BP values in the lower extremities that are lower than BP values in the upper extremities may indicate coarctation of the aorta	Compare the upper and lower extremities: 15–20 mm Hg difference between them is significant and requires consultation with and referral to a cardiologist. Evaluate preductal (right hand) and postductal (right foot) PO oxygenation values. If oxygen saturations for both hand and foot are greater than 95% and there is less than a 3% difference between the hand and foot saturations, *no cardiac consultation and referral is necessary.* Consultation with and referral to pediatric cardiology.
Pulses	Bounding pulses in any extremity. Whether a pulse is bounding may be difficult to determine, but even the smallest premature infant should *not* have a palmar pulse. Presence of a palmar or digital pulse is indicative of a bounding pulse in any neonate.	PDA and other aortic runoff lesions such as truncus arteriosus or systemic arterio-venous fistula	Evaluate respiratory rate, pulses, blood pressures, and PO oxygenation. Consultation with and referral to neonatology and/or pediatric cardiology.

Abbreviations: PDA, patent ductus arteriosus; PO, pulse oximetry.

Table 4-3: Common Murmurs of the Newborn

Cardiac Defect	Pathology	Murmur	Other Findings	Action Required
Patent ductus arteriosus (PDA)	Failure of the ductus arteriosus to close after birth	Heard best at the fourth intercostal space left of the sternal border Machine-like sound	Bounding pulses Wide pulse pressure Active point of maximum intensity	Consultation with and referral to pediatric cardiology
Atrial septal defect (ASD)	Opening between the atria of the heart with left-to-right shunting Commonly occurs in the area of the foramen ovale Closure of the pulmonic valve is delayed	Heard best in the pulmonic area	May hear a widely split S_2	Consultation with and referral to pediatric cardiology
Ventricular septal defect (VSD)	Opening between the two ventricles of the heart	Heard best at the lower-left sternal border Harsh systolic murmur	May be a sign of congestive heart failure Pulmonary hypertension	Consultation with and referral to pediatric cardiology
Coarctation of the aorta	Narrowing of the aorta resulting in left-to-right shunting and possibly left-sided failure	Systolic murmur	Third heart sound that sounds like "Ken-tuck-ee" Unequal, diminished pulses in lower versus upper extremities Blood pressure lower in lower than upper extremities Oxygenation on pulse oximetry better pre-than postductally	Consultation with and referral to pediatric cardiology

Many hospitals routinely screen all newborns for CCHDs. However, CCHD screening is not currently included in all states' newborn screening panels.

Newborn Skin Assessment

Newborn skin should be pink and well perfused, with a capillary refill of less than 2 seconds. Skin turgor is assessed by slightly pinching the skin of the newborn. Well-hydrated skin should be elastic and immediately return to normal. Mucous membranes should be pink and moist. In a postmature infant, it is normal to see cracked, dry skin on the abdomen, hands, and feet. Variations in newborn skin are identified in **Table 4-4**. **Table 4-5** lists abnormal findings in the newborn skin and indicates how these conditions should be managed.

Table 4-4: Variations in Newborn Skin

Skin Presentation	Definition	Comments
Acrocyanosis	Bluish discoloration of the hands and feet after birth.	Peripheral cyanosis is normal in the first 24–48 hours due to the immature cardiac circulation. Presence after 24–48 hours is usually due to cold stress.
Harlequin sign	Unilateral color change on one side of the body. Half of the newborn turns red, with a line of demarcation appearing down the baby's midline.	Transient, harmless color change lasting for 10–20 minutes. It is more common in low-birth-weight infants. Autonomic vasomotor instability results in a red color on the dependent side of the body and pallor on the superior side of the body.
Erythema toxicum	Normal newborn rash abruptly occurs as yellow or white papules over an erythematous base, usually 1 to 3 mm in diameter, over the baby's body except for palmar surfaces. Occurs in 30–70% of newborns.	Unknown cause, but may be the result of an awakening of the immune system.
Milia	Exposed sebaceous glands that look like whiteheads on the infant's face, nose, or chin.	Disappear within the first month of life. No treatment is needed.

Skin Presentation	Definition	Comments
Mongolian spots (slate-colored spots)	Bluish-gray pigmentation of the skin occurring on the lower back and across the shoulders, hips, and legs.	Due to uneven pigmentation, Mongolian spots are most common in dark-skinned neonates. They resemble bruising, fade over time (months to years), and can be confused with bruising of non-accidental trauma (NAT). Documentation of location and size is necessary.
Strawberry hemangioma	Raised capillary nevi, occurring anywhere on the body, that increases in size for the first few months of life, slowly decreases in size over time, and disappears by 10 years of age.	No referral is necessary unless the hemangioma is near the eye or interferes with vision.
Stork bites	Telangiectatic nevus or nevus simplex that appears as a pale pink or reddish discoloration of the skin at the nape of the neck, the lower axilla, around the nasal bridge, and on the eyelids.	More noticeable when the infant is crying. Usually disappears by the second birthday, and requires no intervention.
Lanugo	Fine, soft hair that covers the newborn's back, shoulders, cheeks, forehead, and scalp. Lanugo is more common in the premature infant and disappears within the first 4 weeks of life.	Normal—no referral is required.
Linea nigra	Line of increased pigmentation from umbilicus to genitalia.	Normal; more common in dark-skinned infants.
Vernix caseosa	Cheesy, gray-white substance covering and protecting the skin during fetal life. Coverage at birth is directly related to gestational age.	Gradually diminishes near term.
Acne neonatorum	Appears at several weeks of age as an acne-like rash; caused by maternal hormones' stimulation of sebaceous glands. More common in males.	Lotions, creams, and ointments worsen the rash.
Petechiae	Pinpoint-sized hemorrhage on the skin.	Normal on the presenting part, but its presence on the body on other than the presenting part may be symptomatic of infection.

Table 4-5: Abnormal Findings in Newborn Skin

Red Flags in Skin Assessment	Examination Findings	Clinical Significance	Action Required
Jaundice	Yellowing of the skin Most visible after blanching Progression is head-to-toe	Physiologic or pathologic jaundice Blood incompatibility (ABO; Rh) Immature liver function Diseases involving the liver	Blood type and Coombs test. Direct and total bilirubin.
Circumoral or periorbital cyanosis; cyanosis of the chest or abdomen	Bluish discoloration around the lips, eyes, or torso and abdomen	Central cyanosis, pathologic cyanosis, caused by hypoxemia Because of fetal hemoglobin, a neonate must have an oxygen saturation $\leq$ 60% to be visibly cyanotic	Requires assessment for respiratory, cardiac, infectious, or neurologic conditions. Evaluation of PO oxygenation—preductally and postductally.
Café-au-lait spots	Hyperpigmented lesions, usually macules; typically irregular in shape and light brown color	Most likely benign Neurofibromatosis Tuberous sclerosis Gaucher disease McCune-Albright syndrome	Any newborn with 6 or more café-au-lait spots greater than 1 cm requires further workup for neurofibromatosis.
Mottling	Marbling or spiderweb appearance of the infant's skin	Hypothermia due to cold stress Baby acts infected—poor feeding, lethargic, hypothermic	Check axillary temperature and maintain in a neutral thermal environment. Check blood pressure—may be hypotensive or in shock.
Pallor	Pale, rather than pink skin color Difficult to evaluate in newborn with darker pigmentation—look at the soles of the feet, the palms of the hand, and around the mouth	Anemia Baby acts infected—poor feeding, lethargic, hypothermic	Check hemoglobin and hematocrit. Check blood pressure—may be hypotensive or in shock.

Head Assessment

Assess the anterior and posterior fontanels. The anterior fontanel is formed at the junction of the two frontal and parietal bones, is diamond shaped, measures between 1 and 4 cm, and is soft and flat. Parents should be educated about this "soft spot"—that it can be touched and cleaned without harm to the infant. The posterior fontanel is located at the junction of the two parietal and occipital bones. It is triangle shaped, smaller than the anterior fontanel (admitting only a finger), and also soft and flat. A third fontanel, located along the sagittal suture between the anterior and posterior fontanels, is either a normal variant, a sign of an infant with congenital infection, or a sign of trisomy 21. During infancy, the posterior fontanel closes before the anterior fontanel.

Palpate all five sutures (frontal, coronal, lambdoidal, sagittal, and parietal) for firmness and mobility. Palpate to determine if the sutures are open or overlapped due to molding of the head during labor and birth. Within 24 to 48 hours after birth, the initial head molding and overlapping of sutures resolves. This results in palpation of a larger anterior fontanel and suture lines that are palpated as depressions (Gardner & Hernandez, 2016).

Table 4-6 lists abnormalities in the head, eye, ear, nose, and throat examination and recommendations for their management.

Cephalohematoma A cephalohematoma is a collection of blood under the periosteum of the skull bone caused by pressure during labor, birth, or an operative vaginal delivery. A cephalo-hematoma does not cross the suture line and resolves without intervention in 6 to 8 weeks.

Caput Succedaneum Caput succedaneum is a localized swelling of the soft tissue of the scalp caused by pressure on the head during labor and birth. The swelling crosses suture lines and resolves spontaneously within 24 to 48 hours. As the molding resolves, the head circumference measurement becomes larger than that taken on the first day of life.

Eye Assessment Eye examination must be done when the infant is in the quiet alert state or is aroused to wakefulness with manipulation. Tipping a newborn backward and raising him or her slowly, or shading the eyes from bright light results in spontaneous eye-opening (Gardner & Hernandez, 2016). Term newborns are able to fix and focus on an object that is 8 to 10 inches from the face and follow horizontally and sometimes vertically. The image reflected in the newborn's pupil is the object or person that the child is seeing.

Assess the eyes for size, shape, and placement on the face. Sclera should be whitish, white, or bluish white, and the iris is often blue or gray in light-skinned newborns and brown in infants with darker skin tones. Permanent eye colors appear by 3 to 6 months of age. Pupils should be equal, round, and reactive to light. A positive red reflex indicates an intact lens and

Table 4-6: Abnormal Findings in the Head, Eye, Ear, Nose, and Throat (HEENT) Examination of a Newborn

Red Flags in HEENT Assessment	Examination Findings	Clinical Significance	Action Required
Head			
Skull	Palpable depression in skull bones	Skull fractures may be linear, depressed, palpable, or nonpalpable	Skull x-ray. Consultation with and referral to neonatologist, pediatrician, or pediatric neurology depending on x-ray results.
	Palpable softening of skull bones	More common with forceps deliveries Craniotabes: Caused by maternal vitamin D deficiency	
Fontanel	Bulging, tense, or full to palpation	Normal finding when infant cries Increased intracranial pressure caused by birth injury, bleeding, infection, or hydrocephalus	Consultation with and referral to neonatologist, pediatrician, or pediatric neurology.
Fontanel	Depressed with palpation	Very late sign of dehydration in the neonate	Consultation with and referral to neonatologist or pediatrician.
Sutures	No movement of sutures when gentle downward pressure is exerted Lack of normal expansion of sutures with growth	Craniosynostosis Microcephaly	Consultation with and referral to neonatologist, pediatrician, or pediatric neurology.
Sutures	Widely separated and/or abnormally rapid expansion	Hydrocephalus Increased intracranial pressure	Consultation with and referral to neonatologist, pediatrician, or pediatric neurology.

Red Flags in HEENT Assessment	Examination Findings	Clinical Significance	Action Required
Eye			
Cornea	Hazy	Glaucoma	Consultation with and referral to neonatologist and/or pediatric ophthalmology.
Red reflex	Unable to elicit a red reflex	Congenital infection	Consultation with and referral to neonatologist, pediatrician, or pediatric infectious disease, and ophthalmology.
	Gray or dull white pupil	Congenital cataracts	
		Retinoblastoma	
Placement of eyes on the face	Eyes should be spaced so that a "third eye" easily sits between the two eyes	Congenital chromosomal anomaly or syndrome	Consultation with and referral to neonatologist and/or genetics.
	Hypotelorism: Eyes are too closely spaced, so that "third eye" will not "fit" between		
	Hypertelorism: Eyes are too widely spaced, so that "third eye" fits between with extra space available		
Palpebral fissures	Small palpebral fissures: Eye openings too small	Congenital chromosomal anomaly or syndrome	Consultation with and referral to neonatologist and/or genetics.
Epicanthal folds	Mongolian slant: Outer canthus of the eye is higher than the inner canthus (eye slants upward)	Congenital chromosomal anomaly or syndrome such as trisomy 21	Consultation with and referral to neonatologist and/or genetics.
	Anti-Mongolian slant: Outer canthus of the eye is lower than the inner canthus (eye slants downward)		

(Continued)

Table 4-6: Abnormal Findings in the Head, Eye, Ear, Nose, and Throat (HEENT) Examination of a Newborn (*Continued*)

Red Flags in HEENT Assessment	Examination Findings	Clinical Significance	Action Required
Eye			
Pupil and iris	Coloboma of the iris: Keyhole-shaped pupil	Congenital chromosomal anomaly or syndrome	Consultation with and referral to neonatologist and/or genetics.
	Constricted pupil, unilaterally dilated pupil	Brain injury	Consultation with and referral to neonatology or pediatrics and pediatric neurology.
	Brushfield's spots: White specks across the entire circumference of the iris	Normal variant / Associated with congenital infection and trisomy 21	Consultation with and referral to neonatology, pediatrics, pediatric infectious disease, or genetics.
Sclera	Blue in color	Osteogenesis imperfect	Consultation with and referral to neonatologist, genetics, pediatrics, and orthopedics.
	Yellow color	Hyperbilirubinemia	
Eye examination	Purulent eye drainage / Injected sclera / Moderate lid edema	Infection: Possibly bacterial, gonococcal, or chlamydial	Culture eye drainage. Possible IV or PO antibiotics based on culture results.
Ear			
Outer ear	Malformed or malpositioned ears	Congenital chromosomal anomaly or syndrome	Consultation with and referral to neonatologist, pediatrics, renal, and/or genetics.
	Preauricular sinuses, skin tags	Outer ear and renal tissue forms at same time in fetal life; associated with renal abnormalities	

Red Flags in HEENT Assessment	Examination Findings	Clinical Significance	Action Required
Nose			
Patency of nose: • Obstruct one nostril, close the mouth, and observe breathing from the open nostril • Place a stethoscope under each nostril and watch for fogging of exhalation • Pass soft catheter (only if necessary)	Choanal atresia: Membranous or bony obstruction in the nasal passage, unilateral or bilateral Noisy breathing, apnea and cyanosis when mouth is closed, but pink with crying (mouth open) Other causes of nasal obstruction: Mucus, infection, tumor, cyst, nasal discharge, drugs	May be associated with congenital chromosomal anomaly or syndrome May be isolated abnormality	Consultation with and referral to neonatologist, pediatrics and pediatric ear/nose/throat specialist.
Throat (Mouth)			
Tongue	Macroglossia: Large tongue that protrudes from the mouth Frenulum too tight so that tongue is not freely moveable	Congenital chromosomal abnormalities and syndromes such as trisomy 21 and Beckwith-Wiedemann syndrome Difficulty latching on and breastfeeding	Consultation with and referral to neonatologist, pediatrics, and pediatric endocrinology. Consultation with and referral to pediatrics and lactation.
Palate: Inspect and palpate the soft and hard palates	Cleft palate: Visible opening in the soft or hard palate Submucous cleft: Palpable lack of the bone at the posterior part of the hard palate High-arched palate: Steep arch to palate with palpation	Isolated abnormality or associated with congenital chromosomal abnormalities or syndromes Often able to breastfeed better than bottle- or formula-feed	Consultation with and referral to neonatologist, pediatrics, pediatric surgery, and lactation specialist.

(Continued)

Table 4-6: Abnormal Findings in the Head, Eye, Ear, Nose, and Throat (HEENT) Examination of a Newborn (*Continued*)

Red Flags in HEENT Assessment	Examination Findings	Clinical Significance	Action Required
Throat (Mouth)			
Copious oral secretions	Not cleared by frequent oral suctioning Distress with feeding: Color changes, choking, coughing, and gagging	Esophageal atresia; tracheoesophageal fistula as isolated anomaly or associated with congenital chromosomal abnormalities or syndromes	Consultation with and referral to neonatologist, pediatrics, pediatric surgery, and lactation specialist.
Neck			
Webbing	Redundant skin, webbing of the neck can be seen and palpated	Associated with congenital chromosomal abnormalities such as trisomy 21, Turner's or Noonan's syndrome	Consultation with and referral to neonatologist, pediatrics, and genetics.
Assumes posture with head tilted back and edematous area at neck	Neonatal goiter	Rare; due to intrauterine deprivation of thyroid hormone	Consultation with and referral to neonatologist, pediatrics, and pediatric endocrinology.
Palpable and/or visible mass in neck	Cystic hygroma: Transilluminates, soft, fluctuates	Most common neck mass in neonate Due to sequestered lymph channel that becomes a cyst Small cysts resolve spontaneously Larger cysts may interfere with breathing and feeding; surgical removal	Consultation with and referral to neonatologist, pediatrics, and pediatric surgery.

retina. In darker-skinned newborns, the red reflex may appear more milky white than red. Subconjunctival or sclera hemorrhages, tearless crying, and strabismus are normal.

Ears A full-term infant should have firm, flexible cartilage in the ear, as well as a normal, well-formed ear shape at birth. Recoil of a term newborn's ear is brisk. Premature infants, including late-preterm infants, may have underdeveloped cartilage resulting in a soft and pliable ear with less recoil.

Assess placement of each ear by evaluating an imaginary line from the inner canthus to the outer canthus of the eye to the occiput. If the top of the pinna of the ear touches the imaginary line, the ear is correctly placed; if the top of the pinna is below the line, the ear is low set. Additionally, the angle of placement of the external ear should be almost vertical; thus, if the angle is greater than 10 degrees from vertical, placement is abnormal. **Table 4-6** lists abnormalities of the ear and indicates their significance and management.

Hearing can be assessed by the newborn's response to voices and noises in the examination room. Newborns recognize the familiar sound of their parent's voices and are able to turn toward them. If the newborn is in a quiet alert state, this ability can be demonstrated for parents. All newborns should have a formal newborn hearing screening with follow-up as indicated (Nelson, Bougatsos, & Nygren, 2008). Infants who do not pass the initial hearing screening at birth should be retested within 1 month.

Nose Assess the size and shape of the nose, which should be symmetrical and midline. Newborns are obligatory nasal breathers and must have patent nasal passages. Sneezing clears the newborn's small nasal passages. Sneezing may also be an avoidance behavior that signals to caregivers that the baby is over-stimulated. Newborns have an acute sense of smell immediately after birth and by 3 days of age are able to discriminate the smell of their mother's breastmilk from that of a stranger. Table 4-6 lists abnormalities of the nose.

Mouth Term and late-preterm newborns should be able to root for food, gag to protect their airway, and suck, swallow, and breathe effectively. Mucous membranes of the mouth should be pink and moist, indicating adequate hydration and oxygenation status. The hard and soft palates should be intact. Epstein or epithelial pearls—small, firm, white cysts that contain keratin—are located on the gums and in the roof of the mouth. Epstein pearls are normal and resolve spontaneously. Natal teeth, another normal variant, are early tooth eruptions, are almost always loose, and should be removed to prevent aspiration.

Neck All newborns should have a short neck that is freely mobile and without webbing. Asymmetry of the neck is usually due to in utero positioning. The thyroid is unable to be palpated unless it is enlarged. Table 4-6 outlines abnormalities of the neonatal neck.

Thorax Assessment

Chest A term newborn's chest should be cylindrical with an anterior–posterior diameter of 1:1. The average chest circumference of a term newborn is 33 cm, or 2 cm less than the head circumference. As a result of maternal hormones, breast engorgement is normal in both male and female newborns in the first 2 weeks of life.

Respirations should be easy, nonlabored, and without the use of accessory muscles so that there is no evidence of grunting, flaring, or retracting. There should be no precordial activity observed.

Clavicles should be inspected for bruising and palpated for crepitus. The clavicle should be smooth and have no separation, and no crepitus should be felt. **Table 4-7** outlines abnormalities of the thorax and abdomen.

Abdomen Inspect the abdomen, which should be round and domed. The umbilical cord should have three vessels: two arteries and one vein. Approximately 1% of babies will have a single artery. The cord begins drying soon after birth, loosens from the skin in 4 to 5 days, and falls off at 7 to 10 days of life. There is no need to apply alcohol or other solution to the cord.

On auscultation, bowel sounds should be present in all four quadrants by 1 or 2 hours of life. On palpation, the abdomen should be soft, and the liver can be palpated at 1 to 2 cm below the right costal margin. The tip of the neonatal spleen can be felt from the left side, 2 to 3 cm below the left costal margin.

Genitalia Assessment

Table 4-8 outlines the assessment of the genitalia in a newborn.

Male The genitalia in newborn boys should be assessed for the placement of the urethral opening, which should be at the tip of the penis. Both testes should be descended and palpable. A hydrocele is a collection of fluid in the scrotal sac around the testes. A hydrocele transilluminates and resolves spontaneously; no intervention is necessary.

Female Assess the size of the labia minora, labia majora, and clitoris. A milky discharge from the vagina is normal. Additionally, blood-tinged mucosa from the vagina at 3 to 4 days after birth is the normal result of the withdrawal of maternal hormones. Presence of a vaginal skin tag is normal and represents a visible hymenal ring.

Assessment of Back, Hips, and Extremities

Spine Place the newborn prone to evaluate the alignment of the spine, which should be straight and flexible. Palpate the spine for any inconsistencies in the vertebrae, and observe

Table 4-7: Abnormalities of the Thorax and Abdomen in the Newborn Examination

Red Flags in Thorax Assessment	Examination Findings	Clinical Significance	Action Required
Asymmetry of the chest	Barrel chest: Anterior–posterior diameter 2:1 rather than the normal dimension of 1:1	Transient tachypnea of the newborn: Hyper-expansion of lung	Consultation with and referral to neonatologist or pediatrician.
	Larger or smaller on one side of the chest	Diaphragmatic hernia, diaphragm paralysis, pneumothorax, emphysema, pulmonary agenesis, or pneumonia	Consultation with and referral to neonatologist or pediatrician
Clavicles	Palpable mass over clavicle	Fractured clavicle	Consultation with and referral to neonatologist or pediatrician.
	Crepitus, bruising, tenderness, limited arm movement, or lack of Moro reflex on affected side		
Abdomen			
Umbilical cord	2 vessels (one artery, one vein)	Associated with congenital anomalies of the renal or cardiovascular system	Consultation with and referral to neonatologist or pediatrician.
	Green or yellow-stained cord	Cord stained by meconium, which indicates intrauterine compromise	
	Skin around cord is red and indurated; discharge and odor from the cord	Omphalitis	Consultation with and referral to neonatologist, pediatrician, or pediatric infectious diseases.
	Persistent drainage from cord without other symptoms of omphalitis	Patent urachus, umbilical fistula, or cyst	Consultation and referral to neonatologist or pediatrician.
Scaphoid abdomen	Sunken abdomen due to the lack of abdominal contents; auscultation of bowel sounds in the chest, not the abdomen	Diaphragmatic hernia	Consultation with and referral to neonatology or pediatric surgery.

(Continued)

Table 4-7: Abnormalities of the Thorax and Abdomen in the Newborn Examination (*Continued*)

Red Flags in Thorax Assessment	Examination Findings	Clinical Significance	Action Required
Abdomen			
Abdominal wall defects	Umbilical hernia: Protrusion of intestine at the base of the umbilical cord	More common in low-birth-weight and African American male infants; hypothyroidism	If hernia is reducible, no immediate therapy is needed.
	Omphalocele: Protrusion of abdominal contents through an abdominal wall defect at the base of the umbilical cord; organs are covered by a membrane	Associated with congenital chromosomal abnormalities (trisomy 13, 18, or 21; Beckwith-Wiedemann syndrome), congenital heart defect	Consultation with and referral to neonatologist, pediatric surgery, or pediatric cardiology.
	Gastroschisis: Protrusion of abdominal contents through an abdominal wall defect that is lateral to the midline; no membrane covers the organs	Isolated anomaly associated with fewer congenital chromosomal abnormalities than omphalocele	Consultation with and referral to neonatologist and pediatric surgery.
	Large, flaccid, wrinkled appearance of the abdomen with various genitourinary malformations	Prune belly syndrome: Congenital absence of the abdominal muscles; almost exclusively seen in males	Consultation with and referral to neonatologist, genetics, pediatric surgery, or pediatric urology.
	Protrusion of the bladder through the abdominal wall due to malformations of the genitourinary, musculoskeletal, and intestinal tracts	Exstrophy of the bladder	Consultation with and referral to neonatologist, genetics, pediatric surgery, or pediatric urology.
Auscultate abdomen	Abdominal distention and lack of bowel sounds	Intestinal obstruction, necrotizing enterocolitis, paralytic ileus, imperforate anus, peritonitis, meconium plug, Hirschsprung's disease	Consultation with and referral to neonatologist and pediatric surgery.

Table 4-8: Abnormalities of the Genitalia in the Newborn Examination

Red Flags in Genitalia Assessment	Examination Findings	Clinical Significance	Action Required
Male			
Penis	Micropenis: Abnormally short or thin penis measured at midshaft on a stretched penis (more than 2 standard deviations below the mean for length/ width for age)	Normal penile width is 0.9–1.3 cm at midshaft; more than 2 standard deviations below the mean for length/ width for age is abnormal	Consultation with and referral to neonatologist, pediatric endocrinology, genetics, or urology.
		May be presentation of ambiguous genitalia	Document.
	Constantly erect penis	Priapism; may be a complication of phototherapy	Consultation with and referral to pediatric urology.
Urethral opening	Hypospadias: Urethral opening on the ventral side of the penis	Do not circumcise	
	Epispadias: Urethral opening is on the dorsal side of the penis	Do not circumcise	
Empty scrotal sac	Undescended testes: Testes palpable in inguinal canal rather than in scrotal sac Unilateral more common than bilateral	Cryptorchidism: Affects 33% of preterm infants and 3% of full-term infants (Connor, 1993); most undescended testes resolve spontaneously by age 3 months	Consultation with and referral to pediatrics and pediatric surgeon.
		May be presentation of ambiguous genitalia	

(Continued)

Table 4-8: Abnormalities of the Genitalia in the Newborn Examination (*Continued*)

Red Flags in Genitalia Assessment	Examination Findings	Clinical Significance	Action Required
Male			
Inguinal or scrotal swelling	Intestinal herniation resulting in swelling	Inguinal hernia: If hernia is easily reducible and non-incarcerated, surgery can be scheduled	Consultation and referral to pediatrics and pediatric surgeon.
	Swelling with discoloration (red/bluish red), palpable masses, and pain/tenderness with palpation	Testicular torsion: Unilateral twisting of the testis on its spermatic cord with compromised blood supply	Urgent/emergency surgery to reestablish blood supply.
		Trauma	
		Tumor	
Female			
Ambiguous genitalia	Enlarged clitoris, labial fusion, and/or urethral opening not ventral to vaginal opening	Inability to determine sex of baby by inspection of the genitalia	Consultation with and referral to pediatrics, endocrinology, genetics, urology, or surgery.
		Urogenital sinus	
Generalized swelling and distension of external genitalia	Distended vagina and imperforate hymen	Hydrocolpos: Distended vagina	Consultation with and referral to pediatrics and pediatric surgeon.
		Hydrometrocolpos: Distended vagina and uterus	
Lower abdominal (pelvic) mass and no voiding			
Localized, reducible swelling of the labia	Inguinal hernia	Palpation of gonad in suprapubic area	Consultation with and referral to pediatrics, endocrinology, genetics, urology, or surgery.
		A female newborn with a prolapsed ovary or a male infant with ambiguous genitalia	

the area at the base of the spine for the presence of a pilonidal dimple. Be sure that the base of the skin is visible and there is no secretion from the base. The incurving reflex is checked as the newborn turns toward the side of the spine that is stroked. **Table 4-9** lists abnormalities of the back, hips, and extremities, and indicates their significance and management.

Upper Extremities

Both the upper and lower extremities should be examined to determine if the infant has full range of motion (i.e., flexion, extension, adduction, internal rotation) and symmetry. Count the fingers and toes (mothers count them!!). Note muscle tone. Palpate brachial pulses for strength, equality, and comparison to strength and quality of femoral pulses.

Lower Extremities

Palpate femoral pulses for strength, equality, and comparison to strength and quality of brachial pulses. Evaluate the infant's hip stability. Perform the Barlow and Ortolani's maneuvers to determine developmental hip dysplasia (**Box 4-2**). Assess the symmetry of skin folds in the gluteal and femoral areas.

Note the size, shape, and symmetry of the newborn's feet. Both feet should be straight. Deviation inward of the metatarsal bones is metatarsus adductus, which may be either positional or structural. Table 4-9 describes abnormalities of the newborn foot, including their significance and management.

Neurologic Examination

Reflexes

Newborns are born with unlearned, instinctual, primitive reflexes for survival and protection. These reflexes disappear as they are integrated into development as the infant grows and matures.

The **rooting reflex** is present at birth and disappears around 3 to 4 months of age. Stroke the baby's cheek, and he or she will turn toward the stimulated side and open the mouth. Stroke the center of the lips, and the baby will open the mouth wide to accept the nipple. If the newborn is sleepy or satiated, there may be no response. If the baby is awake and alert and does not respond, the newborn may have facial paralysis if the lack of response is unilateral. If there is no response bilaterally, the neonate is neurologically depressed and requires a prompt pediatric neurology referral.

Table 4-9: Abnormalities of the Back, Hips, and Extremities in the Newborn Examination

Red Flags in Assessment	Examination Findings	Clinical Significance	Action Required
Back			
Spine	Curvature of the vertebral column	Associated with congenital chromosomal abnormalities or syndromes.	Consultation with and referral to pediatric neurology and genetics.
	Pilonidal dimple	May be surrounded by tufts of hair.	
	Pilonidal sinus	Sinus: Greater than 50% risk of neurologic deficit, intradural tumors, or tethered cords (Ackerman & Menezes, 2003).	Prompt radiologic evaluation and consultation with and referral to pediatric neurology or neurosurgery so that timely intervention preserves or improves neurologic function (Ackerman & Menezes, 2003).
	Spina bifida: Lack of closure or incomplete closure of the posterior portion of the vertebral column	Neural tube defects: Mildest form of neural tube defect. Meninges and spinal cord are normal. Defect is covered with skin and most often occurs in the lumbar and lumbosacral area of the spine.	Immediate latex precautions.
	Meningocele: Bony defect in which meninges protrude	Defect is covered by thin atrophic skin and involves more than one vertebra; spinal roots and nerves are normal.	Consultation with and referral to pediatric neurology or neurosurgery.
	Myelomeningocele: Bony defect with bilateral broadening or absence of vertebrae	Most severe form of neural tube defect, in which meninges, spinal nerves, and roots protrude. Neural tube is exposed. The higher the defect on the spine, the greater degree of paralysis. Frequently associated with hydrocephalus.	

Red Flags in Assessment	Examination Findings	Clinical Significance	Action Required
Upper Extremities			
Arm	Palpable mass over clavicle, crepitus, tenderness at fracture site and with arm movement	Fractured clavicle.	Immobilize affected arm.
	Unilateral limited arm movement or failure of arm to adduct and raise with elicitation of Moro reflex	Palsies due to dislocation, fracture, or injury to brachial plexus.	Consultation with and referral to pediatric orthopedics.
	Crepitus, tenderness, palpable mass, limb shortening, blue sclera	Osteogenesis imperfecta.	
Hands	Count number of fingers: • Polydactyly: More than 5 fingers on each hand • Syndactyly: Fewer than 5 fingers on each hand	May be isolated finding or associated with congenital chromosomal abnormalities or syndromes.	Consultation with pediatrics or genetics.
	Simian crease: Palmar line that courses straight across the palm	Bilateral: Associated with congenital chromosomal abnormalities (trisomy 21). Unilateral: Familial, normal variant.	
Hypotonia	Lack of muscle tone, resulting in the baby being limp and floppy	Neuromuscular disorders, CNS dysfunction, including hypoxic–ischemic encephalopathy, sepsis, perinatal drug intake, congenital chromosomal abnormalities (i.e., trisomy 21, Prader-Willi syndrome).	Consultation with and referral to neonatology, genetics, or infectious disease.
	Test flexion development by checking recoil: Extend arms alongside the body and let go; the arm response is recoil	Flexion develops in upper extremity after lower extremity. Developmental immaturity.	

(Continued)

Table 4-9: Abnormalities of the Back, Hips, and Extremities in the Newborn Examination (*Continued*)

Red Flags in Assessment	Examination Findings	Clinical Significance	Action Required
Upper Extremities			
Hypertonia	Increased muscle tone, resulting in tightly clenched fists, arm flexion	CNS irritability, hemorrhage, infection, seizure, NAS, congenital chromosomal abnormality or syndrome.	Consultation with and referral to neonatologist, genetics, or infectious disease.
Lower Extremities			
Hips	Assess skin folds in gluteal and femoral areas	Asymmetry suggestive of congenital developmental dysplasia of the hip, which is more common in females and breech presentations.	Perform the maneuvers described in Box 4-2.
Hypotonia	Froglike position of legs	Developmental immaturity. Progression to flaccidity indicative of progression of hypoxemia, sepsis, or some other condition.	Consultation with and referral to neonatologist, genetics, or infectious disease.
Hypertonia	Test flexion development by checking recoil: Extend legs and let go; the leg response is recoil. Increased muscle tone resulting in tightly clenched toes and feet and leg flexion	Flexion develops in the lower extremities before the upper extremities. Developmental immaturity. CNS irritability, hemorrhage, infection, seizure, NAS, congenital chromosomal abnormality or syndrome.	Consultation with and referral to neonatologist, genetics, or infectious disease.

Red Flags in Assessment	Examination Findings	Clinical Significance	Action Required
Feet	Count number of toes: • Polydactyly: More than 5 toes on each foot • Syndactyly: Fewer than 5 toes on each foot	May be isolated finding or associated with congenital chromosomal abnormalities or syndromes.	Consultation with pediatrics or genetics.
	Inward rotation of one or both feet	Positional: Flexible deformity due to in utero positioning; forefoot can be abducted to and beyond the midline.	Corrects without treatment. Parental massage and maneuver of the foot to and beyond the midline may be performed.
		Structural: Forefoot cannot be abducted beyond the midline.	Consultation with and referral to pediatric orthopedics for early treatment.
		Clubfoot (talipes equinovarus): Adduction of the forefoot—points medially; pronounced heel varus; downward pointing (equines positioning) of the foot and toes. Affected foot is not able to be abducted to or beyond the midline because the tendons that connect the muscles of the feet and leg are too short.	Consultation with and referral to pediatric orthopedics for early treatment.

Abbreviations: CNS, central nervous system; NAS, neonatal abstinence syndrome.

Box 4-2: Maneuvers to Assess for Developmental Dysplasia of the Hip

Barlow's Maneuver: Place the newborn supine. Adduct the thighs and hips while gently applying pressure to the newborn's knees to detect hip dislocation. Barlow's maneuver is positive if the femur head dislocates, which can be felt and seen.

Ortolani's Maneuver: Do Ortolani's maneuver if Barlow's maneuver is positive, to confirm the dislocation of the affected hip. Place the newborn supine. Flex the infant's knees and hips at a 90-degree angle, and place the flexed knee in the space between the examiner's thumb and index finger, with the examiner's index finger gently putting pressure over the greater trochanter of the newborn. The examiner then gently abducts the infant's legs. If a "clunk" is felt, Ortolani's maneuver is positive. An orthopedic referral is needed in such a case.

The **sucking reflex** is present prior to (begins at 26 to 28 weeks' gestation) and at birth. Test the quality of sucking by placing a nipple or a gloved finger in the infant's mouth and assessing the strength of the suck. Also assess the hard and soft palates for clefts and arching; feel for a submucous cleft. The strength of the sucking reflex is dependent on gestational age: at term, neonates have a strong sucking reflex. A recently fed, satiated baby may not suck vigorously. Absence of a strong suck reflex indicates neurologic depression from CNS conditions, neonatal abstinence syndrome (NAS), and/or developmental immaturity. Late-preterm infants may have a weaker suck, fall asleep during feeding, and have other feeding problems. Depending on the cause of a weak suck, these neonates may need intervention for adequate feeding and referral to pediatric neurology.

The **tonic neck reflex** is present at birth and integrates with the other infant behaviors by 4 to 6 months of age, so that rolling over, reaching, and grasping can occur. Place the newborn supine, gently rotate the head to one side, and hold it in this position for 15 seconds. A positive response occurs when the arm and leg extend on the facial side and flex on the other side.

The **palmar grasp reflex** is present at birth and integrates with the other infant behaviors between 5 and 6 months of age, to allow voluntary grasping of objects. Place a finger in the infant's palm and lightly press on the palm; the infant should wrap the fingers around the examiner's finger. Test this reflex bilaterally: grasp should be equal in both hands and strong enough to raise the newborn's trunk for a few seconds.

The **Galant reflex** is present at birth and disappears by 2 months of age. To evaluate truncal incurvation, suspend the newborn in the prone position, stroke the back 2 to 3 cm from the spinal column, and observe the response. The infant should flex toward the stimulated side. An asymmetric response is abnormal; in such a case, the newborn should be referred to pediatric neurology immediately.

The **Moro reflex** is present at birth and usually integrates with the other infant behaviors at 6 to 8 months of age, to enable sitting and protective extension of the arms and hands.

Make a loud noise or drop the infant's head slightly and observe the reaction of the arms and fingers. In a positive Moro reflex, both arms abduct, then return to the midline while the fingers splay and the thumb and forefinger are positioned as a "C." An asymmetric response is indicative of a brachial plexus injury or a fractured clavicle. Absence of the Moro reflex indicates a severe brain stem problem. The Moro reflex is considered the most critical assessment in an infant to determine if the neurologic system is intact.

The **plantar grasp** is present at birth and does not integrate with the other infant behaviors until 8 to 10 months of age, when standing and walking abilities develop. To test this reflex, press firmly against the base of the toes and watch the toes curl down. Plantar grasp tests the S1 and S2 spinal nerves. An abnormal response requires a pediatric neurology consult.

The **Babinski reflex** is present at birth and integrates with the other infant behaviors at 8 to 9 months of age, to allow standing and walking. Stroke the infant's foot from the heel upward toward the ball of the foot. A positive Babinski reflex results in fanning or hyperextension of the toes, which is a normal response until 2 years of age.

Cranial Nerves

Cranial Nerve I (Olfactory) The sense of smell is well developed in full and preterm infants. At 5 days of age, neonates are able to differentiate their mother's breast pad, stop crying, turn toward it, and begin sucking (Sullivan & Toubas, 1998). Placing an alcohol pad or other noxious scent under the infant's nose should elicit a grimace.

Cranial Nerves II (Optic), III (Oculomotor), IV (Trochlear), and VI (Abducens) Shine a light into the newborn's eyes, and there is rapid eye closure—the optical blink reflex. To assess the newborn's ability to focus and follow, place the newborn at 8 to 10 inches from the examiner's face, see your reflection in the infant's pupils (the baby is looking at you), and then slowly move your head horizontally. The baby's eyes, and then the baby's head, should follow your face.

Another technique to test these cranial nerves is to place a high-contrast object (such as a black-and-white picture) 8 to 10 inches from the baby's face, see the object reflected in the baby's pupil, and slowly move the object horizontally. Some term newborns can also follow for a short distance vertically.

Cranial Nerves V (Trigeminal), IX (Glossopharyngeal), and XII (Hypoglossal) Assess these cranial nerves by observing the rooting and sucking reflexes. Swallowing is assessed by observing the infant latch on and breastfeed or bottle-feed.

Cranial Nerve VII (Facial) The glabella tap tests for blinking. Tap the newborn lightly on the forehead between the eyes—on the bridge of the nose. Facial palsy is assessed in the crying and noncrying infant. Injury to the facial nerve manifests in the crying infant as an inability to close the affected eye, wrinkle the brow, or contort the mouth. Facial weakness and palsy may be caused by central nervous system (CNS) injury, nerve damage, or muscle weakness syndromes, and affect the newborn's ability to feed. Facial symmetry and grimacing are continuously assessed throughout the remainder of the examination.

Cranial Nerve VIII (Auditory) Place the newborn supine in a quiet room to assess the ability to hear and alert to sound. Production of a loud sound (such as a hand clap) should produce the acoustic blink reflex as well as a Moro reflex (until the infant reaches 4 months of age). Speaking to the newborn should elicit a quieting of behavior and sucking; the eyes should turn toward the sound first, followed by the head. Term newborns are able to distinguish and turn toward the familiar sounds of their parents' voices, distinguishing them from the voices of strangers.

All newborns should be screened for hearing loss with otoacoustic emissions or auditory brain stem response testing prior to discharge (Nelson et al., 2008). If born in a birth center, infants should be referred for testing as soon as possible after birth.

Brazelton Examination

The Neonatal Behavioral Assessment Scale (NBAS) was developed by Brazelton in 1979 as a psychological scale to assess an individual neonate's capabilities for social relationships (Brazelton, 1984). Using elements of the Brazelton scale, advanced practice nurses teach parents about their own infant's patterns of behavior, temperament, and newborn states. Aspects of the Brazelton exam are performed at 2 to 3 days of life, at discharge, or on the follow-up visit at 1 to 2 weeks of life.

The neonate must be in the quiet alert state to interact with the examiner. The Brazelton exam assesses the infant's best performance in response to stimulation and handling by the examiner. Selected maneuvers include having the neonate fix, follow, and find the source of noise and a visual stimulus, such as the face or an inanimate object. Demonstrating that their newborn knows their voices and will turn toward them, rather than toward the "strange" voice of the advanced practice nurse, is exciting for parents to see and shows them their baby's innate competency. Strategies for handling, soothing, and comforting their baby can be taught and demonstrated during this exam. Even siblings are able to participate by ringing a bell or rattle and watching their brother or sister respond.

Sleepy, crying, and hungry newborns will not be able to participate in the Brazelton examination. Perinatal use of antidepressants and smoking have been shown to alter the newborn's neurobehavioral examination. Newborns exposed to selective serotonin reuptake inhibitors (SSRIs) in late pregnancy have been shown to exhibit mild and spontaneously resolving behaviors such as tremors and tremulousness, restlessness and irritability, abnormal crying, rigidity, fewer state changes, and more active sleep patterns with startles and arousal (Moses-Kolko et al., 2005; Oberlander, Warburton, Misri, Aghajanian, & Hertzman, C. (2006).

Student Practice Activities

Multiple Choice

1. Transient tachypnea of the newborn develops more often in the infant who is born:
    A) by cesarean section.
    B) after a prolonged first stage of labor.
    C) with intrauterine growth restriction.

2. The physiologic effect of pulmonary surfactant is to:
    A) increase alveolar surface tension.
    B) decrease alveolar surface tension.
    C) improve chest wall compliance.

3. A consequence of hypothermia in the newborn is:
    A) decreased metabolic demand.
    B) hypoglycemia.
    C) metabolic alkalosis.

4. In which of the following cases is it most appropriate to screen for hypoglycemia?
    A) The second of twins, who weighs 3 kg at birth
    B) A male infant born at 38 weeks' gestation
    C) A small-for-gestational-age female infant

5. Physiologic hyperbilirubinemia in the newborn is characterized by serum bilirubin that peaks at:
    A) 24 hours of age.
    B) 48 hours of age.
    C) 72 hours of age.

6. A potential association of hypoglycemia in the newborn infant due to impaired production of glucose is:
    A) cold stress.
    B) infant of a diabetic mother.
    C) infant small for gestational age.

References

Ackerman, L., & Menezes, A. (2003). Spinal congenital dermal sinuses: A 30-year experience. *Pediatrics, 112*, 641–647.

American Academy of Pediatrics (AAP) & American College of Obstetricians and Gynecologists (ACOG). (2012). *Guidelines for perinatal care* (7th ed.). Washington, DC: AAP.

Ballard, J. L., Khoury, J. C., Wedig, K., Wang, L., Eilers-Walsman, B. L., & Lipp, R. (1991). New Ballard score, expanded to include extremely premature infants. *Journal of Pediatrics, 119*(3), 417–423.

Brazelton, T. B. (1984). *Neonatal behavioral assessment scale* (2nd ed.). Philadelphia, PA: Spastics International Medical Publishers/Lippincott.

Connor, G. K. (1993). Genitourinary assessment. In E. P. Tappero & M. E. Honeyfield (Eds.), *Physical assessment of the newborn: A comprehensive approach to the art of physical examination* (pp. 91–100). Petaluma, CA: NICU Ink.

Gardner, S. L., & Hernandez, J. A. (2016). Initial nursery care. In S. L. Gardner, B. S. Carter, M. Enzman Hines, & J. A. Hernandez (Eds.), *Merenstein and Gardner's handbook of neonatal intensive care* (8th ed., pp. 71–104). St. Louis, MO: Mosby-Elsevier.

Haddad, G. G., & Green, T. P. (2014, November 20). Diagnostic approach to respiratory disease. In R. M. Kliegman, R. E. Behrman, H. B. Jenson, & B. F. Stanton (Eds.), *Nelson textbook of pediatrics*. Retrieved from http://www.nlm.nih.gov/medlineplus/ency/article/001562.htm

Moses-Kolko, E. L., Bogen, D., Perel, J., Bregar, A., Uhl, K., Levin, B., & Wisner, K. L. (2005). Neonatal signs after late in utero exposure to serotonin reuptake inhibitors: Literature review and implications for practice. *Journal of the American Medical Association, 293*, 2372–2383.

Nelson, H. D., Bougatsos, C., & Nygren, P. (2008). Universal newborn hearing screening: Systematic review to update the 2001 US Preventive Services Task Force recommendations. *Pediatrics, 122*, e266–e276.

Niremeyer, S., Clarke, S. B., & Hernandez, J. A. (2016). Delivery room care. In S. L. Gardner, B. S. Carter, M. Enzman Hines, & J. A. Hernandez (Eds.), *Merenstein and Gardner's handbook of neonatal intensive care* (8th ed., pp. 47–70). St. Louis, MO: Mosby-Elsevier.

Oberlander, T. F., Warburton, W., Misri, S., Aghajanian, J., & Hertzman, C. (2006). Neonatal outcomes after prenatal exposure to selective serotonin reuptake inhibitor antidepressants and maternal depression using population-based linked health data. *Archives of General Psychiatry, 63*, 898–906.

Sullivan, R., & Toubas, P. (1998). Clinical usefulness of maternal odor in newborns: Soothing and feeding preparatory responses. *Biology of the Neonate, 74*, 402–408.

CHAPTER 5

NEWBORN AND NEONATAL NUTRITION

B. J. Snell and Sandra L. Gardner

Introduction

Once the placenta no longer provides nutrition, a newborn's survival depends on the ability to take in nutrients. The reflex of sucking develops early in gestation; indeed, during pregnancy, ultrasounds have captured the innate ability of the fetus to suck (Petrikovsky, Kaplan, & Pestrak, 1995; Ross & Nijland, 1997). Sucking and suckling, however, are two different actions. Sucking is a primitive reflex that is strong in the newborn. Suckling, in contrast, is the process of not only creating a vacuum in the mouth, but also coordinating a compression or expression of the teat efficiently to retrieve milk, and swallowing to propel the nutrients to the stomach— all while simultaneously coordinating breathing.

The foundational and component parts for oral feeding are present at birth, and healthy, term newborns will transition to such feeding so that they can survive. Suckling is a learned behavior, with learning most effectively occurring when an optimal environment and support are provided. The literature is replete with case studies of newborns who, when placed in their mother's arms immediately after birth and allowed to transition without interference, "crawl" to the breast and initiate suckling. This breast crawl was originally described in Sweden and subsequently named by Dr. Marshall Klaus in 1998 (Chaturvedi, 2008; Widstrom et al., 1987). Generally, the newborns who exhibit this behavior are "naturally born babies" from healthy pregnancies who are born at term. Nevertheless, babies born via cesarean birth and preterm newborns may achieve the same outcome. What appears to make the difference in the ability to make this transition successfully is the environment and support provided. Provision of such an environment requires that the providers present at birth recognize when to intervene and when to remain present and in the assessment/evaluation mode.

For years, midwives have recognized they need to "do nothing, well"—and this mandate includes initiation of feeding at birth (Kennedy, 2000). A mantra of the author has always been "If you can conceive a baby and grow a baby, you can birth a baby and breastfeed a baby." All of these phases take energy and persistence at times, yet collectively they provide the optimal foundation for the newly born baby and family.

Working from physiological, psychological, and environmental perspectives, this chapter discusses neonatal nutrition so as to provide a foundation for assessment and management of the newborn during the first month of life. Some conditions that require additional assessment and management for initiation and maintenance of adequate nutrition to ensure that the newborn thrives are also presented. While this chapter is not an in-depth compendium of breastfeeding issues and management, it does cover conditions commonly encountered during the initiation and early maintenance of breastfeeding. Additionally, for the mother who cannot or declines to breastfeed, a review of formula feeding is provided.

Influences on Breastfeeding Success: Prenatal, Intrapartal, and Postpartal

Provision of adequate nutrition for the newborn requires education of the mother about how her nutrition will affect first her growing fetus and then her newborn. The placenta is a remarkable organ that can filter many toxins to protect a growing fetus, but it is truly governed by the concentration principle. In turn, mothers must be educated to recognize that their baby's exposure to these influences in utero can imprint and provide a foundation for nutrition that is not optimal for a growing child. Women during pregnancy are as motivated as they will ever be to "do their best." Principles of healthy nutrition are critical not only for ensuring the continuation of the pregnancy, but also for growing a child. Providers must begin early in pregnancy and throughout gestation to discuss breastfeeding, encourage breastfeeding, and teach the foundation for breastfeeding. For those mothers who decline to breastfeed or have a condition that precludes breastfeeding, principles of formula feeding need to be provided.

In 2011, the rate of initiation of breastfeeding in the United States was 79%, yet by 6 months after birth, only 49% of mothers continued to breastfeed (Centers for Disease Control and Prevention [CDC], 2014). These statistics represent an improvement from 2010, when the rate of initiating breastfeeding at birth was only 77%. *Healthy People 2020* goal is to increase the rate of breastfeeding at 6 months to 60.5% (Chantry, 2011). Demographics continue to show that non-Hispanic black women have the lowest rates of initiation and maintenance of breastfeeding (CDC, 2010).

Hospital policies and procedures also greatly impact the initiation of breastfeeding. The Baby-Friendly Hospital Initiative (BFHI) is a global effort launched by the World Health Organization (WHO) and UNICEF in 1991 to implement practices that protect, promote, and support breastfeeding (WHO, UNICEF, & Wellstart International, 2009). As part of its work, the BFHI has identified practices that negatively impact breastfeeding and has provided an outline of strategies that have demonstrated improvement in rates of successful initiation and breastfeeding exclusivity (Holmes, McLeod, & Bunik, 2013). Many of the practices that negatively impact breastfeeding involve not just the postpartum and early neonatal periods, but are also present and promulgated at birth (i.e., use of Pitocin for induction and/or stimulation of labor, high cesarean section rates, and high epidural anesthesia usage rates). In the years to come, the BFHI will focus on these practices as opportunities to further improve rates of breastfeeding initiation and continuation.

Prenatal Promotion of Breastfeeding

The promotion of successful breastfeeding begins during pregnancy. Prenatal promotion of breastfeeding as the optimal method for infant feeding gives parents the information they need to make an informed decision. Providing a pregnant woman with "affirmations" that her body and breasts are "made" to be successful creates the mind–body connection necessary for successful breastfeeding. Evidence demonstrates that prenatal education focused on breastfeeding and early postpartum interventions are the most effective strategy to ensure successful breastfeeding initiation and exclusivity (Chung et al., 2008).

Prenatal care includes assessment of any condition that may affect breastfeeding and appropriate consults to prevent problems. All professional societies, both domestic and international, have recommendations for initiation of breastfeeding and provision of breastmilk for the first year of life (American Academy of Pediatrics [AAP] Section on Breastfeeding, 2012; American College of Nurse-Midwives [ACNM], 2011; American College of Obstetricians and Gynecologists [ACOG], 2013; Association of Women's Health, Obstetric and Neonatal Nurses [AWHONN], 2007; National Association of Neonatal Nurses [NANN], 2009). Therefore, care providers involved with birth and the early postnatal period are required to provide information, recommendations, and support for breastfeeding unless there is a true contraindication to this feeding method. "Women will benefit from moderated group discussions, group prenatal visits, systematic case management, or referral to a lay support organization prior to delivery" (ACOG, 2013; Caine, Smith, Beasley, & Brown, 2012; Chung et al., 2008; Rotundo, 2011). There is also good evidence that peer counseling promotes the initiation and maintenance of breastfeeding (Chapman et al., 2010; Sudfeld, Fawzi, & Lahanya, 2012). The ACNM's (2011)

Position Statement on Breastfeeding promotes breastfeeding as the optimal method of feeding a baby, noting that "breastfeeding is a combination of learned and instinctive behaviors of both mother and infant and that the choice to breastfeed is affected by sociocultural factors, including attitudes of health care providers."

Intrapartal Promotion of Breastfeeding

While much work goes into "preparation for labor and birth," the predominant model of intrapartum care (in the United States) focuses on strategies that are not supportive of breastfeeding. Use of oxytocin for labor induction, widespread use of epidural anesthesia, operative delivery (i.e., forceps or vacuum), and cesarean section deliveries actually increase the risk of early cessation of breastfeeding (ACOG, 2013; Beilin et al., 2005; Gizzo et al., 2012; Montgomery, Hale, & Academy of Breastfeeding Medicine [ABM], 2012). Research by Fernandez et al. (2012) found that newborn feeding behavior is suppressed by intrapartum use of oxytocin. Likewise, epidural anesthesia has been found to negatively affect newborn sucking (Montgomery et al., 2012). In contrast, the continuous presence of one or more support persons during childbirth improves outcomes in relation to breastfeeding. A hallmark of midwifery care, of course, is the provision of continuous presence during labor and birth (as per the ACNM's core competencies). Care by a doula has also been shown to positively influence breastfeeding (Kozhimannil, Attanasio, Hardeman, & O'Brien, 2013).

Postpartal Promotion of Breastfeeding

Interventions after birth (i.e., separation of mother and baby; excessive newborn suction) may also negatively impact the newborn transition and breastfeeding. After birth, the healthy newborn should be placed immediately in skin-to-skin contact with the mother and allowed to transition naturally regardless of which method of feeding the mother chooses. Babies should be placed in their mother's arms and remain there until after the first breastfeeding. Care providers can facilitate newborn feeding by teaching mothers how to recognize and respond to their baby's feeding cues (**Box 5-1**). All necessary procedures can be completed while the baby is in the mother's arms. Delaying all initial procedures that are not critical (i.e., weighing, measuring, administration of

Box 5-1: Newborn Hunger Cues

- Wriggling or restless movements
- Mouth movements and sucking
- Tongue protrusion
- Hands to mouth or face
- Rooting with stimulation of legs or cheeks

newborn medications) until after the "golden period: positively influences the newborn's ability to initiate breastfeeding (AAP, Section on Breastfeeding, 2012; Bramson et al., 2010; Christensson et al., 1992; Marin-Gabriel et al., 2010; Mikiel-Kostyra, Mazur, & Boltruszko, 2002; Moore, Abderson, Bergman, & Dowswell, 2012; Preer, Pisegna, Cook, Henri, & Philipp, 2013).

Initial postpartum care also influences breastfeeding, and exclusive rooming-in enhances breastfeeding. Despite some sources' suggestions that babies should be cared for in a nursery because their mothers need rest and sleep, evidence does not support these contentions. Studies over multiple decades have found that mothers obtain similar amounts of sleep when babies are rooming-in compared to when babies are separated from them in a term nursery at night (Ball, Ward-Platt, Heslop, Leech, & Brown, 2006; Keefe, 1988; Waldenstrom & Swenson, 1991). Separating mother and baby at any time interrupts the opportunity for the mother to learn and respond to her baby's cues in a timely fashion.

Support staff should be available to assist breastfeeding mothers and ready to provide assistance. Breastfeeding support is time intensive, however, and many staff do not or are not able to take the time to adequately assess and assist. Postpartally, feeding adequacy must be assessed and documented (Holmes et al., 2013; Kervin, Kemp, & Pulver, 2010; Perez-Escamilla, Pollitt, Lonnerdal, & Dewey, 1994; Renfrew, McCormick, Quinn, & Dowswell, 2012). Assessment and documentation of the effectiveness of breastfeeding should be done every 8 to 12 hours while the mother is in the hospital: "Peripartum care of the dyad should address and document infant positioning, latch, milk transfer, baby's weight, clinical jaundice, and any problems raised by the mother, such as nipple pain or the perception of an inadequate breastmilk supply" (Holmes et al., 2013).

Improvement of long-term breastfeeding rates focuses on the prevention of early discontinuation. A retrospective study of Women, Infants and Children (WIC) recipients in Connecticut found that the most common reasons for discontinuation of breastfeeding were (1) age of child, (2) mother's return to work, (3) sore nipples, (4) lack of access to breast pumps, and (5) free formula provided by WIC (Haughton, Gregorio, & Perez-Escamilla, 2010). The authors of this study noted that lactation support was provided in less than 50% of the primary care offices for mothers having problems. Maternal breastfeeding problems typically met with a recommendation from the care provider to introduce formula, which undermined maternal confidence, generally exacerbated the problem, and resulted in discontinuation of breastfeeding. A meta-analysis by Chung et al. (2008), however, found that professional support—not formula supplementation—improved "immediate" breastfeeding rates.

Physiology and Pathophysiology of Breastfeeding

In utero, the dependent fetus is nourished by maternal glucose, which moves easily across the placenta via facilitated diffusion. Approximately 30% to 40% of the glucose is retained in the placenta for use (Graves & Haley, 2013). Due to its large molecular structure, insulin does not pass through the placental barrier; instead, the fetus produces its own insulin to maintain homeostasis (Csont, Groth, Hopkin, & Guillet, 2014).

When umbilical cord clamping is performed, the fetus must be able to both mobilize indigenous stores of energy and initiate feeding if it is to thrive. Healthy, term newborns transition from the continuous feeding in utero to intermittent feeding after birth when they remain with their mother and are supported by attending staff. The AAP recommends putting the baby to breast within the first hour after birth to enable the newborn to maintain glucose homeostasis (Wight, Marinelli, & ABM, 2014; Csont et al., 2014).

Lactation

In the mother, lactation—that is, milk production—depends on two processes: mammogenesis and lactogenesis. Mammogenesis is the growth and development of glandular tissue in the breast and differentiation of secretory epithelial cells during pregnancy; it is stimulated by hormones (Hartmann, Cregan, Ramsay, Simmer, & Kent, 2003). The milk production system of the breast (alveoli or lactocytes) is stimulated by progesterone, while the milk collection (ductal) system is stimulated by estrogen. At birth, removal of the placenta causes a sudden drop in the woman's levels of estrogen and progesterone, so that milk secretion is initiated.

Nutritive suckling on the maternal breast stimulates the secretion of prolactin. This prolactin enters the bloodstream and travels to the alveoli of the breast, where milk is produced (**Figure 5-1** and **Figure 5-2**).

Nutritive suckling also stimulates the secretion of oxytocin, which enters the bloodstream and travels to the myoepithelial cells in the breast, causing those cells to contract and resulting in the ejection of milk into the ductal system. The establishment of a milk supply depends on adequate secretion of prolactin, as does maintenance of the milk supply. Maintaining an adequate milk supply requires adequate nutritive stimulation of the breast and removal of milk on a regular and frequent basis (Gardner & Lawrence, 2016). Once let-down of milk occurs, breastfeeding is rhythmic: the suck–swallow–breathe (SSB) cycle occurs in a 1 second to 1 second to 1 second (1:1:1) ratio (Lawrence & Lawrence, 2001). Factors that affect milk supply are listed in **Table 5-1**.

Nutritional Composition of Breastmilk

At birth, the infant gut is sterile and contains suboptimal enzyme systems to manage large or complex proteins; it becomes colonized with maternal bacteria through contact and breastfeeding. Seventy percent of a newborn's developing immune system is found within the neonatal gastrointestinal system (Vighi, Marcucci, Sensi, Cara, & Frati, 2008). Colonizing the

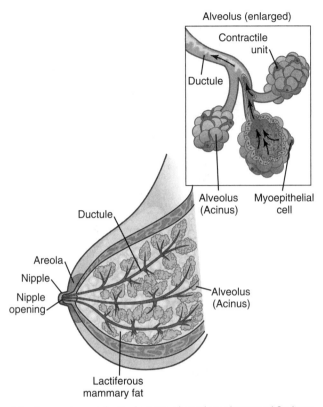

Figure 5-1: Structure of the human breast during lactation based on ultrasound findings.

newborn gut, especially with beneficial bacteria, is paramount to development and maturation of the immune system. Breastmilk contains a variety of components—including prebiotics, probiotics, long-chain polyunsaturated fatty acids, and immunoglobulins—that enhance colonization of the gut (Venter & Dean, 2008). In addition, breastmilk assists in proliferation and colonization with *Bifidobacterium* and *Lactobacillus* organisms through fermentation of nondigestible oligosaccharides to promote gut health (Gardner & Lawrence, 2016). Secretory immunoglobulin A (IgA) is passed from mother to infant through breastmilk and captures larger molecules and pathogens to prevent absorption and protect the infant from infection. Nucleotides in breastmilk have anti-inflammatory properties and protect the newborn against bacteria, viruses, and fungi.

Lactogenesis occurs in several stages, including production of colostrum, followed by transitional milk and mature milk. Colostrum—the first milk produced—has been noted to be present in women as early as 3 months' gestation (King et al., 2015). Its composition is mostly protein with concentrated immunoprotective properties (Venter & Dean, 2008). Colostrum is

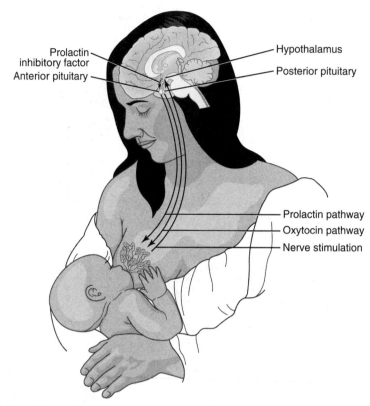

Figure 5-2: Ejection reflex arc, also known as the let-down reflex.

low in fat, carbohydrates, and glucose, and its intake by the newborn stimulates the development of ketones in the newborn, which in turn promotes stabilization of blood glucose (Wight et al., 2014).

The volume of colostrum varies by individual mother, but the average amount present on the initial day of birth is 50 mL (Lawrence & Lawrence, 2011); it is yellow-gold in color. The newborn's stomach capacity at the first feeding is in the range of 1–2 mL/kg, so the volume of colostrum at the first feedings is ideal. With an energy content of 67 kcal/dL (Lawrence & Lawrence, 2011), colostrum enables the newborn to normalize its blood sugar during the transition from the placenta and intrauterine environment to the extrauterine environment. As a concentrated solution, colostrum encourages the newborn to focus on learning the skill of sucking and expression with a small amount of liquid, rather than being overwhelmed with large boluses. With each nursing session, milk volume increases, physiologically stretching the neonatal stomach. At birth, term neonates have 10% more fluid volume that they diurese, making them thirsty and eager to feed.

Table 5-1: Factors That Enhance or Disrupt Successful Breastfeeding

Enhance Breastfeeding	Disrupt Breastfeeding
Early initiation (within the first hour of life) of breastfeeding	Mother and newborn are separated (i.e., maternal or neonatal illness, cesarean section delivery) and breastfeeding within the first hour of life is disrupted
Mother knows newborn hunger cues in Box 5-1.	Mother does not know newborn hunger cues and waits for newborn to cry for feeding—crying is a late sign of newborn/neonatal hunger
Frequent breastfeeding: 10–12 times/day in the first 24 hours; 8–10 times/day in the first month of life	Infrequent breastfeeding
Exclusive breastfeeding	Supplementation with an artificial nipple (ABM, 2009)
Complete expression of breastmilk with each nursing session	Inadequate emptying of breast with nursing sessions
Offering both breasts with each feeding	Mother is impatient and prohibits baby from completing the feeding on the first breast before moving to the second breast
Maternal rest and relaxation	Maternal fatigue, stress, and/or anxiety
	Visitors who are disruptive to rest/sleep and need to be "entertained"
	Sick or preterm newborn
Skin-to-skin (kangaroo) care provides warmth, improves milk supply, facilitates bonding and frequent breastfeeding	Hospital "routines": keeping newborns in central nursery; not individualizing care; continuous disruptions for care rather than efficient care that minimizes disturbance of the mother or newborn
Rooming-in of mothers and newborns	
Adequate maternal diet and fluid intake: advise to "eat to hunger and drink to thirst"	Lack of adequate caloric and fluid intake
Milk production and let-down results in significant maternal thirst; keep fluids close at hand and drink an increased amount (8–12 glasses/day)	
Vegan diets require a continuation of vitamin B_{12} supplementation while breastfeeding	

(Continued)

Table 5-1: Factors That Enhance or Disrupt Successful Breastfeeding (*Continued*)

Enhance Breastfeeding	Disrupt Breastfeeding

Maternal drugs that enhance milk supply include galactogogues:
• Herbal: available at natural food stores
  – Fenugreek: 2–3 capsules or teas a day until milk production is adequate
  – More Milk Plus (fenugreek, blessed thistle, nettle, and fennel): 1 capsule 4 times/day until milk production is adequate
• Prescription:
  – Metoclopramide: 10 mg orally 3 times/day for 10 days
    ○ Tiered dosing: 1 tablet on day 1; increase from 1 tablet/day to 3 tablets/day for days 3–10; then reduce to 2 tablets on day 11 and 1 tablet on day 12
    ○ Medication is a central dopamine antagonist and can make the mother sleepy and fatigued
  – Domperidone: not available in the United States because of cardiac arrhythmias as a side effect
	Maternal drugs that reduce milk supply include bromocriptine, antihistamines, and oral contraceptives (especially estrogen–progesterone combinations)

Discharge teaching that emphasizes the need for visitors to be coordinated so that the mother receives adequate rest and privacy for frequent breastfeeding	Constant disruptions with frequent visitors so that the mother, father, and newborn are stressed and exhausted and breastfeeding is not often enough.

Transitional milk appears at 5 to 10 days to the first 2 weeks of life (Lawrence & Lawrence, 2011) after vaginal birth, though its emergence may be delayed following cesarean birth. This process of "the milk coming in" is heralded by breast fullness and some degree of engorgement. Engorgement occurs as a result of both milk production and the shift of fluids from the uterine/abdominal area to the breast; it is increased in women who receive intrapartal intravenous (IV) fluids. Transitional milk, which is higher in volume and protein than colostrum, is white with a blue tint. It is also lower in fat than colostrum, with a higher concentration of lactose, the primary carbohydrate in breastmilk.

A mature milk supply should be established by 10 to 14 days after birth. Mature milk is bright white in color and emerges in two phases during each breastfeeding session: foremilk and hindmilk. The first milk expressed by the breast when breastfeeding begins (foremilk) is lower in fat than the milk expressed after let-down (hindmilk).

Establishing an adequate milk supply is critical for successful breastfeeding. Lactogenesis occurs naturally once the baby is born, as long as the mother is healthy. Maintenance of milk (i.e., galactopoesis) relies on the symbiotic relationship between mother and baby, through a positive feedback system between nutritive suckling on the maternal nipple and the pituitary gland (Figure 5-2). Babies should nurse as needed and not be time limited. Limitation of time on either breast impedes the baby's opportunity to imprint in the early breastfeeding period and causes the infant to lose out on the benefits of the high-fat hindmilk (Riordan & Wambach, 2010).

Most normal newborns are active feeders during the early hours after birth. Following the initial feeding, they typically experience a quiet sleep period (for as long as 8 to 12 hours) before exhibiting active feeding cues. Even so, mothers should offer the breast every 2 to 3 hours during the days before their "milk comes in" because newborns will arouse and suckle if offered. Typically sleepy in the first 24 to 36 hours after birth, the normal term baby will generally begin demand feeding after that time. Some newborns will cluster feed every 1.5 to 2 hours and then take a longer sleep time (4 to 5 hours). When satiated, newborns will stop actively suckling and unlatch from the breast.

Supplemental feedings are not necessary in term, healthy newborns. In fact, supplemental feedings are associated with both maternal engorgement and milk supply problems. Formula supplements alter the development of intestinal flora, enhance the development of allergies, impact bonding, and interfere with infant weight gain (ABM, 2009; Blomquist, Jonsbo, Serenius, & Persson, 1994; Bystrova, Widstrom, Mathhiesen, Ransjo-Arvidson, & Uvnas-Moberg, Perrine, Scanlon, Li, Odem, & Grummer-Strawn, 2012). Use of water or glucose-in-water as a supplement should be avoided because their potential enhancement of hyperbilirubinemia (AAP, Subcommittee on Hyperbilirubinemia, 2004). In the first few days after birth, new mothers may worry that their baby is not "getting enough" because of the normal cluster feeding pattern. Care providers often interpret the mother's concern as a desire to supplement with formula, when instead they should support and educate a new mother and empower her with strategies such as skin-to-skin contact, which often soothe a "fussy" baby. "No supplements" should be a standing order. Supplements should be prescribed *only* when medically necessary, after a thorough neonatal assessment and evaluation of feeding adequacy and competency (ABM, 2009).

The evidence about pacifier use is contradictory. Using pacifiers for pain control, for alerting infants prior to feeding, and for preterm infants in the neonatal intensive care unit (NICU) is supported by evidence (Gardner, Goldson, & Hernandez, 2016; Gardner & Hernandez, 2016). In contrast, in healthy term breastfeeding newborns, pacifier use appears to counterproductive to establishing successful, exclusive breastfeeding (Howard et al., 2003). However, a recent Cochrane review concluded that pacifier use did not significantly affect prevalence or duration of exclusive or partial breastfeeding (Jaafar, Jahanfar, Angolkar, & Ho, 2012).

Contradictions to Breastfeeding

There are few contraindications to breastfeeding. Most maternal drugs and therapeutics transfer into human milk, but drug levels in breastmilk rarely exceed 1% to 2% of the drug ingested by the mother (Lawrence & Lawrence, 2001). The most comprehensive information about drugs and breastfeeding is available at LactMed (http://www.toxnet.nlm.nih.gov) and from the Infant Risk Center (http://infantrisk.com/). Maternal substance abuse (i.e., cocaine, which concentrates in human milk and has resulted in neonatal intoxication and death; Chaney, Franke, & Wadlington, 1988; Chasnoff, Lewis, & Squires, 1987) and use of some maternal medications (e.g., cytotoxic and immunosuppressive drugs) may contraindicate breastfeeding.

Maternal infectious diseases—including active tuberculosis (TB), herpes simplex (HS), varicella, and human immunodeficiency virus (HIV) infection—may alter or contraindicate breastfeeding in some mother–baby dyads. Active TB requires separation of mother and newborn until the mother is treated and has negative sputum. Pumped milk from mothers with active TB can be fed to their infant because the tubercle bacillus is not passed through breastmilk but rather through respiratory contact (Lawrence & Lawrence, 2001). HS lesions on the breast contraindicate breastfeeding until the lesions have healed. In the interim, breastmilk should be pumped and dumped because of the possibility that it might become contaminated during the pumping process. Active varicella infection (AAP, Section on Breastfeeding, 2012) requires separation of mother and infant, but the baby can be fed pumped breastmilk until the mother's active skin lesions are healed. In developed countries, breastfeeding by HIV-infected mothers is contraindicated because safe alternatives are available (AAP, Committee on Pediatric AIDS, 2013; Lawrence & Lawrence, 2001, 2011). In the developing world, WHO (2010) recommends one of three options for mothers who want to breastfeed who are HIV positive: (1) that mothers receive antiviral therapy while breastfeeding, (2) not breastfeed, or (3) if breastfeeding without antiretroviral therapy to breastfeed exclusively for 12 months.

Neonatal galactosemia, the inborn error of metabolism that prohibits the breakdown of galactose, contraindicates breastfeeding.

Common Problems with Breastfeeding

Breastfeeding difficulties may be a maternal problem, a neonatal problem, or a combination of maternal and neonatal problems. Providers caring for mothers and their newborns must be able to assess, diagnose, and treat common maternal and neonatal problems for breastfeeding to succeed. If they do not have these capabilities, care providers must be able to refer mothers and their newborns with problems for safe and effective lactation counseling.

Maternal Problems

Sore Nipples A common complaint of breastfeeding mothers is sore/painful nipples. During the first 6 weeks after birth, sore nipples affect as many as 96% of nursing mothers. Early assessment and education of the nursing mother can prevent or correct many of the problems that might create or worsen sore nipples. Demonstrating the newborn infant's ability to open the mouth widely (by stimulating the root reflex with nipple stimulation of the center of the mouth) facilitates a healthy latch-on. Bringing the baby to the breast enhances a higher latch above the nipple, thereby avoiding the case in which the baby makes a shallow latch and then "chews" his or her way up the areola.

Positioning on the maternal breast is critical. Teaching the mother to change the newborn's position on the breast will prevent persistent pressure in one area of the nipple and areola and facilitates emptying of all quadrants of the breast. The various positions for breastfeeding include cradled tummy-to-tummy (**Figure 5-3**); the football/modified cradle, which enables the mother to control the baby's head in bringing the baby to the breast (**Figure 5-4**); and side-lying, which enables a mother who has undergone a cesarean section to breastfeed comfortably. Breastfeeding twins is also possible with the football and cradled holds (**Figure 5-5**).

Other strategies to prevent sore nipples include avoiding pacifiers and artificial nipples; these devices encourage a "biting" pattern that differs from the nutritive sucking of breastfeeding. Teaching the mother the correct technique for breaking the seal/suction before removing her infant from her breast can also prevent breast trauma.

Once nipples have become sore and tender, several interventions are available to enhance maternal comfort and salvage breastfeeding efforts. Breast shells prevent tender, sore nipples from touching clothes and causing further irritation (**Figure 5-6**). Nipple shields are not indicated for sore nipples and significantly reduce milk transfer (McKechnie & Eglash, 2010). Available evidence does not support the widespread use of nipple shields as is often seen in the United States. McKechnie and Eglash (2010) conclude that nipple shields have unknown risks and that mothers should be followed closely, with use of these devices remaining limited, until better evidence of long-term outcomes is available.

Use of nipple creams has produced mixed results: some women obtain relief with these creams, whereas others do not. If a mother is using or wants to use a cream, lanolin is effective and easy to obtain. The appropriate application of cream is to put a small amount on the nipple only, not the entire areola. Placing cream on the areola may contribute to poor latch-on because the baby is likely to slide off the areola, is unable to retain a high latch, and as a result sucks only on the nipple. Prior to recommending the use of lanolin, assess the mother for allergy to wool. Women with a wool allergy (i.e., "wool makes me itch") can have an allergic reaction to lanolin.

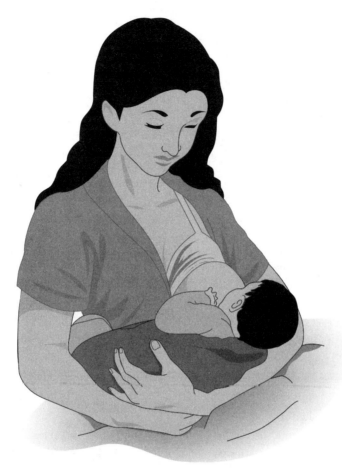

Figure 5-3: Cradled in the tummy-to-tummy position.

Structural Abnormalities

Flat/Inverted Nipples Flat nipples can occur even if the nipple prior to birth appears to be everted (**Figure 5-7**). With engorgement, nipples may flatten. An important assessment of maternal nipples by the provider should occur when the "milk comes in." Interventions to assist the mother with flat/inverted nipples are listed in **Box 5-2**.

Engorgement Engorgement—that is, excessive fullness of the breast—presents early in the postpartum period, generally by days 2 to 5. Breast engorgement is experienced as fullness, tenderness, and pain that stretches and firms the areola as well as flattens the nipple, making latch-on difficult. Mothers may also experience hot flashes and a low-grade fever. Initial engorgement occurs during the first week but may occur at any time if there is a delay in nursing or pumping. During lactogenesis, frequent breast emptying is necessary; otherwise,

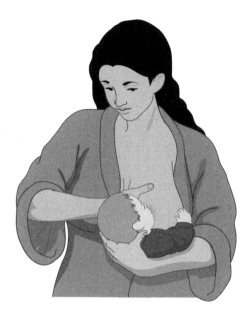

Figure 5-4: Football hold.

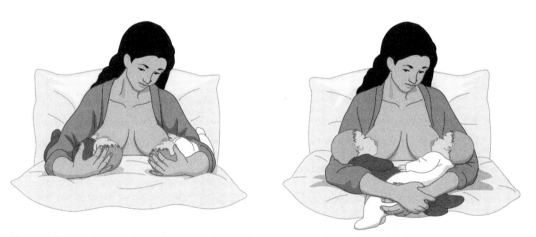

Figure 5-5: Breastfeeding twins: football hold position (left) and cradle position (right).

a prolactin-inhibiting factor is released, resulting in a decrease in milk production. Elevated pressure in the alveoli of the breast also inhibits continued milk production, and plugged ducts and/or mastitis may occur. Recommendations for managing engorgement are listed in **Box 5-3**.

Insufficient Milk Supply Inability to make sufficient milk is very rare, with causes generally being limited to those listed in **Box 5-4**. A complete breast exam during prenatal care should

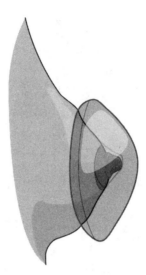

Figure 5-6: Breast shell.

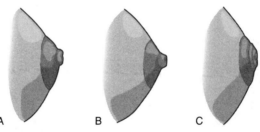

A   B   C

Figure 5-7: Inverted nipples. A. A normal and an inverted nipple are similar in appearance when the nipple is not stimulated. B. A normal nipple protrudes when stimulated. C. An inverted nipple retracts when stimulated.

Box 5-2: Interventions for Flat/Inverted Nipples

- Instruct the mother to use cold compresses or roll the nipple to elicit an eversion of the nipple.
- Use an electric breast pump to draw out the nipple before offering the breast to the infant.
- Wear a breast "shell" between feedings.
- Work to get the infant's mouth open as wide as possible; teach chin stimulation.

identify breast asymmetry that may indicate insufficient tissue. Assessment of insufficient breast tissue includes a specific history about breast changes during pregnancy and the first few days after birth. Points to investigate include whether the breasts became enlarged or tender during pregnancy, and whether the breasts became full or engorged during the postpartum period.

Box 5-3: Interventions for Engorgement

- Frequent feedings at least every 2 to 3 hours
- No limitation of nursing time
- Apply warm, moist compresses before nursing
- Use reverse pressure softening to soften the areola so that the baby can latch on easier (La Leche League International, 2005)
- Use electric breast pump to remove enough milk so that the nipple/areola are softened for newborn latch
- Use a mild analgesic such as ibuprofen or naproxen
- Wear a supportive bra 24 hours a day
- Cold compresses—may provide relief and can be used after nursing

Box 5-4: Etiology of Insufficient Milk Supply

- Congenital insufficiency of glandular breast tissue (rare; more common with history of infertility)
- Breast surgery (augmentation/reduction): Severance of the mammary nerve with reduction interrupts the neural communication between the nipple and the pituitary resulting in the potential for reduced milk supply
- Uncorrected hypothyroidism
- History of polycystic ovary syndrome (Hurst, 2007)
- Retained placental fragments
- Significant postpartum hemorrhage
- Anemia

Box 5-5: Neonatal Signs of Insufficient Maternal Milk Supply

- Restlessness or irritability during or between feedings
- Infant acts "hungry all the time" (fussy, rooting, restless)
- Lack of audible swallowing during nursing
- Weight loss is more than expected
- Urine output or bowel movements are inadequate

Neonatal signs of an insufficient milk supply are listed in **Box 5-5**. Babies who are not growing appropriately require intensive assessment, time, and frequent follow-up because infancy is a critical period of brain growth. The primary provider should either invest the time to help lactation succeed or refer the mother with an insufficient milk supply to a lactation consultant who can work with her more intensively.

Box 5-6: Neonatal Signs of Adequate Milk Supply/Intake

- Awakens to feed every 1.5 to 2 hours; feeds and goes to sleep
- After let-down occurs, audible swallowing is heard
- Infant sleeps restfully between feedings
- Starts gaining weight at the end of the first week of life (or sooner)
- Gains ½ to 1 ounce/day
- Regains birth weight by 2 weeks of age; doubles birth weight by 6 months; triples birth weight by 1 year of age
- Full, tense breasts and milk glands are soft and empty after breastfeeding
- After let-down, newborns/neonates/infants ingest 70% to 80% of their feeding in the first 6 minutes of nursing (Nyqvist, Farnstrand, Eeg-Olofsson, & Ewald, 2001)
- There is no correlation between the 15 to 20 minutes mothers need to pump to empty their breasts and the efficiency of the breastfeeding infant
- Urine output and bowel movements are adequate

Mothers need to know how to assess if their newborns/infants are getting enough milk. Neonatal signs of adequate milk intake are listed in **Box 5-6**. Early assessment and intervention is needed to preserve the opportunity for breastfeeding. Galactogogues, which can be recommended to boost milk supply, are listed in Table 5-1.

Candidiasis   Candidiasis—that is, infection of the nipple (and the infant's mouth) with *Candida albicans*—usually becomes evident 1 to 2 weeks after breastfeeding has been initiated, but can occur at any time during breastfeeding. Candidiasis affects the nipple and ductal system in both breasts, may be present before the mother is symptomatic, and occurs in as many as 20% of lactating women. Although the lactoferrin found in breastmilk inhibits growth of *C. albicans*, total inhibition of *Candida* is not assured. Recent antibiotic treatment is a risk factor for breast candidiasis. Laboring women who receive prophylactic treatment for group B *Streptococcus* (GBS) have a higher incidence of candidiasis with breastfeeding; they should be advised to take probiotics for 3 weeks after a course of antibiotics to rebalance their normal flora. Maternal and neonatal symptoms of candidiasis are listed in **Box 5-7**.

Interventions begin with a thorough, detailed history and examination of the breasts, as well as examination of the oral cavity of the infant and rectal/perineal area for diaper rash. The treatment must target both mother and baby, which may require a collaborative effort between providers. Failure to treat both members of the mother–baby dyad is likely to result in continual reinfection. Traditional and complementary treatments are listed in **Table 5-2**. If candidiasis persists after adequate treatment, a milk culture should be sent to determine if another pathogen is present and treatment changed as indicated (Betzold, Laughlin, & Shi, 2007).

Box 5-7: Symptoms of Candidiasis

Maternal

- Nipples/areolas may be itchy, burning, cracked, red/pink, or shiny/flaky. In severe cases, weeping blisters may be present.
- Acute pain occurs during and after nursing, which is generally described as "shooting" inside the breast or breasts that feel "like they are on fire/burning."
- The mother may have a vaginal infection.
- The mother experiences fatigue.

Neonatal

- Oral thrush: White plaques on mucous membranes of the mouth that do not wipe off and bleed when attempting to remove; mouth pain and refusal to feed.
- Monilial diaper rash: Intense inflammation that is bright red, sharply demarcated in the inguinal folds, thighs, buttocks, abdomen, and genitalia. Satellite lesions may extend the rash over the infant's trunk.

Mastitis Mastitis is a bacterial infection in breast tissue but not in breastmilk. Although the highest incidence of mastitis occurs during the first 6 to 7 weeks after birth, such infection can also occur earlier, during the first month after birth. Approximately 10% to 33% of breastfeeding women develop mastitis. The pathophysiology of this condition includes milk stasis due to plugged ducts or irregular/incomplete emptying of the breast, nipple trauma, overabundant milk supply, maternal fatigue and stress, and a prior history of mastitis. Women typically experience a sudden unilateral onset of a localized, red, hot, swollen area of the breast that is tender to touch. They often report flu-like symptoms, including chills, fever with a temperature of greater than 101°F (38.5°C), headache, and body aches.

Treatment includes antibiotic therapy and supportive care. Because the most common infecting organism is *Staphylococcus aureus,* penicillin is the most effective prescription. The first line of treatment is dicloxicillin 500 mg 2 times daily for 10 to 14 days. If the mother has a penicillin allergy, alternative therapies include clindamycin 300 mg or erythromycin 250 to 500 mg 2 times daily for 10 to 14 days. Mothers are advised to begin probiotics and continue using them throughout the antibiotic course and for at least 3 weeks following treatment. Supportive care such as rest, analgesics (ibuprofen) for pain and edema, and frequent breastfeeding is critical. If breastfeeding on the affected breast is painful, the mother can pump this breast to prevent engorgement. Infants may refuse to nurse on the affected breast because of the increased sodium level in the milk. If nipple trauma is present, referral to a lactation consultant is an important aspect of treatment to prevent recurrence.

Table 5-2: Traditional and Complementary Therapies for Candidiasis

Therapy	Dose	Comments
Traditional		
Mycostatin Oral Suspension for baby		Topical oral therapy Treat for 10–14 days
Maternal breasts	1 drop Mycostatin Oral Suspension on nipples after breastfeeding	
Keep maternal nipples as dry as possible/open to air		
Boil pacifiers and breast pump parts daily, if being used		
Avoid application of breastmilk to nipples after feeding		
Expressed milk should not be stored for later use because freezing does not kill *Candida* and reinfection is likely		
All-Purpose Nipple Ointment: • Mupirocin 2% ointment, 15 g • Betamethasone 0.1% ointment, 15 g • Miconazole powder to final concentration of 2% miconazole	Total volume is 30 g Sparingly apply to nipples after each feeding	Compounding pharmacy Limit use to 5–7 days
Fluconazole (Diflucan)	Loading dose: 200–400 mg PO Maintenance dose: 100–200 mg PO daily for 14–21 days	Used for severe cases as off-label use and not approved by FDA for this indication Recommendation that use until asymptomatic for 7 days, then discontinue Minimal side effects Minimal excretion into breastmilk (1% of maternal dose; safe for breastfeeding baby) (Wiener, 2006)
Complementary		
Grapefruit seed extract	500 mg PO 3 times/day	

Newborn/Neonatal Conditions

Feeding Refusal Table 5-3 identifies the most common reasons why newborns and neonates refuse to nurse, and recommendations to correct these problems. Assessment of breastfeeding refusal begins with an observation by the provider of a breastfeeding session to identify the reason(s) for the refusal. Poor feeding and feeding refusal may be signs of hypoglycemia or neonatal infection/sepsis. The care provider must *always* assess and screen late-preterm and term infants for these causes of feeding refusal, especially if none of the etiologies in Table 5-3 is found to be present. Hypoglycemia is discussed in more depth later in this section.

Late-Preterm Infant Late-preterm infants (LPIs)—those born between 34 0/7 and 36 6/7 weeks' gestation—represent 75% of all preterm births (Davidoff et al., 2006). These infants have increased morbidities when compared to term infants, including those related to feeding.

Table 5-3: Etiology and Interventions for Feeding Refusal

Etiology	Interventions
Incorrect positioning of baby at the breast	Position correctly using proper body alignment.
Flat/inverted nipples	Demonstrate milk expression to soften nipple/areola and enhance nipple erection. Use electric breast pump.
Breast engorgement	Initiate early and frequent breastfeeding (offer breast every 2–3 hours). Placing warm packs on the breast prior to feeding to encourage milk flow and softening of nipples is controversial, but is an option.
Infant's nose may be blocked	Review positioning to adjust baby's alignment at the breast. Thick secretions may be diluted with saline drops and removed with bulb syringe suctioning.
"Nipple confusion" if baby has received artificial feeding with bottles	Review positioning. Eliminate any artificial feeding. Educate family that bottle-feeding is unnecessary. Refer to a lactation specialist as needed.
Tight frenulum (see the discussion of ankyloglossia)	Assess the mother's nipples for any trauma. Refer to a provider who will assess and "clip" the frenulum, if needed.

In fact, one study cited feeding difficulties among 76% of LPIs compared to 28.6% of full-term newborns (Wang et al., 2004). Both the AAP (Engle, Tomashek, Wallman, & Committee on Fetus and Newborn of AAP, 2007) and AWHONN (2005, 2014) identify feeding, feeding concerns, and assessment for adequacy of intake and weight gain as important issues in the discharge and follow-up of the LPI.

Although the LPI has intact digestive and absorptive functions, intestinal motility and colonization may be delayed (Brown, Hendrickson, Evans, Davis, & Hay, 2016). Developmental immaturity of the LPI's oromotor tone, function, and neural integration may contribute to poor feeding, falling asleep during feeding, and failure to awaken when hungry (Brown et al., 2016; Meier, Furman, & Degenhardt, 2007; Radtke, 2011). Because of these issues, many LPIs are poor feeders regardless of the method of feeding—breast or bottle. They have uncoordinated suck–swallow–breathe patterns, awaken less frequently, exhibit fewer cues of feeding readiness, are easily fatigued, and fall asleep before completing a feeding (Gardner, 2007; Gardner & Lawrence, 2016; Meier et al., 2007). These behaviors result in poor breast stimulation and incomplete breast emptying, which in turn lead to inadequate milk production. Just being an LPI is an independent risk factor for breastfeeding difficulties, readmission for hyperbilirubinemia or jaundice, and lack of exclusive breastfeeding at 4 months of age (Lucas, Gupton, Holditch-Davis, & Brandon, 2014; Meier et al., 2007; Nagulesapillai, McDonald, Fenton, Mercader, & Tough, 2013).

LPIs are in a critical period of brain growth. At 34 weeks' gestation, the LPI's brain weighs 65% of a full-term infant's brain (Guihard-Costa & Larrosche, 1990). At 36 weeks' gestation, the LPI's brain weighs 80% of the full-term infant's brain (Meier et al., 2007). Between 34 weeks' and 40 weeks' gestation, the LPI's brain increases its cortical volume by 50% (Guihard-Costa & Larrosche, 1990; Huppi et al., 1998). Recent systematic reviews of follow-up data on LPIs have found more school/behavior problems, less advanced cognitive functioning, higher prevalence of psychiatric problems, and subtle intellectual and neuropsychological deficits compared to children born at full term (Baron, Litman, Ahronovich, & Baker, 2012; DeJong, Vorhoeven, & Van Baar, 2012).

A feeding plan that parents are involved in creating and are committed to complying with needs to be established prior to discharge from either a hospital or birth center (ABM, 2011; AWHONN, 2010; Engle et al., 2007; Meier et al., 2007). In addition, LPIs need a follow-up visit for assessment of feeding and other issues at 24 to 48 hours after discharge (AWHONN, 2005, 2014; Engle et al., 2007).

Strategies to facilitate breastfeeding in LPIs are listed in **Box 5-8**. Extra time and lactation consultation are necessary to assist breastfeeding mothers until their infants mature and are able to nurse effectively. As the LPI matures, feeding ability is likely to improve. The challenge for care providers and the breastfeeding mother is to persevere while supporting nutrition and hydration until 40 weeks' gestation when the majority of LPIs have matured enough to breastfeed without difficulty.

Box 5-8: Strategies to Facilitate Breastfeeding in Late-Preterm Infants

- Proper positioning
- Use breast pump
- Use Lact-Aid Nursing supplementer
- Use nipple shield
- Awakening every 2 to 3 hours to feed (for 8 to 12 breastfeedings/day)
- Use of skin-to-skin care
- Weighing the baby before and after breastfeeding
- Alternative methods of enteral nutrition

Data from Academy of Breastfeeding Medicine. (2011). ABM clinical protocol #10: Breastfeeding the late preterm infant (33 0/7 to 36 6/7 weeks gestation). *Breastfeeding Medicine, 6*(3), 151–157; Gardner, S. L. (2007). Late-preterm ("near-term") newborns: A neonatal nursing challenge. *Nurse Currents, 1,* 1; Lucas, R., Gupton, S., Holditch-Davis, D., & Brandon, D. (2014). A case study of a late preterm infant's transition to full at breast feedings at 4 months of age. *Journal of Human Lactation, 30,* 28–30; Meier, P. P., Furman, L. M., & Degenhardt, M. (2007). Increased lactation risk for late preterm infants and mothers: Evidence and management strategies to protect breastfeeding. *Journal of Midwifery and Women's Health, 52,* 579–587.

Research into poor growth and neurodevelopmental outcomes in extremely low-birth-weight (ELBW) premature infants shows that early, aggressive nutrition improves outcomes for these babies (Ehrenkranz et al., 2006; Lucas, Morley,& Cole, 1998; Stephens et al., 2009). Using a postdischarge preterm infant formula has been shown to also improve neurodevelopmental outcomes in larger preterm infants when compared to feeding these infants a term formula after discharge (Lucas, Morley, & Cole, 1998; Lucas et al., 1990). More aggressive nutritional support for LPIs may improve their outcomes as well.

Fortification of human milk (both mother's own and donor milk) and use of preterm rather than term formula is a reasonable plan for feeding the LPI. Preterm discharge formulas contain more nutrients than term formula, but less than preterm infant formulas (**Table 5-4**). Preterm discharge formulas for the LPI are especially important if growth is compromised and/or until the LPI is taking full enteral feedings appropriate for a term infant (Brown et al., 2016; Phillips et al., 2013). LPIs must be wakened at night to feed because they are unable to add more volume to their daytime feedings to accommodate the loss of nighttime intake (AWHONN, 2014; Wessel, 2011). Adequate hydration and caloric intake is measured by the parameters in **Table 5-5**.

Structural Abnormality

Ankyloglossia (Tongue-Tie) Ankyloglossia is a congenital condition of newborns in which the inferior lingual frenulum is attached to the tip of the tongue (**Figure 5-8**). While the incidence of ankyloglossia is only 2.8% to 10.7% of all infants, it is implicated in 25% of infants with breastfeeding

Table 5-4: Comparative Nutritional Composition of Postdischarge Preterm Formulas (Feedings per 100 kcal)

	Postdischarge Formulas	
	Enfamil Enfacre [†]	**Similac Expert Care Neosure‡**
Nutrient density, (kcal/oz)	22	22
Energy (kcal)	100	100
Protein		
Amount (g)	2.8	2.8
% Total calories	11	11
Source	Nonfat milk, whey protein concentrate	Nonfat milk, whey protein concentrate
Fat		
Amount (g)	5.3	5.5
% Total calories	47	49
Source	High oleic, soy, MCT, and coconut oils; Single cell oil products (DHA and ARA)	Soy, coconut, and MCT oil; Single cell oil products (DHA and ARA)
Oil ratio (approximate)	34:29:20:14:2.2:0.8	44.7:29:24.9:0.25:0.4
Linoleic acid (mg)	950	750
Carbohydrate		
Amount (g)	10.4	10.1
% Total calories	42	40
Source	Corn syrup solids, lactose	Corn syrup solids, lactose
Minerals		
Calcium (mg)	120	105
Phosphorous (mg)	66	62
Ca:P ratio	1.8:1	1.7:1
Sodium mg (mEq)	35 (1.5)	33 (1.4)
Potassium mg (mEq)	105 (2.7)	142 (3.6)
Chloride mg (mEq)	78 (2.2)	75 (2.1)
Iron (mg)	1.8	1.8
Zinc (mg)	1.25	1.2
Magnesium (mg)	8	9
Vitamins		
Vitamin A		
(mcg RE)	135	105
(international units)	(450)	(350)
Vitamin D (international units)	80	70
Vitamin E (international units)	4	3.6
Vitamin K (mcg)	8	11
Vitamin Cascorbic acid (mg)	16	15
Vitamin B_1—thiamine (mcg)	200	175
Vitamin B_2—riboflavin (mcg)	200	150
Vitamin B_6 (mcg)	100	100
Folic Acid (mcg)	26	25
Other Characteristics		
Potential renal solute (mOsm)	24.5	25.2
Osmolality (mOsm/kg water)	250	250

Modified from Brown, L. D., Hendrickson, K., Evans, R., Davis, J., Anderson M. S., & Hay, W. W. (2015). Enteral nutrition. In S. L. Gardner, B. S. Carter, M. Enzman Hines, & J. A. Hernandez (Eds.), *Merenstein and Gardner's handbook of neonatal intensive care* (8th ed., pp. 377–418). St. Louis, MO: Mosby-Elsevier.

Table 5-5: Parameters to Assess to Evaluate Adequate Hydration and Caloric Intake in Term Infants or Preterm Infants Corrected* to Term

Parameter	Significance
Caloric intake: intake/day	100–110 kcal/kg/day
Hydration state: output/day	By 3 days of age: 3 voids and 3 stools/day
	By 4 days of age: 4 voids and 4 stools/day
	By 6 days of age and thereafter: 6 voids and 3 stools/day
	(Phillips et al., 2013)
Weight gain/day	25–35 g/day (½–1 oz/day)
Length gain/week	2.5–3.5 cm/week
Head circumference increase/week	0.5 cm/week (Foman, Haschke, Ziegler, & Nelson, 1982)

* Calculating corrected gestational age: (Weeks premature + weeks old) – 40 weeks = Corrected gestational age (CGA) in weeks

Example: An infant is born at 36 weeks' gestational age and is now 5 weeks old.

(36 weeks + 5 weeks) – 40 weeks = 1-week-old CGA—on a growth chart this baby would be plotted at 1 week to correct for prematurity. The CGA is used to measure attainment of developmental milestones, growth, and feeding, rather than the preterm infant's chronological age, for at least the first year of life.

problems (Edmunds, 2012). This condition interferes with forward movement of the newborn's tongue, which is needed to support and cup the nipple/areola so that the breast will express milk effectively. Mothers of newborns and neonates with ankyloglossia complain of significant nipple soreness and may have an insufficient milk supply. Infants have poor weight gain.

Palate Abnormality A high, arched (but intact) palate is an anatomic variation. Usually infants with a high arched palate have the ability to breastfeed effectively. Mothers of such infants may develop very sore nipples, however. Once this structural abnormality is identified, appropriate referral to a therapist who is knowledgeable in assisting with breastfeeding is helpful for both mother and baby. The ABM has a clinical protocol for facilitating breastfeeding in infants with cleft lip, cleft palate, and cleft lip and palate (Reilly, Reid, Skeat, & ABM, 2013).

Hypoglycemia Transient hypoglycemia—that is, low blood glucose concentration—occurs in healthy term newborns in the first few hours after birth. Transient hypoglycemia is very common, "occurring in almost all mammalian newborns," and is self-limiting (Wight et al., 2014). No studies have shown that treating transiently low blood glucose levels results in better short- or long-term outcomes compared with no treatment (Bolyut, vanKempen, & Offringa, 2006; Koivisto, Blanco-Sequeiros, & Krause, 1972). In addition, evidence indicates that in the term, healthy, appropriately grown newborn without clinical signs, treatment is detrimental

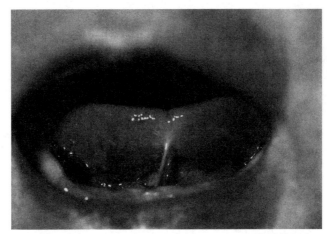

Figure 5-8 : Ankyloglossia (tongue-tie).   © SPL / Science Source

and significantly impacts the successful initiation and maintenance of breastfeeding (Cole & Peevy, 1994; Durand et al., 1997; Heck & Erenberg, 1987; Hoseth, Joergensen, Ebbesen, & Moeller, 2000; Sexson, 1984; Swenne, Ewald, Gustafsson, Sandberg, & Ostenson, 1994).

The initial blood glucose of a term, healthy newborn should be approximately 60% to 70% of the maternal glucose level (King et al., 2015). At birth, most women will be in a fasting state, so that their infant's blood glucose level will be approximately 40 to 60 mg/dL at birth. After birth, all infants follow a pattern of initial decline in glucose level over the first 2 hours, with a gradual rise then occurring in the first 3 to 4 days of life, regardless of feeding method (**Figure 5-9**). Initiation of feeding within the first hour of life and continuation of on-demand feeding facilitates the normal transition from in utero to extrauterine life. Even infants of diabetic mothers (IDM) have less hypoglycemia and stabilize blood glucose faster when breastfeeding is initiated within 30 minutes of birth (Straussman & Levisky, 2010, cited in Csont et al., 2014).

The level of blood glucose that denotes hypoglycemia remains controversial:

> There is no absolute correlation between blood or plasma glucose concentrations, clinical signs or symptoms, and either short-term or long-term sequelae. Instead, "reference" glucose concentrations generally reflect the lower limit of the normal range in a specific population of newborn infants, determined by statistical analysis of data collected in that population. (Rozance, McGowan, Price-Douglas, & Hay, 2016, p. 339)

Consequently,

> [A] number of current references use 40 to 45 mg/dl as the lower limit of "normal" plasma glucose concentrations in the first 72 hours of life. By 72 to 96 hours of age mean plasma glucose concentrations are very similar to those seen in older children and adults. (Rozance et al., 2016, p. 339)

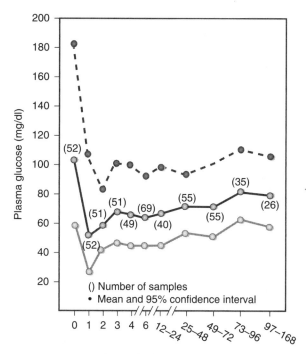

Figure 5-9: Plasma glucose concentrations during the first week of life in healthy appropriate-for-gestational-age term infants.
Reproduced from Srinivasan, G., Pildes, R. S., Cattamanchi, G., Voora, S., & Lilien, L. D. (1986). Plasma glucose values in normal neonates: a new look. *Journal of Pediatrics, 109*(1): 114–117. Copyright 1986, with permission from Elsevier.

Neonates at risk for hypoglycemia (**Table 5-6**) should be monitored and treated when necessary. If screening is determined to be needed based on risk or signs of hypoglycemia, blood glucose detection should begin by 2 hours of life. According to Hawdon, Platt, and Aynsley-Green (2006), obtaining a blood glucose too early after birth can lead to confusion about the normal physiologic fall in levels, leading to a result that is difficult to interpret and/or overtreatment. Routine monitoring of blood glucose in neonates is not recommended, however, and has been found to be unnecessary and potentially harmful. Organizations such as WHO (Williams, 1997), AAP (2012), and the National Childbirth Trust of the United Kingdom (1997) do not recommend routine monitoring of blood glucose because it is harmful to successful initiation of breastfeeding patterns (Wight et al., 2014).

In 2011, the AAP published a clinical report entitled "Postnatal Glucose Homeostasis in Late-Preterm and Term Infants" (Adamkin & Committee on Fetus and the Newborn of the AAP, 2011). This report identified the following aspects of care related to hypoglycemia in neonates: (1) identification of infants at risk, (2) assessment of blood glucose levels that require intervention, (3) treatment criteria for intravenous (IV) and/or oral nutrition, (4) frequency of

Table 5-6: Term Newborns from Low-Risk Pregnancies at Increased Risk for Hypoglycemia

Small for gestational age (SGA): < 10th percentile in United States; < 2% in United Kingdom	Perinatal stress requiring significant resuscitation
Large for gestational age (LGA): > 90th percentile for weight and macrosomic appearance*	Cold stress: unable to maintain temperature
Discordant twin: weight 10% < weight of larger twin	Polycythemia
All infants of diabetic mothers, especially if poorly controlled	Suspected infection
Low birth weight: < 2500 g	Respiratory distress
Prematurity	Maternal drug treatment (e.g., terbutaline, beta blockers, oral hypoglycemic)

* ABM guidelines note that it is unnecessary to screen all LGA babies. Glucose monitoring is recommended for infants from maternal populations who were unscreened for diabetes during the pregnancy where LGA may represent undiagnosed and untreated maternal diabetes.

blood glucose monitoring, and (5) delineation of neonatal symptoms of hypoglycemia. According to the AAP guidelines, glucose screening should be performed only if the infant is at risk and individualized based on the factors involved with the individual infant. The AAP (Adamkin & Committee on Fetus and the Newborn of the AAP, 2011) advises the following glucose thresholds based on infant age:

- Birth to 4 hours of age: ≥ 25 mg/dL
- After 4 hours and up to 24 hours of age: ≥ 45 mg/dL

If glucose falls below these levels, then IV therapy should be initiated while awaiting laboratory confirmation of hypoglycemia in infants with clinical signs. Monitoring should be continued until normalized based on two consecutive satisfactory measurements taken prior to feeding. Laboratory confirmation of bedside testing should be done, as bedside testing may not always be reliable.

Although the blood glucose level that defines hypoglycemia remains controversial, there is consensus that the symptomatic infant needs treatment. Sequelae of hypoglycemia include neurologic symptoms that may result in childhood seizures or childhood metabolic syndrome (Boney, Verma, Tucker, & Vohr, 2005; Burns, Rutherford, Boardman, & Cowan, 2008; Straussman & Levisky, 2010, cited in Csont et al., 2014).

Asymptomatic newborns with documented hypoglycemia are managed by breastfeeding every 1 to 2 hours or fed 1 to 5 mL/kg of expressed milk or substitute, and their glucose level is rechecked until normalized. Term babies should not be given nasogastric (NG) feeds, as they will fight this feeding method, which increases their risk of aspiration. If glucose levels remain low, begin IV glucose therapy and consult with and collaborate with other care providers as indicated.

Breastfeeding should be continued during IV therapy. Extra effort to support breastfeeding may be necessary because mother and baby may be separated by cesarean section birth or by management of the neonate in the NICU. If the baby is transferred to the NICU, the mother must be provided with the support and equipment necessary to stimulate initial lactogenesis and ongoing milk supply. Double-pumping electric breast pumps yield more milk production than their manual counterparts (AAP, Section on Breastfeeding, 2012; WHO et al., 2009). Supporting the mother is critical to initiating production of breastmilk as well as mediating the "inadequacy" that many mothers feel when their baby needs additional support. Encouraging skin-to-skin care in the NICU supports the mother's contribution to her newborn's care, facilitates breastfeeding, and is not contraindicated with IV therapy.

If collaboratively managing the infant with hypoglycemia, carefully document physical examination, screening values, laboratory confirmation, treatment, and changes in clinical condition (i.e., response to treatment). The infant should not be discharged until reasonable levels of blood glucose are maintained through a fast of 3 to 4 hours. Monitoring must be recommenced if adverse changes (i.e., low glucose level, development of hypoglycemia symptoms) occur when the infant goes without feeding for 3 to 4 hours.

Hyperbilirubinemia and Jaundice Effective, frequent breastfeeding does not alter bilirubin levels in the first 5 days of life, but infrequent nursing and delayed initiation of breastfeeding may. **Table 5-7** shows research findings on the relationship between the number of feedings in 24 hours and bilirubin levels.

Breastfeeding prevents hyperbilirubinemia because colostrum's laxative effect stimulates the passage of meconium and prevents the reabsorption of bilirubin from the intestine. The earlier passage of meconium decreases the risk of significant jaundice.

Poor Weight Gain Prior to and after discharge, breastfeeding behavior needs to be assessed by the care provider. Patterns of suckling may have changed from the initial assessment. **Box 5-9** lists conditions in which consultation with a lactation specialist may be helpful.

Table 5-7: Relationship Between Number of Feedings per Day and Bilirubin Levels

Number of Feedings in 24 Hours	Bilirubin Level
6 feeds/day	11
7 feeds/day	9.3 ± 3.5
8 feeds/day	6.5 ± 4.0
12 feeds/day	5.0

Box 5-9: Conditions for Referral to a Lactation Specialist/Consultant

Maternal
- Maternal anxiety
- Previous difficulty with breastfeeding
- Flat/inverted nipples
- History of breast surgery
- Multiple gestation
- Difficulty establishing breastfeeding after first few feedings (e.g., poor latch, sore nipples, sleepy baby)

Neonatal
- Late preterm (34 6/7 to 36 6/7 weeks' gestation)
- "Early term" (37 to 38.6 weeks' gestation)
- Congenital anomaly
- Hyperbilirubinemia/jaundice

Data from Holmes, A., McLeod, A., & Bunik, M. (2013). ABM clinical protocol #5: Peripartum breastfeeding management for the healthy mother and infant at term. *Breastfeeding Medicine, 8,* 469–473.

Babies with planned early discharge or birth at home or in a birth center require early evaluation to prevent delayed diagnosis of feeding problems. Early identification facilitates early intervention, which results in breastfeeding success, adequate neonatal weight gain, and avoidance of supplements (ABM, 2009).

All infants should be seen between 3 and 5 days of age or within 24 to 72 hours of discharge to evaluate the infant and determine how the infant is doing with breastfeeding (AAP, 2015; AAP, Committee on the Fetus and Newborn, 2010; AAP, Section on Breastfeeding, 2012).

Standard of Care/National Guidelines for Care

Throughout this chapter, the national and international guidelines regarding breastfeeding that represent the most current standards of care have been used and referenced. The Academy of Breastfeeding Medicine has developed guidelines (with the caveat that they are not to be considered the standard of care) for management of common medical problems that may impact successful breastfeeding. ABM protocols are available without charge at the organization's website (http://www.bfmed.org). The AAP is also a valuable resource for practice guidelines on breastfeeding (AAP, Section on Breastfeeding, 2012), breastfeeding and HIV (AAP, Committee on Pediatric AIDS, 2013), and hypoglycemia (Adamkin & Committee on Fetus and Newborn of the AAP, 2011).

In the United Kingdom, the National Institute for Health Care and Excellence (NICE) provides national guidance and advice to improve health and social care throughout the

National Health Service. NICE guidelines to maximize the use of evidence in clinical practice are available on this organization's website (http://www.nice.org.uk). NICE's quality statement # 5 about breastfeeding indicates that women should receive breastfeeding support from a service that uses an evaluated, structured program.

Teaching/Counseling About Breastfeeding

Focus on the benefits of breastfeeding begins prenatally, especially in first-time mothers, and continues throughout the intrapartal and postpartal periods. "Breast is best" for both mother and newborn is not just an opinion, but an evidence-based fact. Educating mothers about the dynamic quality of mother's own milk to prevent and protect the newborn/infant against all diseases that the mother has had or been immunized against is important. The significant importance of skin-to-skin care, avoidance of mother–baby separation, and initiation of breastfeeding in the first hour of life needs to be emphasized. Parent education materials about breastfeeding should not be provided by companies that produce and market breastmilk substitutes; such materials are inappropriate sources of breastfeeding information and have been shown to negatively impact the success of breastfeeding (ABM, 2009; Howard et al., 2000; Snell, Krantz, Keeton, Delgado, & Peckham, 1992).

Discharge instructions and follow-up care with breastfeeding mothers should address pumping and storage of breastmilk (Evans, Marinelli, Taylor, & ABM, 2014). Many mothers will pump milk for an occasional feeding or to have available when returning to work. As a benefit of the Patient Protection and Affordable Care Act in the United States, breastfeeding mothers are able to rent a breast pump that is covered by insurance.

Safe pumping, handling, and storage of human milk is important to prevent contamination and the risk of infection. Pumped milk that is not used immediately must be refrigerated or frozen to prevent proliferation of bacteria. Breastmilk storage guidelines for healthy babies are listed in **Table 5-8**. Freezing milk results in changes to the composition of the milk including (1) reduction of antioxidant properties, (2) rupture of the fat globules, (3) alteration of the casein component of protein, and (4) decrease in fat and caloric content. Deterioration occurs with freezing and thawing and is cumulative over time (Garcia-Lara et al., 2012).

Formula Feeding

Many mothers choose to feed formula to their infants from birth, to supplement breastfeeding with formula, or to wean early from breastfeeding and transition their infant to formula feeding. Reasons for the choice of formula, rather than breastfeeding, are listed in **Box 5-10**. A recent study showed that 73.6% of mothers who discontinued breastfeeding did so in the first 6 weeks postpartum (Brown et al., 2014). Research shows that only 18.8% of infants

Table 5-8: Breastmilk Storage Guidelines for Healthy Babies

	Freshly Expressed Breastmilk	Thawed Breastmilk (Previously Thawed)
Room temperature	4–6 hours at 66–78°F	Do not store
Cooler with ice packs	24 hours at 59°F	Do not store
Refrigerator	3–8 days at 32–39°F	24 hours
Freezer (separate compartment)	3–4 months at –4°F	Never refreeze thawed breastmilk
Deep freezer	6–12 months at 0°F	Never refreeze thawed breastmilk

Data from La Leche League International. (2014). What are the LLLI guidelines for storing my pumped milk? Retrieved from http://www.lalecheleague.org/faq/milkstorage.html.

Box 5-10: Reasons Mothers Choose to Feed Their Infants with Formula

- Problems with breastfeeding/lack of confidence in breastfeeding ability
- Infant feeding difficulty
- Inconvenience
- Infant weight and nutrition
- Going back to full-time work or school
- Concerns about quantity or quality of breastmilk
- Fatigue
- Postpartum depression
- Maternal need for medication

Data from Brown, C. R. L., Dodds, L., Legge, A., Bryanton, J., & Semenic, S. (2014). Factors influencing the reasons why mothers stop breastfeeding. *Canadian Journal of Public Health, 105,* e179–3185; Dias, C. C., & Fiqueiredo, B. (2015). Breastfeeding and depression: A systematic review of the literature. *Journal of Affective Disorders, 171,* 142–154; Flaherman, V. J., Hicks, K. G., Cabana, M. D., & Lee, K. A. (2012). Maternal experience of interactions with providers among mothers with milk supply concerns. *Clinical Pediatrics, 51,* 778–784; Hamdan, A., & Tamin, H. (2012). The relationship between postpartum depression and breastfeeding. *International Journal of Psychiatry in Medicine, 43,* 243–259; Mandal, B., Roe, B. E., & Fein, S. B. (2010). The differential effects of full-time and part-time work status on breastfeeding. *Health Policy, 97,* 79–86; Odom, E. C., Li, R., Scanlon, K. S., Perrine, C. G., & Grummer-Strawn, L. (2013). Reasons for earlier than desired cessation of breastfeeding. *Pediatrics, 131,* e726–e732; Taveras, E., Capra, A. M., Braveman, P. A., Jensvold, N. G., Escobar, G. J., & Lieu, T. A. (2003). Clinical support and psychosocial risk factors associated with breastfeeding discontinuation. *Pediatrics, 112,* 108–115; Wagner, E. A., Chantry, C. J., Dewey, K. G., & Nommsen-Rivers, L. A. (2013). Breastfeeding concerns at 3 and 7 days postpartum and feeding status at 4 months. *Pediatrics, 132,* e865–e875; Williamson, I., Leeming, D., Lyttle, S., & Johnson, S. (2012). "It should be the most natural thing in the world": Exploring first-time mothers' breastfeeding difficulties in the UK using audio diaries and interviews. *Maternal and Child Nutrition, 8,* 434–447.

who were begun on breastfeeding are still exclusively breastfeeding at 6 months of age. By 6 months of age, 49% of infants are receiving a combination of breastmilk and formula (CDC, 2014). British mothers interviewed about their feeding practices expressed relief that infant formula was available and provided a reasonable alternative to breastfeeding (Lee, 2007).

Mothers choosing formula feeding often encounter a lack of professional support and education about their choice of formula and its preparation (Lee, 2007). This lack of support and education is especially prevalent in the delivering hospital, such that the parents often leave the hospital without proper education on safe formula preparation, storage, and use (Cairney & Barbour, 2007; Labinar-Wolfe, Fein, & Shealy, 2008; Lee, 2007; Tarrant, 2007). One study showed that 77% of new parents did not receive instruction on formula preparation and 73% received no education on formula storage from a health professional (Labinar-Wolfe et al., 2008). Younger women often receive support for formula feeding from friends and relatives who may, or may not, be adequately knowledgeable to provide safe assistance (Cairney & Barbour, 2007).

"Well parents can read the formula instructions on the label," some providers might protest. In fact, research shows that mothers do *not* consistently read or follow the formula-package labels for safe preparation or handling of formula (Herbold & Scott, 2008; Labinar-Wolfe et al., 2008). Unsafe practices related to formula preparation and storage are listed in **Table 5-9**.

Table 5-9: Unsafe Practices and Consequences in Formula Preparation and Storage

Unsafe Practice	Consequence
Lack of proper hand hygiene (hand washing/hand rubs) before preparing formula	Infection Diarrhea
Using the wrong amount of water to dilute powdered formula	Fluid and electrolyte imbalance Undernutrition Decreased weight gain Dehydration
Leaving formula at room temperature longer than recommended	Infection Diarrhea
Reusing bottles/nipples without proper cleaning	Infection Diarrhea
Heating formula in a microwave	Oral burns from "hot spots" in microwaved liquids

Formula Choices

Modern formulas are designed and supplemented with nutrients to mimic the composition of human milk as well as the outcomes of the breastfed infant. The composition of infant formula provides 40% to 45% of calories from carbohydrates, 5% to 6% of calories from protein, and 50% of calories from fat (Joeckel & Phillips, 2009). Infant formulas are commercially available as ready-to-feed versions, which require no dilution, and as concentrates (either liquid or powder), which require dilution with water.

Cow's Milk–Based Formula　Healthy full-term newborns are most often started on standard cow's milk–based formulas at birth. Although based on cow's milk, formulas vary in their composition of macronutrients such as protein, fats, and carbohydrates and of micronutrients such as vitamins and minerals. To provide formula-fed newborns with nutrition that is similar to the nutrition found in breastmilk, the caloric content of formula is similar to that of breastmilk, approximately 19 to 20 calories per fluid ounce (Oski, Bennett, & Campbell, 1980). Full-term formula-fed infants require caloric intake of 100 to 110 kcal/kg/day for adequate growth of ½ to 1 ounce/day (20 to 30 grams/day) (Brown et al., 2016).

Cow's milk–based formulas contain cow-milk proteins—that is, whey/casein mixtures that approximate human milk. As in human milk, lactose is the major carbohydrate in formula. Vegetable oil blends of fat mimic the fatty acid content of human milk. Additives to formulas include (1) long-chain polyunsaturated fats (docosahexaenoic acid [DHA] and arachidonic acid [ARA]), (2) iron, (3) nucleotides, (4) lutein, and (5) vitamin D (Joeckel & Phillips, 2009). To prevent iron-deficiency anemia and the consequences of developmental delay that accompany it, all infants should receive iron-fortified formulas (Martinez & Ballew, 2011; O'Connor, 2009). Contrary to popular myths, iron-fortified formulas do not increase colic-like or gastrointestinal symptoms such as constipation (Oski et al., 1980; Singhal et al., 2000).

Table 5-10 compares commercially available formulas for full-term infants, including cow's milk-based, lactose-free, and soy protein-based products.

Soy Protein–Based Formula　Approximately 25% of the total infant formula sales in the United States are attributable to soy protein–based formulas (Bhatia & Greer, 2008). Although clinical indications for soy protein–based formulas are few, their increasing use in the first year of life is largely driven by mothers' decisions rather than by healthcare providers (Berger-Achituv et al., 2005). Soy formulas are cow's milk protein and lactose free; their protein source is soy, and formulas are supplemented with amino acids such as L-carnitine, L-methionine, and taurine (Bhatia & Greer, 2008; Martinez & Ballew, 2011). Fat content is provided by vegetable oil blends.

Soy protein–based formulas provide the macronutrients and micronutrients necessary to support adequate growth rates and bone mineralization in healthy full-term neonates. For strict vegan and vegetarian families, soy protein–based formulas are an acceptable alternative to breastfeeding or as supplements to breastfeeding (Zeno, Hosley, & Steward, 2015). For infants requiring strict lactose restriction (i.e., those with congenital lactase deficiency or galactosemia), these formulas are used because they are lactose free. Lactose intolerance is rare in infants because they digest lactose easily. Some infants, however, may develop a transient lactose intolerance after an acute gastrointestinal illness accompanied by diarrhea. Formula change is usually not necessary in such a case.

Parents may turn to soy protein–based formula if they believe that symptoms of gas, regurgitation, and fussiness are due to cow's-milk protein allergy (CMPA). True CMPA is estimated to occur in only 2% to 7.5% of healthy infants (Berseth, Johnston, Stolz, Harris, & Mitmesser, 2009). By comparison, sensitization to cow's-milk protein is often (in 10% to 14% of infants with an immunoglobulin E [IgE]–mediated CMPA; Bhatia & Greer, 2008; Zeigler et al., 1999) accompanied by sensitization to soy protein in infants younger than 6 months of age (Klemola et al., 2002). This cross-sensitization is due to the structural similarities of cow's milk protein and soy protein (Kattan, Cocco, & Jarvinen, 2011). In addition, 30% to 64% of infants with a non-IgE allergic enteropathy or colitis because of CMPA have allergic reactions to soy protein (Martinez & Ballew, 2011). Infants with IgE-mediated CMPA may be able to tolerate soy protein–based formulas. In contrast, infants who are sensitive to both cow's-milk protein and soy protein can be fed extensively hydrolyzed formula, which enables them to obtain relief from symptoms of rash, vomiting, diarrhea, abdominal pain, and bloody stools (Bhatia & Greer, 2008; O'Connor, 2009).

Hydrolyzed Formulas Formulas in which the casein and whey have been partially, extensively, or completely hydrolyzed are marketed for infants with feeding issues characterized by fussiness, gas, and colic (**Table 5-11**). The casein and whey of these cow's milk–based formulas are subjected to heat and enzymatically hydrolyzed into peptide chains and free amino acids that are less likely to stimulate antibody production in the presence of protein (Joeckel & Phillips, 2009; O'Connor, 2009). Although little research supports the efficacy of the hydrolyzed formulas in relieving infant symptoms, a recent meta-analysis of use of partially hydrolyzed 100% whey protein formulas found these products to be efficacious in preventing or reducing allergy symptoms, particularly atopic dermatitis (Alexander & Cabana, 2010). Use of extensively hydrolyzed formulas is recommended for those infants unable to tolerate or digest intact cow's-milk protein. In addition, some infants with colic have been shown in a double-blind randomized study to have less daily crying when fed extensively hydrolyzed infant formula (Lucassen, Assemdelft, Gubbles, van Eijk, & Douwes, 2000).

Amino Acid Formula Formulas that contain 100% amino acids are hypoallergenic; the majority of their fat source is medium-chain triglycerides (MCT) oil, and many are also lactose free. Amino acid formulas are best used for those infants with malabsorption, abnormal gastrointestinal (GI) tracts (e.g., short bowel syndrome), or persistent symptoms of extreme protein sensitivity after a trial of extensively hydrolyzed formula (Brown et al., 2016; Joeckel & Phillips,

Table 5-10: Comparative Nutritional Composition of Term Infant Feedings per 100 kcal

	Cow's Milk–Based With Intact Protein						Lactose Free	Soy Protein–Based	
	Mature Human Milk (28 Days)	Enfamil Newborn	Enfamil Infant†	Similac Advance Stage 1‡	Similac Advance Stage 2‡	Similac Sensitive	Enfamil Prosobee Lipil†	Similac Isomil Advance‡	
Nutrient density (kcal/oz)	20	20	20	20	19	19	20	19	
Energy (kcal)	98-110	100	100	100	100	100	100	100	
Protein									
Amount (g)	1.8	2.1	2	2.07	2.07	2.14	2.5	2.45	
% Total calories	7	8	8	8	8	8.5	10	10	
Source	Human milk	Nonfat milk, whey protein concentrate	Nonfat milk, whey protein concentrate	Nonfat milk and whey protein concentrate	Nonfat milk and whey protein concentrate	Milk protein isolate	Soy protein isolate and L-methionine	Soy protein isolate and L-methionine	
Fat									
Amount (g)	4.3-4.9	5.3	5.3	5.4	5.6	5.4	5.3	5.46	
% Total calories	50	48	48	49	50	49	48	49	
Source	Triglycerides	Palm olein Soy oil Coconut oil High oleic sunflower oil Single cell oil products (DHA and ARA)	Palm olein soy oil Coconut oil High oleic sunflower oil Single cell oil products (DHA and ARA)	High oleic safflower oil Soy oil Coconut oil Single cell oil products (DHA and ARA)	High oleic safflower oil Soy oil Coconut oil Single cell oil products (DHA and ARA)	High oleic safflower oil Soy oil Coconut oil Single cell oil products (DHA and ARA)	Palm olein Soy oil Coconut oil High oleic sunflower oil Single cell oil products (DHA and ARA)	High oleic safflower oil Soy oil Coconut oil Single cell oil products (DHA and ARA)	
Linoleic acid (mg)	440-1500	860	800	1000	1000	1000	860	1000	
Carbohydrate									
Amount (g)	10-11	11.2	11.3	10.8	10.7	10.7	10.6	10.4	
% Total calories	40-44	45	45	43	43	43	42	42	
Source	Lactose and glucose	Lactose	Lactose	Lactose	Lactose	Maltodextrin and sugar	Corn syrup solids	Corn syrup and sucrose	
Minerals									
Calcium (mg)	39-45	73	78	78	82	88	105 (5.2)	110 (5.5)	
Phosphorus (mg)	18-24	43	43	42	44	59	69	79	

Ca:P ratio	1.9-2.1	1.8	1.8	1.8	1.8	1.5	1.5	1.4
Sodium (mg [mEq])	18-26 [0.8-1.1]	27 [1.2]	27 [1.2]	24 [1]	25 [1.1]	32 [1.4]	36 [1.6]	44 [1.9]
Potassium (mg [mEq])	60-80 [1.5-2]	108 [2.8]	108 [2.8]	105 [2.7]	110 [2.8]	110 [2.8]	120 [3.1]	110 [2.8]
Chloride (mg [mEq])	55-63 [1.6-1.8]	63 [1.8]	63 [1.8]	65 [1.8]	68 [1.9]	68 [1.9]	80 [2.3]	65 [1.8]
Iron (mg)	0.05-0.75	1.8	1.8	1.8	1.9	1.9	1.8	1.9
Zinc (mg)	0.2-0.3	1	1	0.75	0.79	0.79	1.2	0.79
Magnesium (mg)	4.5-5	8	8	6	6	6	8-11	7.9
Vitamins								
Vitamin A (international units)	110-320	300	300	300	300	300	300	300
Vitamin D (international units)	3-3.2	75	60	60	75	60	60	60
Vitamin E (international units)	0.3-0.6	2	2	1.5	1.5	1.5	2	1.5
Vitamin K (mcg)	0.3	9	9	8	8	8	8-9	11
Vitamin C—ascorbic acid (mg)	5.6-6	12	12	9	9	9	12	9
Vitamin B1—thiamine (mcg)	29-31	80	80	100	100	100	80	63
Vitamin B2—riboflavin (mcg)	49-51	140	140	150	160	160	90	95
Vitamin B6 (mcg)	10-46	60	60	60	63	63	60	63
Folic acid (mcg)	2.5-18	16	16	15	16	16	16	16
Other Characteristics								
Potential renal solute load (mOsm)	14	19.1	18.6	18.7	20.5	20.3	23	23.2
Osmolality (mOsm/kg water)	290-305	300	300	310	310	200	200	200

† Mead Johnson Nutritionals, Evansville, Indiana.

‡ Abbott Nutrition, Columbus, Ohio

Reproduced from Brown, L. D., Hendrickson, K., Evans, R., Davis, J., Anderson, M. S., & Hay, W. W. (2015). Enteral nutrition. In S. L. Gardner, B. S. Carter, M. Enzman Hines, & J. A. Hernandez (Eds.), Merenstein and Gardner's handbook of neonatal intensive care (8th ed., pp. 377–418). St. Louis, MO: Mosby-Elsevier.

Table 5-11: Comparative Nutritional Composition of Hydrolyzed Infant Feedings per 100 kcal

	Partially Hydrolyzed		Extensively Hydrolyzed				Completely Hydrolyzed	
	Enfaml Gentlease	Similac Total Comfort	Enfamil Nutramigen	Similac Expert Cearali-mentum	Enfamil Pregestimil	Enfamil Puramino	Elecare (For Infants)	Nutricia Neocate Infant Dha/Ara
Nutrient density (kcal/oz)	20	19	20	20	20	20	20	20
Energy (kcal)	100	100	100	100	100	100	100	100
Protein								
Amount (g)	2.3	2.32	2.8	2.75	2.8	2.8	3.1	2.8
% Total calories	9	9	11	11	11	11	15	11
Source	Partially hydrolyzed nonfat milk and whey protein concentrate solids (soy)	Whey protein hydrolysate	Casein hydrolysate, L-cystine, L-tyrosine, L-tryptophan	Casein hydrolysate, L-cystine, L-tyrosine, L-tryptophan	Casein hydrolysate, L-cystine, L-tyrosine, L-tryptophan	Free L-amino acids	Free L-amino acids	Free L-amino acids
Fat								
Amount (g)	5.3	5.4	5.3	5.54	5.6	5.3	4.8	5.1
% Total calories	48	49	48	48	48	48	43	46
Source	Palm olein, soy, coconut, and high oleic sunflower oils Single cell oil products (DHA and ARA)	High oleic safflower oil, soy and coconut oil Single cell oil products (DHA and ARA)	Palm olein, soy, coconut and high oleic sunflower oils Single cell oil products (DHA and ARA)	Safflower oil, MCT oil, soy oil Single cell oil products (DHA and ARA)	MCT oil, soy oil, corn oil, and high oleic safflower oil or sunflower oil Single cell oil products (DHA and ARA)	Palm olein, coconut, soy and high oleic sunflower oils Single cell oil products (DHA and ARA)	Safflower oil, MCT, soy oil Single cell oil products (DHA and ARA)	MCT, high oleic sunflower oil, sunflower oil, canola oil Single cell oil products (DHA and ARA)
Oil ratio (approximate)	44:19.5:19.5:14.5	40:30:29	44:19.5:19.5:14.5	38:33:28	55:25:10:7.5	44:19.5:14.5	39:33:28	N/A
Linoleic acid (mg)	800–860	1000	860	1900	940	860	840	738
Carbohydrate								
Amount (g)	10.8	11	10.3	10.2	10.2	10.3	10.7	10.8
% Total calories	43.5	42	41	41	41	41	42	43
Source	Corn syrup solids	Corn syrup solids, sugar, galactoo-ligosac-charides	Corn syrup solids	Sugar, modified tapioca starch	Corn syrup solids	Corn syrup solids, modified tapioca starch	Corn syrup solids	Corn syrup solids

Minerals

Constituent								
Calcium (mg)	116	116	94	94	105	94	105	82
Phosphorus (mg)	82.2	84.2	52	52	75	52	70	46
Ca:P ratio	1.4:1	1.4:1	1.8:1	1.8:1	1.4:1	1.8:1	1.5:1	1.8:1
Sodium mg (mEq)	39.1 (1.7)	45 (2)	47 (2)	47 (2)	44 (1.9)	47 (2)	46 (2)	36 (1.6)
Potassium mg (mEq)	109 (2.8)	150 (3.9)	110 (2.8)	110 (2.8)	118 (3)	110 (2.8)	121 (3.1)	108 (3.1)
Chloride mg (mEq)	79.9 (2.2)	60 (1.7)	88 (2.5)	86 (2.4)	80 (2.3)	86 (2.4)	68 (1.9)	63 (1.8)
Iron (mg)	1.5	1.8	1.8	1.8	1.8	1.8	1.9	1.8
Zinc (mg)	1.1	1.15	1	1	0.75	1	0.79	1
Magnesium (mg)	10.3	8	11	8	7.5	8–11	6	8

Vitamins

Constituent								
Vitamin A (international units)	280	273	300	350	300	300	300	300
Vitamin D (international units)	72.9	60	50	50	45	50	60	60
Vitamin E (international units)	1.4	2.1	2	4	3	2	1.5	2
Vitamin K (mcg)	8.8	13	8	12	15	8–9	8	9
Vitamin C—ascorbic acid (mg)	10.7	9	12	12	9	12	9	12
Vitamin B$_1$—thiamine (mcg)	140	210	80	80	60	80	100	80
Vitamin B$_2$—riboflavin (mcg)	110	105	90	90	90	90	160	140
Vitamin B$_6$ (mcg)	112	84.2	60	60	60	60	63	60
Folic acid (mcg)	13.3	29.5	16	16	15	16	16	16

Other Characteristics

Constituent								
Potential renal solute load (mOsm)	16.8	18.7	25	25	25.3	25	22.5	21
Osmolality (mOsm/kg water)	340	350	350	260–280	370	260–320	200	220–230

This table lists the major constituents; refer to product inserts for a complete listing of vitamins, minerals, and trace elements.

ARA, Arachidonic acid; DHA, docosahexaenoic acid; MCT, medium-chain triglycerides.

Reproduced from Brown, L. D., Hendrickson, K., Evans, R., Davis, J., Anderson, M. S., & Hay, W. W. (2015). Enteral nutrition. In S. L. Gardner, B. S. Carter, M. Enzman Hines, & J. A. Hernandez (Eds.), Merenstein and Gardner's handbook of neonatal intensive care (8th ed., pp. 377–418). St. Louis, MO: Mosby-Elsevier.

2009). After introduction of the amino acid formula, success is evaluated by a reduction in the infant's symptoms (Hill, Heine, & Cameron, 2000).

Prethickened Formulas   Milk-based formulas with rice starch added as a thickener are marketed for the management of infants with gastroesophageal reflux (GER) or regurgitation. These formulas have the consistency of regular formula and flow easily through a standard bottle nipple; their viscosity increases only when they come in contact with stomach acid (Joeckel & Phillips, 2009; Moukarzel, Abdelnour, & Akatcherian, 2007; Vandenplas et al., 1998). The thickener does not alter the caloric or nutrient balance of the formula (Moukarzel et al., 2007).

In contrast to these prethickened formulas, just adding "rice cereal" to formula results in unwanted consequences:

- The viscosity of the formula in the bottle is increased.

- The more viscous formula needs a larger nipple hole.

- Difficulty in regulating flow of the viscous formula results in increased air/formula intake through the enlarged nipple hole.

- Regurgitation and GER are exacerbated (Moukarzel et al., 2007; Vandenplas et al., 1998).

A meta-analysis of randomized, controlled trials reviewed the use of various thickeners for the treatment of GER and found no thickener to be superior to the others (Horvath, Dziechciarz, & Szajewska, 2008). The same meta-analysis also noted that thickeners were only moderately effective in relieving GER symptoms and that, compared to standard formula, there was a decrease in regurgitation, vomiting, crying, and irritability. Two studies showed that use of a prethickened formula (Enfamil AR) reduced symptoms (i.e., fewer feedings with regurgitation, less volume regurgitated, fewer feedings with choking–gagging and coughing, better sleep) by the end of the first week of use of the thickened formula (Moukarzel et al., 2007; Vanderhoof, Moran, Harris, Merkel, & Orenstein, 2003). "Off label" use of these formulas has been reported by mothers who use thickened formulas to promote their infant's sleeping through the night (Nevo, Rubin, Tamir, Levine, & Shaoul, 2007).

Reduced-Lactose Formulas   Although formulas containing non-lactose carbohydrates are used for infants with congenital lactase deficiency and galactosemia, their use for treating formula intolerance has not been well studied. Recently, a prospective, randomized clinical trial compared tolerance of a standard cow's milk–based formula with tolerance of a lactose-free formula in full-term healthy newborns (Lasekan et al., 2011). Both groups receiving the standard and lactose-free formulas grew well and tolerated their feedings, but the lactose-free group had fewer episodes of regurgitation and softer stools.

A more recent study compared lactose-free milk-based and soy-based formulas to intake of milk-based formula with lactose (Sherman, Anderson, & Rudolph, 2015). Use of both lactose-free formulas did not decrease infant behaviors (i.e., crying, fussiness, need for attention) or caregiver distress because of the infant's behaviors. Rather, caregiver distress and infant's distressing behaviors improved over a few weeks' time, without a change in formula.

Formula Intolerance

The lack of parental education about infant formula may contribute to poor decisions about formula changes. Research shows that in the first 6 to 7 months of life, approximately 38% to 47% of formula-fed infants experience at least one formula change (Nevo et al., 2007; Polack, Khan, & Maisels, 1999). The majority of these formula changes are made by parents without discussion with the baby's healthcare providers. Only 4% of formula changes are initiated by healthcare providers (Nevo et al., 2007).

Parental formula changes are typically based on parents' interpretation of the infant's behavior as "not tolerating" the formula (Nevo et al., 2007). Parents tend to rely on advice from family and friends, previous experience, or marketing information in making decisions to change their infant's formula (Huang, Labinar-Wolf, Huang, Choiniere, & Fein, 2013; Tarrant, 2007). When parents, rather than healthcare providers, change the formula, there is an increased likelihood of further unnecessary changes during infancy (Huang et al., 2013). A consensus-based algorithm for management of infant fussiness, crying, and gassiness in formula-fed infants is provided in **Figure 5-10.**

When a formula change is initiated by parents for a benign, self-limiting symptom that represents normal neonatal physiology and developmental immaturity, and the infant's behavior improves over time, the parents may attribute this response to their successful treatment of

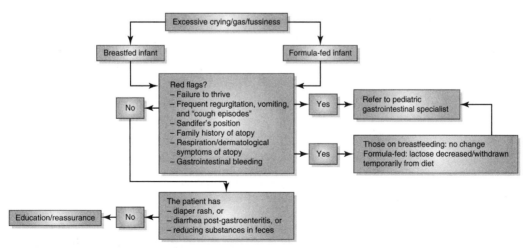

Figure 5-10 : Algorithm for the management of gassiness in formula-fed infants.
Reproduced from Vandenplas, Y., & Alarcon, P. (2015). Updated algorithms for managing frequent gastro-intestinal symptoms in infants. *Beneficial Microbes, 6*(2): 199–208. Reproduced with permission of Wageningen Academic Publishers.

formula intolerance. In reality, the improvement in the infant's behavior may be the result of neurologic and gastrointestinal maturation. If symptoms persist after a formula change, further evaluation for an organic cause may be warranted (Berseth et al., 2009).

Normal Neonatal Physiology, Pathology, or Formula Intolerance?

Regurgitation and Gastroesophageal Reflux

Approximately 73% of healthy term infants experience at least one episode of regurgitation in the first month of life (Hegar et al., 2009). Regurgitation occurring more than once a day has been estimated to occur in 67% of young infants (Neu, Corwin, Lareau, & Marcheggiani-Howard, 2012). Regurgitation, which is a normal physiologic phenomenon in infants, is an involuntary return of swallowed formula or secretions into or out of the mouth. Gastroesophageal reflux (GER) is the movement of stomach contents into the esophagus and possibly the mouth. The developmental immaturity of the neonate's gastrointestinal tract contributes to the "normality" of regurgitation/GER, prompting the label "happy spitters" for infants with this condition (Hegar et al., 2009). Regurgitation is distinguished from vomiting by the central nervous system origin of vomiting, the forceful expulsion of gastric contents, and the irritability and discomfort that accompany vomiting.

Diagnostic criteria for normal, physiologic, regurgitation are listed in **Box 5-11** and criteria for "troublesome regurgitation" are listed in **Box 5-12**. Regurgitation that is "troublesome" to

Box 5-11: Diagnostic Criteria for Regurgitation in Healthy Infants (3 Weeks to 12 Months of Age)

- Regurgitation episodes 2 to 3 times per day for 3 weeks or longer
- Absence of:
  - Nausea
  - Hematemesis
  - Aspiration
  - Apnea
  - Failure to thrive
  - Difficulty in feeding or swallowing
  - Abnormal posture

Modified from Hyman, P. E., Milla, P. J., Benninga, M. A., Davidson, G. P., Fleisher, D. F., & Taminiau, J. (2006). Childhood functional gastrointestinal disorders: neonate/toddler. *Gastroenterology, 130*(5): 1519–1526. Copyright 2006, with permission from Elsevier.

Box 5-12: Diagnostic Criteria for "Troublesome Regurgitation"

- Regurgitation episodes 4 or more times per day for 2 weeks or longer
- Infant age greater than 3 weeks but less than 6 months

parents occurs in approximately 20% of all infants and requires a history and physical examination to rule out pathologic causes (Hegar et al., 2009; Vandenplas & Alarcon, 2015). Even though healthcare providers know that regurgitation is normal, parents perceive regurgitation as abnormal. Indeed, regurgitation and vomiting are cited by parents as the most common reason for changing an infant's formula (Nevo et al., 2007; Vandenplas et al., 1998). In a prospective study, regurgitation resulted in a change in formula for 62% of the infants (Iacono et al., 2005), yet reduction of regurgitation does not necessarily occur after a formula change (Hyman et al., 2006).

Extensively hydrolyzed formula and anti-regurgitation formula (AR-formula) have both been shown to be effective in treating "troublesome regurgitation" and vomiting. Although use of AR-formula may or may not decrease the number of reflux episodes that occur each day, the volume of regurgitation is reduced, which improves the quality of life for infants and their care givers (Vandenplas et al., 2009). Use of AR-formulas has also been shown to reduce crying and improve sleep and weight gain.

When there is no improvement with use of these formulas, the infant may have CMPA. In the infant with CMPA, elimination of cow's protein–based formulas for a 2-week period decreases regurgitation, whereas reintroduction causes symptoms to recur (Vandenplas et al., 2009). For most infants, antisecretory drugs and prokinetic agents are not efficacious in remedying CMPA (Horvath et al., 2008).

Figure 5-11 presents a consensus-based algorithm for management of regurgitation in formula-fed infants.

Gastroesophageal Reflux Disease

Gastroesophageal reflux disease (GERD) occurs when the reflux of gastric contents and acid results in complications or a decreased quality of life (Vandenplas et al., 1998). Symptoms of GERD and formula intolerance (**Table 5-12**) are similar, and distinguishing them is challenging for both healthcare providers and parents. Additionally, during early infancy, symptoms of irritability, crying, clenched fists, and extending legs or flexing legs onto the abdomen are common and occur without apparent reason, although mothers often attribute them to abdominal pain (Neu et al., 2012; Vandenplas et al., 1998). Generally there is no evidence to support the belief that the baby has abdominal pain or an organic cause for the distress; over time, such symptoms typically resolve spontaneously (Hill et al., 2000). Use of acid-reducing medications relieves symptoms of GERD.

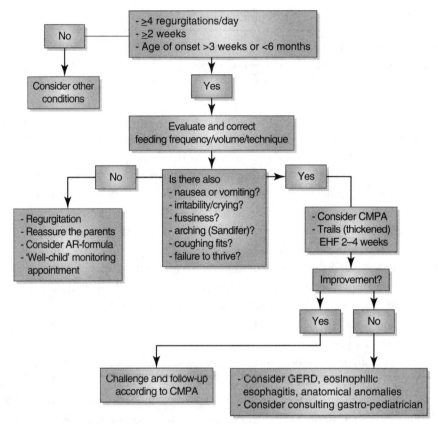

Figure 5-11: Algorithm for the management of regurgitation in formula-fed infants.
AR=anti-regurgitation; CMPA= cows milk protein allergy; EHF= Extensive hydrolysate formula.
Reproduced from Vandenplas, Y., & Alarcon, P. (2015). Updated algorithms for managing frequent gastro-intestinal symptoms in infants. *Beneficial Microbes, 6*(2): 199–208. Reproduced with permission of Wageningen Academic Publishers.

Constipation or Diarrhea

The stools of newborns and neonates reflect the type of feeding they are receiving, their hydration state, and the presence of a gastrocolic reflex. The gastrocolic reflex enables newborns and neonates to stool every time they feed—as something comes in at the mouth, it comes out from their intestine! The uneducated parent calls this "diarrhea." Breastfed infants have the softest and most frequent stools, produced as often 7 to 12 times per day to as infrequently as 1 time per week or once every 3 to 4 weeks (Hyman et al., 2006; Tabbers et al., 2014). Harder stool consistency is seen in formula-fed infants (those not receiving formulas supplemented with prebiotics or probiotics) than those who are breastfed (9.2% versus 1.1%) (Tunc, Camurdan, Ilhan, Sahin, & Beyazova,

Table 5-12: Gastrointestinal Symptoms Associated with Parent Distress

Symptom	GERD[1]	Formula Intolerance[2]
Irritability	X	X
Crying	X	X
Vomiting (distress*)	X	X
Regurgitation		X
Painful swallowing	X	
Abnormal posture: frequent arching of the back	X	
Colic-type symptoms: fussy and gassy		X
Bowel changes (constipation, diarrhea, bloody stools)		X
Refusal to feed	X	X
Apnea	X	
Aspiration	X	

* Distressing to both infant and parents.

Data from [1]Bhatia, J., & Parish, A. (2009). GERD or not GERD: The fussy infant. *Journal of Perinatology, 29,* S7–S11; Hyman, P. E., Milla, P. J., Benninga, M. A., Davidson, G. P., Fleisher, D. F., & Taminiau, J. (2006). Childhood functional gastrointestinal disorders: Neonate/toddler. *Gastroenterology, 130,* 1519–1526. [2] Berseth, C. L., Johnston, W. H., Stolz, S. I., Harris, C. L., & Mitmesser, S. H. (2009). Clinical response to 2 commonly used switch formulas occurs within 1 day. *Clinical Pediatrics, 48,* 58–65; Ewing, W., & Allen, P. (2005). The diagnosis and management of cow milk protein intolerance in the primary care setting. *Pediatric Nursing, 31,* 486–493; Nevo, N., Rubin, L., Tamir, A., Levine, A., & Shaoul, R. (2007). Infant feeding patterns in the first 6 months: An assessment in full-term infants. *Journal of Pediatric Gastroenterology and Nutrition, 45,* 234–239; Vandenplas, Y., Lifshitz, J. Z., Orenstein, S., Lifshitz, C. H., Shepherd, R. W., Casaubon P. R., & Lifshitz, F. (1998). Nutritional management of regurgitation in infants. *Journal of the American College of Nutrition, 17,* 308–316.

2008). When infant formula contains palm oil or palm olein oil as the main source of fat, stool consistency is firmer (Tunc et al., 2008). As the neonate matures, stool frequency normally decreases, and firmer, harder, less frequent stools accompany a change from breastfeeding to formula feeding. The uneducated parent defines these stool changes as "constipation."

In infants, constipation is actually defined as "difficult or rare defecation lasting for 2 weeks" (Biggs & Dery, 2006). **Figure 5-12** provides a consensus-based algorithm for management of constipation in formula-fed infants. Failure to pass meconium in the first 24 to 48 hours of life is abnormal, and the newborn should be referred for diagnostic workup for imperforate anus (high obstruction is possible in the presence of anal opening), Hirschsprung's disease, or meconium ileus or plug (Biggs & Dery, 2006; Tabbers et al., 2014).

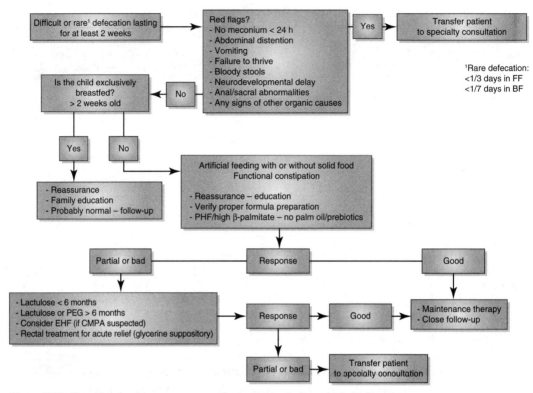

Figure 5-12: Algorithm for the management of constipation in formula-fed infants.
BF= breastfeeding; CMPA=cow's milk protein allergy; EHF=extensive hydrolysate formula; FF=formula feeding; PEG=polyethene glycol; PHF=partial hydrolysate formula.
Reproduced from Vandenplas, Y., & Alarcon, P. (2015). Updated algorithms for managing frequent gastro-intestinal symptoms in infants. *Beneficial Microbes, 6*(2): 199–208. Reproduced with permission of Wageningen Academic Publishers.

Colic

Colic is a common occurrence in the first 1 to 3 months of life. This condition is characterized by episodes of extended crying (usually in the late afternoon or early evening) and difficult-to-soothe behavior, lasting at least 3 hours per day, at least 3 days per week for at least 3 weeks (Hyman et al., 2006). The incidence of colic ranges from 5% to 30%, and it occurs equally in breastfed and bottle-fed infants and in both sexes (Shergill-Bonner, 2010). The etiology of colic is unknown but postulated causes include immature GI function, intolerance to food, transient low lactase activity, CMPA, GER or GERD, and immaturity or imbalance of intestinal flora. After ruling out pathologic causes for the crying, parents should be educated that colic is a self-limiting condition. They should be given strategies for parental coping and taught strategies for soothing a crying baby.

Formula changes are often made in an attempt to treat infant colic. A systematic review found that use of a hydrolyzed protein–based formula or a soy protein–based formula may reduce the symptoms of infant colic (Iacovou, Ralston, Muir, Walker, & Truby, 2012). Colicky babies may be overfed as mothers try to soothe their distressed baby with feeding attempts (Anzman-Frasca et al., 2013; Worobey, Pena, Ramos, & Espinosa, 2014). **Figure 5-13** provides a consensus-based algorithm for management of infant colic in formula-fed infants.

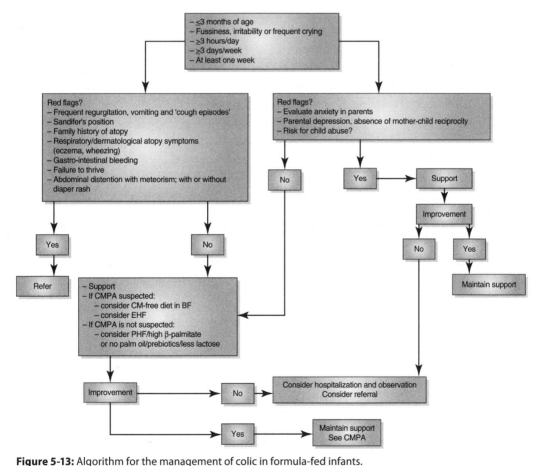

Figure 5-13: Algorithm for the management of colic in formula-fed infants.
AR=anti-regurgitation; CMPA= cows milk protein allergy; BF=breastfeeding; EHF=extensive hydrolysate formula; PHF=partial hydrolysate formula.
Reproduced from Vandenplas, Y., & Alarcon, P. (2015). Updated algorithms for managing frequent gastro-intestinal symptoms in infants. *Beneficial Microbes, 6*(2): 199–208. Reproduced with permission of Wageningen Academic Publishers.

Summary

Regardless of the method of feeding, parents need to be fully educated on how to feed their neonate or infant, the frequency of feeding, abnormal gastrointestinal signs and symptoms, normal urine and stool patterns, and who to call with concerns.

Student Practice Activities

Case Study 1

You are a midwife who is assessing a G1P1 who had an uncomplicated vaginal birth 2 days ago. Her postpartum course has been uncomplicated, and she is now ready to go home. Upon physical examination, you note that her breasts are moderately firm and nipples are everted. She reports that her "milk feels like it is coming in" because her breasts feel so hard. Inspection of the nipples reveals bilateral cracks that are ½ cm in length. The mother reports bleeding from the nipples when she is nursing. Upon more discussion, she reports that nursing is very painful, especially initially with latch-on. She calls her baby a "barracuda baby" and says the nurse told her that her baby just has a strong suck. The cracks appeared within 10 hours of the birth. The mother does not want to supplement her baby but is concerned because of the pain with breastfeeding.

1. What would be your initial plan and what would you assess (be as specific as possible)?
2. What would be your initial plan and what would you assess if the baby has a "heart-shaped tongue" that has difficulty extending over lower gum line?

Case Study 2

You are seeing a formula-fed 2-week-old baby in an office visit who has regained his birth weight plus 8 ounces. His mother complains that he is constipated.

1. How would you deal with this situation?
2. The mother states that the baby's formula contains iron, and iron causes constipation. How do you deal with this statement?

References

Academy of Breastfeeding Medicine (ABM). (2009). ABM clinical protocol #3: Hospital guidelines for the use of supplementary feedings in the healthy term breastfed neonate. *Breastfeeding Medicine, 4,* 175–182.

Academy of Breastfeeding Medicine (ABM). (2011). ABM clinical protocol #10: Breastfeeding the late preterm infant (33 0/7 to 36 6/7 weeks gestation). *Breastfeeding Medicine, 6*(3), 151–157.

Adamkin, D. H., & Committee on Fetus and the Newborn of the American Academy of Pediatrics (AAP). (2011). Postnatal glucose homeostasis in late preterm and term infants. *Pediatrics, 127,* 575–579.

Alexander, D. D., & Cabana, M. D. (2010). Partially hydrolyzed 100% whey protein infant formula reduced risk of atopic dermatitis a meta-analysis. *Journal of Pediatric Gastroenterology and Nutrition, 50,* 422–430.

American Academy of Pediatrics (AAP). (2015). Bright futures. Retrieved from http://brightfutures.aap.org

American Academy of Pediatrics (AAP), Committee on the Fetus and Newborn. (2010). Hospital stay for healthy term newborns. *Pediatrics, 125,* 405–409.

American Academy of Pediatrics (AAP), Committee on Pediatric AIDS. (2013). Infant feeding and transmission of human immunodeficiency virus in the United States. *Pediatrics, 131*(2), 391–396.

American Academy of Pediatrics (AAP), Section on Breastfeeding. (2012). Breast feeding and the use of human milk. *Pediatrics, 129*(3), e827–e841.

American Academy of Pediatrics (AAP), Subcommittee on Hyperbilirubinemia. (2004). Management of hyperbilirubinemia in the newborn infant 35 or more weeks of gestation. *Pediatrics, 11,* 297–316.

American College of Nurse-Midwives (ACNM). (2011). *ACNM position statement on breastfeeding.* Silver Spring, MD: Author.

American College of Obstetricians and Gynecologists (ACOG). (2013). Breastfeeding in underserved women: Increasing initiation and continuation of breastfeeding. ACOG Committee Opinion No. 570, *Obstetrics & Gynecology, 122,* 423–428.

Anzman-Frasca, S., Liu, S., Gates, K. M., Paul, I. M., Rovine, M. J., & Birch, L. L. (2013). Infants' transitions out of a fussing/crying state are modified and are related to weight to weight status. *Infancy, 18,* 662–686.

Association of Women's Health, Obstetric and Neonatal Nurses (AWHONN). (2005). *Near term infant initiative.* Washington, DC: Author.

Association of Women's Health, Obstetric and Neonatal Nurses (AWHONN). (2007). *Breastfeeding.* Washington, DC: Author.

Association of Women's Health, Obstetrics and Neonatal Nurses (AWHONN). (2010). *Assessment and care of the late-preterm infant guideline.* Washington, DC: Author.

Association of Women's Health, Obstetric, and Neonatal Nurses (AWHONN). (2014). *Assessment and Care of the Late Preterm Infant.* Washington, DC: AWHONN.

Ball, H. L., Ward-Platt, M. P., Heslop, E., Leech, S. J., & Brown, K. A. (2006). Randomised trial of infant sleep location on the postnatal ward. *Archives of Disease in Childhood, 91,* 1005–1010.

Baron, I. S., Litman, F. R., Ahronovich, M. D., & Baker, R. (2012). Late preterm birth: A review of medical and neuropsychological childhood outcomes. *Neuropsychology Review, 22*(4), 438–450.

Beilin, Y., Bodian, C. A., Weiser, J., Houssain, S., Arnold, I., Feierman, D. E., & Holzman, I. (2005). Effect of labor epidural analgesia with and without fentanyl on infant breastfeeding: A prospective, randomized, double-blind study. *Anesthesiology, 103,* 1211–1217.

Berger-Achituv, S., Shohat, T., Romano-Zelekha, O., Ophir, E., Rachmani, S., Malovizky, D., & Garty, B. Z. (2005). Widespread use of soy-based formula without clinical indication. *Journal of Pediatric Gastroenterology and Nutrition, 41,* 660–666.

Berseth, C. L., Johnston, W. H., Stolz, S. I., Harris, C. L., & Mitmesser, S. H. (2009). Clinical response to 2 commonly used switch formulas occurs within 1 day. *Clinical Pediatrics, 48,* 58–65.

Betzold, C. M., Laughlin, K. M., & Shi, C. (2007). An update on the recognition and management of lactational breast inflammation. *Journal of Midwifery and Women's Health, 52*(6), 595–605.

Bhatia, J., & Greer, F. (2008). Use of soy protein-based formulas in infant feeding. *Pediatrics, 121,* 1062–1068.

Biggs, W. S., & Dery, W. H. (2006). Evaluation and treatment of constipation in infants and children. *American Family Physician, 73,* 469–477.

Blomquist, H. K., Jonsbo, F., Serenius, F., & Persson, L. A. (1994). Supplementary feeding in the maternity ward shortens the duration of breast feeding. *Acta Paediatrica, 83,* 1122–1126.

Bolyut, N., vanKempen, A., & Offringa, M. (2006). Neurodevelopment after neonatal hypoglycemia: A systematic review and design of an optimal future study. *Pediatrics, 117,* 2231–2243.

Boney, C. M., Verma, A., Tucker, R., & Vohr, B. R. (2005). Metabolic syndrome in childhood: Association with birth weight, maternal obesity, and gestational diabetes mellitus. *Pediatrics, 1,* e291–e296.

Bramson, L., Lee, J. W., Moore, E., Montgomery, S., Neish, C., Bahjri, K., & Melcher, C. L. (2010). Effect of early skin-to-skin mother–infant contact during the first three hours following birth on exclusive breastfeeding during the maternity hospital stay. *Journal of Human Lactation, 26,* 130–137.

Brown, C. R. L., Dodds, L., Legge, A., Bryanton, J., & Semenic S. (2014). Factors influencing the reasons why mothers stop breastfeeding. *Canadian Journal of Public Health, 105,* e179–3185.

Brown, L. D., Hendrickson, K., Evans, R., Davis, J., & Hay, W. W. (2016). Enteral nutrition. In S. L. Gardner, B. S. Carter, M. Enzman Hines, & J. A. Hernandez (Eds.), *Merenstein and Gardner's handbook of neonatal intensive care* (8th ed., pp. 377–418). St. Louis, MO: Mosby-Elsevier.

Burns, C. M., Rutherford, M. A., Boardman, J. P., & Cowan, F. M. (2008). Patterns of cerebral injury and neurodevelopmental outcomes after symptomatic neonatal hypoglycemia. *Pediatrics, 122,* 65–76.

Bystrova, K., Widstrom, A. M., Mathhiesen, A. S., Ransjo-Arvidson, A. B., & Uvnas-Moberg, K. (2007). Early lactation performance in primiparous and multiparous women in relation to different maternity home practices: A randomized trial in St. Petersburg. *International Breastfeeding Journal, 2,* 9.

Caine, V. A., Smith, M., Beasley, Y., & Brown, H. L. (2012). The impact of prenatal education on behavioral changes toward breast feeding and smoking cessation in a healthy start population. *Journal of the National Medical Association, 104,* 258–264.

Cairney, P., & Barbour, R. (2007). A research study of sources of support for bottle feeding in new mothers. *Community Practice, 80,* 30–34.

Centers for Disease Control and Prevention (CDC). (2010). Racial and ethnic differences in breastfeeding initiation and duration, by state- National Immunization Survey, United States, 2004–2008. *Morbidity and Mortality Weekly Report, 59*(11), 327–334.

Centers for Disease Control and Prevention (CDC). (2014). Breastfeeding report card—United States, 2012. Retrieved from http://www.cdc.gov/breastfeeding/pdf/2012BreastfeedingReportCard.pdf

Chaney, N. E., Franke, J., & Wadlington, W. B. (1988). Cocaine convulsions in a breast feeding baby. *Journal of Pediatrics, 112*(1), 134–135.

Chantry, C. (2011). Supporting the 75%: Overcoming barriers after breastfeeding initiation. *Breastfeeding Medicine, 6,* 337–339.

Chapman, D. J., Morel, K., Anderson, A. K, Damio, G., & Perez-Escamilla, R. (2010). Review: Breastfeeding peer counseling: From efficacy through scale-up. *Journal of Human Lactation, 26,* 314–332.

Chasnoff, I. J., Lewis, D. E., & Squires, L. (1987). Cocaine intoxication in a breast feeding infant., *Pediatrics, 80,* 836–838.

Chaturvedi, P. (2008). "Breast crawl" to initiate breastfeeding within half an hour after birth. *Journal of Mahatma Gandhi Institute of Medical Sciences, 13,* 9–14.

Christensson, K., Siles, C., Moreno, L., Belaustequi, A., De la Fuente, P., Lagercranz, H., & Winberg, J. (1992). Temperature, metabolic adaptation and crying in healthy full term newborns cared for skin-to-skin or in a cot. *Acta Paediatrica, 81,* 488–493.

Chung, M., Ip, S., Yu, W., Raman, G., Trikalinos, T., DeVine, D., & Lau, J. (2008). *Interventions in primary care to promote breastfeeding: A systematic review.* AHRQ publication number 08-05125-EF-1. Rockville, MD: Agency for Healthcare Research and Quality.

Cole, M. D., & Peevy, K. (1994). Hypoglycemia in normal neonates appropriate for gestational age. *Journal of Perinatology, 14,* 118–120.

Csont, G. L., Groth, S., Hopkin, P., & Guillet, R. (2014). An evidence-based to breastfeeding neonates at risk for hypoglycemia. *Journal of Obstetric, Gynecologic, and Neonatal Nursing, 43,* 71–81.

Davidoff, M. J., Dias, T., Damus, K., Russell, R., Bettegowda, V. R., Dolan, S., & Petrini, J. (2006). Changes in the gestational age distribution among US singleton births: impact on rates of preterm birth, 1992 to 2002. *Seminars in Perinatology, 30,* 8–15.

De Jong, M., Vorhoeven, M., & Van Baar, A. L. (2012). School outcome, cognitive functioning, and behavior problems in moderate and late preterm children and adults: A review. *Seminars in Fetal and Neonatal Medicine, 17,* 163–169.

Durand, R., Hodges, S., LaRosck, S., et al. (1997, March–April). The effect of skin-to-skin breast-feeding in the immediate recovery period on newborn thermoregulation and blood glucose values. *Neonatal Intensive Care,* 23–209.

Edmunds, J. (2012). Tongue-tie. *Journal of Human Lactation, 28,* 17.

Ehrenkranz, R. A., Dusick, A. M., Vohr, B. R., Wright, L. L., Wrage, L. A., & Poole, W. K. (2006). Growth in the neonatal intensive care unit influences neurodevelopmental and growth outcomes of extremely low birthweight infants. *Pediatrics, 117,* 1253–1261.

Engle, W., Tomashek, K. M., Wallman, C., & Committee on Fetus and Newborn of the American Academy of Pediatrics (AAP). (2007). "Late-preterm": A population at risk. *Pediatrics, 120*(6), 1390–1401.

Evans, A., Marinelli, K., Taylor, J., & Academy of Breastfeeding Medicine (ABM). (2014). ABM clinical protocol #2: Guidelines for hospital discharge of the breastfeeding term newborn and mother: The going home protocol. *Breastfeeding Medicine, 9,* 3–8.

Olza Fernandez, I., Marin Gabriel, M., Malalana Martinez, A., Fernandez-Canadas Morillo, A., Lopez Sanchez, F., & Costarelli, V. (2012). Newborn feeding behavior depressed by intrapartum oxytocin: A pilot study. *Acta Paediatrica, 101,* 749–754.

Foman, S. J., Haschke, F., Ziegler, E. E., & Nelson, S. E. (1982). Body composition reference children from birth to age 10 years. *American Journal of Clinical Nutrition, 35,* 1169.

Garcia-Lara, N. R., Escuder-Vieco, D., Garcia-Algar, O., De la Cruz, J., Lora, D., & Pallas-Alonso, C. (2012). Effect of freezing time on macronutrients and energy content of breastmilk. *Breastfeed Medicine, 7,* 295–301.

Gardner, S. L. (2007). Late-preterm ("near-term") newborns: A neonatal nursing challenge. *Nurse Currents, 1,* 1.

Gardner, S. L., Goldson, E., & Hernandez, J. A. (2016). The neonate and the environment: Impact on development. In S. L. Gardner, B. S. Carter, M. Enzman Hines, & J. A. Hernandez (Eds.), *Merenstein and Gardner's handbook of neonatal intensive care* (8th ed., pp. 419–463). St. Louis, MO: Mosby-Elsevier.

Gardner, S. L., & Hernandez, J. A. (2016). Initial nursery care. In S. L. Gardner, B. S. Carter, M. Enzman Hines, & J. A. Hernandez (Eds.), *Merenstein and Gardner's handbook of neonatal intensive care* (8th ed., pp. 419–463). St. Louis, MO: Mosby-Elsevier.

Gardner, S. L., & Lawrence, R. A. (2016). Breastfeeding the neonate with special needs. In S. L. Gardner, B. S. Carter, M. Enzman Hines, & J. A. Hernandez (Eds.), *Merenstein and Gardner's handbook of neonatal intensive care* (8th ed., pp. 419–463). St. Louis, MO: Mosby-Elsevier.

Gizzo, S., DiGangi, S., Saccardi, C., Patrelli, T. S., Paccagnella G., Sansone L., & D'Antona, D. (2012). Epidural analgesia during labor: Impact on delivery outcome, neonatal well-being, and early breastfeeding. *Breastfeed Medicine, 7,* 262–268.

Graves, B. W., & Haley, M. M. (2013). Newborn transition. *Journal of Midwifery and Women's Health, 58,* 662–670.

Guihard-Costa, A. M., & Larrosche, J. C. (1990). Differential growth between the fetal brain and its infratentorial part. *Early Human Development, 23,* 27–40.

Hartmann, P., Cregan, M., Ramsay, D., Simmer, K., & Kent, J. C. (2003). Physiology of lactation in preterm mothers: Initiation and maintenance. *Pediatric Annals, 32*, 351–355.

Haughton, J., Gregorio, D., & Perez-Escamilla, R. (2010). Factors associated with breastfeeding duration among Connecticut Special Supplemental Nutrition Program for Women, Infants, and Children (WIC) participants. *Journal of Human Lactation, 201*, 266–273.

Hawdon, J. M., Platt, M. P., & Aynsley-Green, A. (2006). Prevention and management of neonatal hypoglycemia. *Archives of Disease in Childhood—Fetal and Neonatal Edition, 70*, F60–F64.

Heck, L. J., & Erenberg, A. (1987). Serum glucose levels in term neonates during the first 48 hours of life. *Journal of Pediatrics, 110*, 119–122.

Hegar, B., Dewanti, N. R., Kadim, M., Alatas, S., Firmansyah, A., & Vanderplas, Y. (2009). Natural evolution of regurgitation in healthy infants. *Acta Paediatrica, 98*, 1189–1193.

Herbold, N. H., & Scott, E. (2008). A pilot study describing infant formula preparation and feeding practices. *International Journal of Environmental Health Research, 18*, 451–459.

Hill, D. J., Heine, R. G., & Cameron, D. J. S. (2000). Role of food protein intolerance in infants with persistent distress attributed to reflux esophagitis. *Journal of Pediatrics, 136*, 641–647.

Holmes, A., McLeod, A., & Bunik, M. (2013). ABM clinical protocol #5: Peripartum breastfeeding management for the healthy mother and infant at term. *Breastfeeding Medicine, 8*, 469–473.

Horvath, A., Dziechciarz, P., & Szajewska, H. (2008). The effect of thickened-feed intervention on gastroesophageal reflux in infants: Systematic review and meta-analysis of randomized, controlled trials. *Pediatrics, 122*, e1268–e1277.

Hoseth, E., Joergensen, A., Ebbesen, F., & Moeller, M. (2000). Blood glucose levels in a population of healthy, breast fed, term infants of appropriate size for gestational age. *Archives of Disease in Childhood—Fetal and Neonatal Edition, 83*, F117–F119.

Howard, C. R., Howard, F. M., Lanphear, B., Eberly, S., deBlieck, E. A., Oakes, D., & Lawrence, R. A. (2003). Randomized clinical trial of pacifier use and bottle-feeding or cup feeding and their effect on breastfeeding. *Pediatrics, 111*, 511–518.

Howard, C., Howard, F., Lawrence, R. Andresen, E., DeBlieck, E., & Wietzman, M. (2000). Office prenatal formula advertising and its effect on breast-feeding patterns. *Obstetrics & Gynecology, 95*, 296–303.

Huang, Y., Labinar-Wolfe, J., Huang, H., Choiniere, C. J., & Fein, S. B. (2013). Association of health profession and direct-to-consumer marketing with infant formula choice and switching. *Birth, 40*, 24–31.

Huppi, P. S., Warfield, S., Kikinis, R., Barnes, P. D., Zientara, G. P., Jolesz, F. A., & Volpe, J. J. (1998). Quantitative MRI of brain development in premature and mature brain. *Annals of Neurology, 43*, 224–236.

Hurst, N. (2007). Recognizing and treating delayed or failed lactogenesis II. *Journal of Midwifery and Women's Health, 52(6)*, 588–594.

Hyman, P. E., Milla, P. J., Benninga, M. A., Davidson, G. P., Fleisher, D. F., & Taminiau, J. (2006). Childhood functional gastrointestinal disorders: Neonate/toddler. *Gastroenterology, 130*, 1519–1526.

Iacono, G., Merolla, R., D'Amico, D., Bonci, E., Cavataio, F., DiPrima, L., & Paediatric Study Group on Gastrointestinal Symptoms in Infancy. (2005). Gastrointestinal symptoms in infancy: A population-based prospective study. *Digest of Liver Disease, 37*, 432–438.

Iacovou, M., Ralston, R., Muir, J., Walker, K. Z., & Truby, H. (2012). Dietary management of infantile colic: A systematic review. *Maternal and Child Health, 16*, 1319–1331.

Jaafar, S. H., Jahanfar, S., Angolkar, M., & Ho, J. J. (2012). Effect of restricted pacifier use in breastfeeding term infants for increasing duration of breastfeeding. *Cochrane Database of Systematic Reviews, 7*, CD007202.

Joeckel, R. J., & Phillips, S. K. (2009). Overview of infant and pediatric formulas. *Nutrition in Clinical Practice*, 24, 356–362.

Kattan, J. D., Cocco, R. R., & Jarvinen, K. M. (2011). Milk and soy allergy. *Pediatric Clinics of North America*, 58, 407–426.

Keefe, M. R. (1988). The impact of infant rooming-in on maternal sleep at night. *Journal of Obstetric, Gynecologic, and Neonatal Nursing, 17*, 122–126.

Kennedy, H. P. (2000). A model of exemplary midwifery practice: Results of a Delphi study. *Journal of Midwifery and Women's Health, 45*, 4–19.

Kervin, B. E., Kemp, L., & Pulver, L. J. (2010). Types and timing of breastfeeding support and its impact on mother's behaviours. *Journal of Paediatric and Child Health, 46*, 85–91.

King, T., Brucker, M. C., Kriebs, J., Fahey, J., Gegor, C., & Varney, H. (2015). *Varney's midwifery* (5th ed.). Burlington, MA: Jones & Bartlett Learning.

Klemola, T., Vanto, T., Juntunen-Backman, K., Kalimo, K., Korpela, R., & Varjonen, E. (2002). Allergy to soy formula and to extensively hydrolyzed whey formula in infant's with cow's milk allergy: A prospective, randomized study with a follow-up to the age of 2 years. *Journal of Pediatrics, 140*, 219–224.

Koivisto, M., Blanco-Sequeiros, M., & Krause, U. (1972). Neonatal symptomatic and asymptomatic hypoglycemia: A follow-up study of 151 children. *Developmental Medicine and Child Neurology, 14*, 603–614.

Kozhimannil, K. B., Attanasio, L. B., Hardeman, R. R., & O'Brien, M. (2013). Doula care supports near-universal breastfeeding initiation among diverse, low-income women. *Journal of Midwifery and Women's Health, 58*, 378–382.

Labinar-Wolfe, J., Fein, S. B., & Shealy, K. R. (2008). Infant formula-handling education and safety. *Pediatrics, 122*, Suppl 2: S85-S90.

La Leche League International. (2005). My breasts feel extremely full and uncomfortable. What is happening and what can I do about it? Retrieved from http://www.llli.org/faq/engorgement.html

Lasekan, J. B., Jacobs, J., Reisinger, K. S., Montalto, M. B., Frantz, M. P, & Blatter, M. M. (2011). Lactose-free milk protein–based infant formula: Impact on growth and gastrointestinal tolerance in infants. *Clinical Pediatrics, 50*, 330–337.

Lawrence, R. A., & Lawrence, R. M. (2001). *Breastfeeding: A guide for the medical profession* (6th ed.). New York, NY: Saunders.

Lawrence, R. A., & Lawrence, R. M. (2011). *Breastfeeding: A guide for the medical profession* (7th ed.). New York, NY: Saunders.

Lee, E. (2007). Health, morality and infant feeding: British mothers' experiences of formula milk use in the early weeks. *Social Health and Illness, 29*, 1075–1090.

Lucas, A., Morley, R., & Cole, T. J. (1998). Randomised trial of early diet in preterm babies and later intelligence quotient. *British Medical Journal, 31*, 1481–1487.

Lucas, A., Morley, R., Cole, T. J., Gore, S. M., Lucas, P. J., Crowle, P., & Powell, R. (1990). Early diet in preterm babies and developmental status at 18 months. *Lancet, 335*, 1477–1481.

Lucas, R., Gupton, S., Holditch-Davis, D., & Brandon, D. (2014). A case study of a late preterm infant's transition to full at breast feedings at 4 months of age. *Journal of Human Lactation, 30*, 28–30.

Lucassen, P., Assendelft, W., Gubbles, J., van Eijk, J. T., & Douwes, A. C. (2000). Infantile colic: Crying time reduction with whey hydrolysate: A double-blind randomized, placebo-controlled trial. *Pediatrics, 106*, 1349–1354.

Marin-Gabriel, M. A., Llana-Martin, I., Lopez-Escobar, A., Fernandez Villalba, E., Romero Blanco, I., & Touza Pol, P. (2010). Randomized controlled trial of early skin-to-skin contact: Effects on the mother and newborn. *Acta Paediatrica, 99*, 1630–1634.

Martinez, J. A., & Ballew, M. P. (2011). Infant formulas. *Pediatric Review, 32*, 179–189.

McKechnie, A. C., & Eglash, A. (2010). Nipple shields: A review of the literature. *Breastfeeding Medicine, 5,* 309–314.

Meier, P. P., Furman, L. M., & Degenhardt, M. (2007). Increased lactation risk for late preterm infants and mothers: Evidence and management strategies to protect breastfeeding. *Journal of Midwifery and Women's Health, 52,* 579–587.

Mikiel-Kostyra, K., Mazur, J., & Boltruszko, I., (2002). Effect of early skin-to-skin contact after delivery on duration of breastfeeding: A prospective cohort study. *Acta Paediatrica, 91,* 1301–1306.

Montgomery, A., Hale, T. W., & Academy of Breastfeeding Medicine (ABM). (2012). ABM clinical protocol #15: Analgesia and anesthesia for the breastfeeding mother, revised 2012. *Breastfeed Medicine, 7,* 547–553.

Moore, E. R., Abderson, G. C., Bergman, N., & Dowswell, T. (2012). Early skin-to-skin contact for mothers and their healthy newborn infants. *Cochrane Database of Systematic Reviews, 5,* CD003519.

Moukarzel, A. A., Abdelnour, H., & Akatcherian, C. (2007). Effects of a pre-thickened formula on esophageal pH and gastric emptying of infants with GER. *Journal of Clinical Gastroenterology, 41,* 823–829.

Nagulesapillai, T., McDonald, S. W., Fenton, T. R., Mercader, H. F., & Tough S. C. (2103). Breastfeeding difficulties and exclusivity among late preterm and term infants: results from the all babies study. *Canadian Journal of Public Health, 104*(4), e351–e356.

National Association of Neonatal Nurses (NANN). (2009). *Position statement #3046: The use of human milk and breastfeeding in the neonatal intensive care unit.* Glenview, IL: Author.

National Childbirth Trust, United Kingdom. (1997). Hypoglycemia of the newborn: Guidelines for appropriate blood glucose screening and treatment of breast-fed and bottle-fed babies in the UK. *Midwives, 110,* 248–249.

Neu, M., Corwin, E., Lareau, S. C., & Marcheggiani-Howard, C. (2012). A review of non-surgical treatment for the symptoms of irritability in infants with GERD. *Journal for Specialists in Pediatric Nursing, 17,* 177–192.

Nevo, N., Rubin, L., Tamir, A., Levine, A., & Shaoul, R. (2007). Infant feeding patterns in the first 6 months: An assessment in full-term infants. *Journal of Pediatric Gastroenterology and Nutrition, 45,* 234–239.

Nyqvist, K. H., Farnstrand, C., Eeg-Olofsson, K. E., & Ewald, U. (2001). Early oral behavior in preterm infants during breastfeeding: An electromyographic study. *Acta Paediatr, 90*(6): 658–663.

O'Connor, N. R. (2009). Infant formula. *American Family Physician, 79,* 565–570.

Oski, F. A., Bennett, R., & Campbell, J.(1980). Iron-fortified formulas and gastrointestinal symptoms in infants: A controlled study. *Pediatrics, 66,* 168–1

Perez-Escamilla, R., Pollitt, E., Lonnerdal, B., & Dewey, K. G. (1994). Infant feeding policies in maternity wards and their effect on breastfeeding success: An analytical overview. *American Journal of Public Health, 84,* 89–97.

Perrine, C. G., Scanlon, K. S., Li, R., Odem, E., & Grummer-Strawn, L. M. (2012). Baby-friendly hospital practices and meeting exclusive breastfeeding intention. *Pediatrics, 130,* 54–60.

Petrikovsky, B. M., Kaplan, G. P., & Pestrak, H. (1995). The application of color Doppler technology to study of fetal swallowing. *Obstetrics & Gynecology, 86,* 605–608.

Phillips, R. M., Goldstein, M., Hougland, K., Nandyal, R., Pizzica, A., Santa-Donato, A., & National Perinatal Association. (2013). Multidisciplinary guidelines for the care of late preterm infants. *Journal of Perinatology, 33*(suppl 2), S5–S22.

Polack, F. P., Khan, N., & Maisels, M. J. (1999). Changing partners: The dance of infant formula changes. *Clinical Pediatrics, 38,* 703–708.

Preer, G., Pisegna, J. M., Cook, J. T., Henri, A. M., & Philipp, B. L. (2013). Delaying the bath and in-hospital breastfeeding rates. *Breastfeeding Medicine, 8,* 485–490.

Radtke, J. V. (2011). The paradox of breastfeeding associated morbidity among late preterm infants. *Journal of Obstetric, Gynecologic, and Neonatal Nursing, 40*, 9–24.

Reilly, S., Reid, J., Skeat, J., & Academy of Breastfeeding Medicine (ABM). (2013). Guidelines for breastfeeding infants with cleft lip, cleft palate and cleft lip and palate. *Breastfeeding Medicine, 8*(4), 349–353.

Renfrew, M. J., McCormick, F. M., Quinn, W. A., & Dowswell, T. (2012). Support for healthy breastfeeding mothers with healthy term babies. *Cochrane Database of Systematic Reviews, 5*, CD001141.

Riordan, J., & Wambach, K. (2010). *Breastfeeding and human lactation* (4th ed.). Sudbury, MA: Jones and Bartlett.

Ross, M. G., & Nijland, M. J. M. (1997). Fetal swallowing: Relationship to amniotic fluid regulation. *Clinical Obstetrics and Gynecology, 40*, 352–365.

Rotundo, G. (2011). Centering pregnancy: The benefits of group prenatal care. *Nursing for Women's Health, 15*, 508–517.

Rozance, P. J., McGowan, J. E., Price-Douglas, W., & Hay, W. W., Jr. (2016). Glucose homeostasis. In S. L. Gardner, B. S. Carter, M. Enzman Hines, & J. A. Hernandez (Eds.), *Merenstein and Gardner's handbook of neonatal intensive care* (8th ed., pp. 337–359). St. Louis, MO: Mosby-Elsevier.

Sexson, W. R. (1984). Incidence of neonatal hypoglycemia: a matter of definition. *Journal of Pediatrics, 105*, 149–150.

Shergill-Bonner, R. (2010). Infantile colic: Practicalities of management, including dietary aspects. *Journal of Family Health Care, 20*, 206–209.

Sherman, A. L., Anderson, J., & Rudolph, C. D. (2015). Lactose-free milk or soy-based formulas do not improve caregivers' distress or perceptions of difficult infant behavior. *Journal of Pediatric Gastroenterology and Nutrition, 61*(1), 119–124.

Singhal, A., Morley, R., Abbott, R., Fairweather-Tait, S., Stephenson, T., & Lucas, A. (2000). Clinical safety of iron-fortified formulas. *Pediatrics, 105*, e38.

Snell, B. J., Krantz, M., Keeton, R., Delgado, K., & Peckham, C. (1992). The association of formula samples given at hospital discharge with the early duration of breastfeeding. *Journal of Human Lactation, 8*, 67–72.

Stephens, B. E., Walden, R. V., Gargus, R. A., Tucker, R., McKinley, L., Mance, M., & Vohr, B. R. (2009). First week protein and energy intakes are associated with 18 month developmental outcomes in extremely low birthweight infants. *Pediatrics, 123*, 1337–1343.

Straussman, S., & Levisky, L. L. (2010). Neonatal hypoglycemia. *Current Opinion in Endocrinology, Diabetes & Obesity, 17*, 20–24.

Sudfeld, C. R., Fawzi, W. W., & Lahanya, C. (2012). Peer support and exclusive breastfeeding duration in low and middle-income countries: A systematic review and meta-analysis. *PLoS One, 7*, e45143.

Swenne, I., Ewald, U., Gustafsson, J., Sandberg, E., & Ostenson, C. G. (1994). Inter-relationship between serum concentrations of glucose, glucagon, and insulin during the first two days of life in healthy newborns. *Acta Paediatrica, 83*, 915–919.

Tabbers, M. M., DiLorenzo, C., Berger, M. Y., Faure, C., Langendam, M. W., Nurko, S., . . . Benninga, M. A. (2014). Evaluation and treatment of functional constipation in infants and children: Evidence-based recommendations from ESPGHAN and NASPGHAN. *Journal of Pediatric Gastroenterology and Nutrition, 58*, 258–274.

Tarrant, R. (2007). Safety first. *World of Irish Nursing and Midwifery, 15*, 28–29.

Tunc, V. T., Camurdan, A. D., Ilhan, M. N., Sahin, F., & Beyazova, U. (2008). Factors associated with defecation patterns in 0–24-month-old children. *European Journal of Pediatrics, 167*, 1357–1362.

Vandenplas, Y., & Alarcon, P. (2015). Updated algorithms for managing frequent gastrointestinal symptoms in infants, *Beneficial Microbes, 6*(2), 199–208.

Vandenplas, Y., Lifshitz, J. Z., Orenstein, S., Lifshitz, C. H., Shepherd, R. W., Casaubon, P. R., & Lifshitz, F. (1998). Nutritional management of regurgitation in infants. *Journal of the American College of Nutrition, 17,* 308–316.

Vandenplas, Y., Rudolph, C. D., DiLorenzo, C., Hassall, E., Liptak, G., Mazur, L., Sondheimer, J., & North American Society for Pediatric Gastroenterology, Hepatology, and Nutrition; & European Society for Pediatric Gastroenterology, Hepatology, and Nutrition. (2009). Pediatric gastroesophageal reflux clinical practice guidelines: Joint recommendations of the North American Society for Pediatric Gastroenterology, Hepatology, and Nutrition (NASPGHAN) and the European Society for Pediatric Gastroenterology, Hepatology, and Nutrition (ESPGHAN). *Journal of Pediatric Gastroenterology and Nutrition, 49,* 498–547.

Vanderhoof, J. A., Moran, J. R., Harris, C. L., Merkel, K. L., & Orenstein, S. R. (2003). Efficacy of a pre-thickened infant formula: A multicenter, double-blind, randomized, placebo-controlled parallel group trial in 104 infants with gastroesophageal reflux. *Clinical Pediatrics, 42,* 483–495.

Venter, C., & Dean, T. (2008). Caring for the newborn: Infant nutrition part 1. *British J Midwifery, 16,* 726–733.

Vighi, G., Marcucci, F., Sensi, L., Cara, G., & Frati, F. (2008). Allergy and the gastrointestinal system. *Clinical Experiments in Immunology, 145*(suppl 1), 3–6.

Waldenstrom, U., & Swenson, A. (1991). Rooming-in at night in the postpartum ward. *Midwifery, 7,* 82–89.

Wang, M., Dorer, D., Fleming, M., et al. (2004). Clinical outcomes of near-term infants. *Pediatrics, 114*(6), 372–392.

Wessel, J. J. (2011). Nutrition and the late preterm infant. *NICU Currents,* (3), 1–6.

Widstrom, A. M., Lilja, G., Aaltomaa-Michalias, P., Dahllof, A., Lintula, M., & Nissen, E. (2011). Newborn behavior to locate the breast when skin-to-skin: A possible method for enabling early self-regulation. *Acta Paediatrica, 100,* 79–85.

Widstrom, A. M., Ransjo-Arvidson, A. B., Christensson, K., Matthiesen, A. S., Winberg, J., & Uvnas-Moberg, K. (1987). Gastric suction in healthy newborn infants: Effects on circulation and developing feeding behaviour. *Acta Paediatrica Scandinavica, 76,* 566–572.

Wiener, S. (2006). Diagnosis and management of candida of the nipple and breast. *Journal of Midwifery and Women's Health, 51(2),* 125<n dash>128.

Wight, N., Marinelli, K., & Academy of Breastfeeding Medicine (ABM). (2014). ABM clinical protocol #1: Guidelines for blood glucose monitoring and treatment of hypoglycemia in term and late-preterm neonates. *Breastfeeding Medicine, 9,* 173–179.

Williams, A. F. (1997). *Hypoglycemia of the newborn: Review of the literature.* Geneva, Switzerland: World Health Organization.

World Health Organization (WHO), UNICEF, & Wellstart International. (2009). Baby-friendly hospital initiative: Revised, updated and expanded for integrated care. Retrieved from http://www.unicef.org/nutrition/files/BFHI_2009_s1.pdf

World Health Organization (WHO). (2010). *Guidelines on HIV and infant feeding.* Geneva, Switzerland: World Health Organization.

Worobey, J., Pena, J., Ramos, I., & Espinosa, C. (2014). Infant difficulty and early weight gain: Does fussing promote overfeeding? *Maternal and Child Nutrition, 10,* 295–303.

Zeigler, R. S., Sampson, H. A., Bock, S. A., Burks, A. W., Jr., Harden, K., Noone, S., & Wilson, G. (1999). Soy allergy in infants and children with IgE-associated cow's milk allergy. *Journal of Pediatrics, 134*(5), 614–622.

Zeno, R., Hosley, S., & Steward, D. (2015). Formula intolerance: Pathology or normal neonatal physiology? *Pediatric Currents, 7,* 1–6.

CHAPTER 6

DEVELOPMENTAL CARE OF THE WELL NEWBORN

Barbara A. Overman and Dorinda L. Welle

Developmental care facilitates optimal newborn development and maternal–newborn intimacy. Maternal–child nursing brings a substantial history of promoting care for the maternal–infant dyad, including the processes of acquaintance and parental role attainment (Mercer, 1995; Rubin, 1967). Pediatric medical learning from the devastating outcomes of prolonged maternal–newborn separation in the early days of neonatal intensive care (Klaus & Kennell, 1976) further laid the foundation for maternal–newborn care models that include "rooming-in" and its associated staffing—that is, "couplet care," in which a single nurse is assigned to care for one dyad.

In this chapter, we describe a psychodynamic approach to developmental care, with an appreciation of the term newborn's impressive capacities not only for behavior but also for awareness, emotion, and relating. A rich heritage of maternal–child nursing theory and practice, midwifery and psychoanalytic theory, and clinical research informs the psychological dimension of physiological processes (Winnicott, 1960, 1965) and the dyadic (mother–baby) context of newborn states and newborn behavior.

This approach to developmental care also draws on an exciting body of neurologic research that challenges old views of infant development as the achievement of *self-regulation* and demonstrates the numerous ways that newborns and mothers engage in *co-regulation* (for a review, see Trevarthen & Aiken, 2001). Newborn development depends on the successful orchestration of physiological processes not only through maternal care but also through the emerging relationship between mother and infant. In this chapter, we apply psycho-analytic concepts to inform ways that developmental care providers can effectively support co-regulation and maternal–newborn wellness through the sometimes organized and some-times disorganized periods of newborn development in the first 28 days of life. Similar to the ways that midwifery philosophy and practice "hold" the space for physiological birth and "hold aside" those aspects of medical intervention that may interfere with the birth process, this approach to developmental care aims to "hold" the space for the newborn's emergence into an infant (Mahler, Pine, & Bergman, 1999) and the dyad's emergence into the family (Winnicott, 1960). An approach that highlights the emotional dimensions of maternal–newborn care might seem like a luxury in many of today's efficiency-oriented and task-intensive healthcare systems and households. Nevertheless, we argue that the substantial evidence base on the relational nature of newborn development and the significant challenges to successful co-regulation of newborn states and developmental processes introduces a compelling ethical dimension to developmental care.

This chapter emerged from an interprofessional dialogue between a midwife with clinical and academic engagement in newborn care and an anthropologist trained in psychoanalytic parent–infant observation. Each of us was curious about the foundational concepts that "the other" brings to understanding mothers and newborns. What does each of us "see" when we encounter or think about a mother and baby in the context of parent–infant observation or midwifery practice? Initially and for quite a while, we listened—and spoke—from a place of "not knowing" (see Trevarthen, 2011) how our different approaches might meet or how they might gain meaning for the other. In the process, we began to "see" an approach to develop-mental care of the well newborn that could take both newborn and mother into account. We also began to "see" newborn behavior and newborn states in a different light. As we present this conceptual foundation and this description of newborn development in the first month of life, practitioners might recognize in our descriptions things they already do and phenomena they have already observed. We offer this chapter as an invitation to think together and further elaborate this approach to developmental care.

Conceptual Foundations of Developmental Care of the Well Newborn

The notion that human development is characterized by periods of stability punctuated by periods of instability and change has informed multidisciplinary understandings of the devel-opment of species (Eldredge, 1985; Gould & Eldredge, 1977), the social organization of groups (Gersick, 1988, 1989, 1991), and the development of infants and children (Brazelton & Sparrow,

2003). In 1934, the educational theorist Vygotsky (1998) described "the crisis of the newborn" in its brand-new developmental phase, introducing the concept of "regression" as a normal feature of successful developmental processes:

> At this time, the child regresses at first even with respect to physical development: in the first days after birth, the newborn loses weight. Adaptation to the new form of life places such high demands on the vitality of the child that, in the words of Blonsky (1930, p. 85), man never stands as close to death as in the hours of his birth. (1998 [original 1934], p. 194)

Contemporary clinical knowledge assures us that newborn weight loss is normal—hardly representing a "crisis"—but this was exactly Vygotsky's (1998) point: that loss of some kind, whether it be weight loss soon after birth, or the temporary loss of recently gained developmental capabilities, is a hallmark and often a predictor of subsequent physiological, emotional, cognitive, and/or social maturation of the infant.

More than half a century later, Brazelton and Sparrow (Brazelton, 1992; Brazelton & Sparrow, 2001, 2003) popularized the notion of normal moments of infant or toddler "regression" that are then followed by "bursts" in developmental gains as a normal and continuous developmental sequence. During a "touchpoint"—defined as the moment of disorganization preceding a developmental leap forward—the infant reverts to behavior patterns (such as inconsolable crying or frequent night waking) that he or she recently "outgrew," while preparing to consolidate new behaviors and cognitive abilities. When the infant takes "one step back" in his or her development, the accompanying behavior changes can generate considerable concern and stress in parents, who may have been counting on the infant's developmental gains to normalize their own everyday routines. Thus Brazelton and Sparrow note that "children's spurts in development (can) result in disruption in the family system" (2003, p. 1).

Newborn development can be considered as occurring within the family as an interpretive system. Interpretation of newborn behavior is informed by many sources, including cultural beliefs, accumulated knowledge from raising other children, the lens of depression or other mental health conditions, and spoken and unspoken feelings about the conception, pregnancy, birth, and presence of a particular baby. Parents are not only trying to "read" or interpret their newborn's "cues," but newborns are also busy frowning, staring, peeking, and feeling their way through their mother's "cues" (Mahler et al., 1999). Developmental care seeks less to offer expert interpretations of the newborn and more to support empathy (Winnicott, 1960) and "alive communication" (Fogel & Garvey, 2007) for the baby's needs, qualities, and developmental experiences.

Parents can sometimes impose adult intentions and motivations on newborn behavior (Kamel & Dockrell, 2000), particularly when the baby is taking that one step back before moving two steps forward in the development trajectory. For example, parents may believe that the infant is rejecting parental caregiving or leveling a criticism of parents' competence. At these moments, providers may reassure parents that the infant is simply going through a growth spurt that will soon resolve (Brazelton & Sparrow, 2001).

While offering anticipatory guidance is appropriate and can reassure parents, listening to the specific interpretations that parents generate to explain the infant's behavior or the infant's change in responsiveness to parental caregiving can be illuminating. Interpretations (Pancheri, 1997) can be informed by cultural orientation, trauma history of the mother, religious beliefs, the experience of and expectations surrounding this particular baby's birth, and the clinical advice of providers: each of these factors infuses the interpretive environment of newborn development. A parent's particular ideas about the infant's intentions or the infant's feelings toward specific parents or siblings have meaning and consequence for that infant's development, that parent's own development, and the quality of the parent's relationship with the infant.

Although the "family system" may experience social disruption during an infant's growth spurt, such moments can help illuminate individual parents' and siblings' psychological barriers to adaptation and empathy, which may be reinforced or activated by the infant's disorganization and distress during normal developmental processes. These developmental crunch points for the infant may trigger parallel disorganization and distress in parents and siblings, particularly in a family member coping with depression, substance abuse, lack of support, or other challenges. The presence of a newborn in the family can be understood as launching a new chapter in the developmental journey of each family member, a journey specific to that person's own life history and identity that also activates the family as an interpretive system, with implications for the quality of caregiving for the newborn. How do particular family members call out the newborn's behaviors, and which emotions and ideas do the newborn's changes in behavior call up in different family members?

Compared to the touchpoints approach, with its focus "on caregiving themes that matter to parents (e.g., feeding, discipline), rather than traditional [infant development] milestones" (Brazelton & Sparrow, 2001; Sparrow & Brazelton, 2009), developmental care in the neonatal period aims to describe the key newborn development processes in a way that guides providers to help parents to "see" these foundational processes, sustain empathy, and provide the caregiving that needs to attend them. Providers have a unique opportunity during the neonatal period to help parents understand and imagine some of the invisible developmental processes that the newborn and the mother separately and together are working to achieve. Being able to "see" the newborn's completion of a distinct maturational process can allow parents to reinterpret the baby's behaviors and their own effectiveness and tolerate the distress that can accompany difficult-to-observe developmental processes.

Midwives and pediatricians have advocated for the centrality of the supportive birth environment, challenging the assumption that "controlled" hospital-based environments optimally support birth. Although popular wisdom associates home birth and water birth with physically and socially supportive environments, these settings were promoted as ideal psychological environments to facilitate the alteration of the birthing woman's consciousness as labor progresses. Michel Odent (1983, 1986) refers to this "lowering"—or *"abaissement"*—of the birthing woman's consciousness as a necessary condition for allowing and tolerating the "primal states"—both physical and emotional—involved in birth.

Fahey and colleagues (Fahey, Foureur, & Hastie, 2008; Fahey & Hastie, 2008; Fahey & Parratt, 2006; Hastie, 2008) advance a similar premise in their midwifery theory of birth territory and midwifery guardianship, arguing that the alteration in the mother's consciousness during birth creates vulnerability that demands "ethical guardianship" of the birthing woman's environment (Fahey & Hastie, 2008, p. 31). This guardianship involves "holding open" the space for physiologic or normal birth by, on the one hand, securing the physical and social features of a facilitative environment and, on the other hand, "holding out" those persons or stimuli that might interfere with *abaissement* and successful completion of birth.

Developmental care extends this framework to the neonatal period, during which providers can help "hold" the developmental environment at a particularly vulnerable phase for mother and newborn. Psychoanalyst and pediatrician Donald Winnicott (1960) considered the newborn's earliest phase of development to be the "holding phase," when the newborn is "maximally dependent" on maternal care. This "holding" informs developmental care of the well newborn:

> The term "holding" here is used to denote not only the actual physical holding of the infant, but also the total environmental provision prior to the concept of [the infant] "living with" [her/his parents]. . . . It includes the management of experiences that are inherent in existence, such as the *completion* (and therefore the *non-completion*) of processes: processes which from the outside may seem to be purely physiological but which belong to infant psychology and take place in a complex psychological field, determined by the awareness and empathy of the mother. (Winnicott, 1960, pp. 43–44)

These key developmental processes during the neonatal period or "holding phase" are, as we will describe in detail later, characterized by moments of organization and pattern, disorganization and distress—making them amenable to unobtrusive "holding" by the developmental care provider. As with developmental care, "when [maternal care] goes well it is scarcely noticed [by the baby], and is a continuation of the physiological provision that characterizes the prenatal state" (Winnicott, 1960, p. 592).

Developmental care aims to provide the mother and newborn with the supportive conditions that will enable the newborn to emerge during the neonatal period as a human infant (Mahler et al., 1999) whose potential can begin to be realized in the context of maternal care.

The developmental care approach to "holding" the maternal–newborn dyad involves a certain "holding back" of performances of professional expertise, demonstrations of caregiving, and predictions of developmental process resolution. It aims instead to "hold" the mother and newborn in a way that allows them to orchestrate the awareness, responsiveness, and adaptability for a lifetime of developmental flow that includes, over and again, moments of completion, organization, and new abilities, eventually followed by phases of temporary loss of these celebrated or taken-for-granted gains and the distressing, yet vital work of reorganization for new capabilities and new maturity.

In the era of evidence-based care, exerting professional restraint may seem like a "step back" for providers who have come to take for granted the didactic, information-based approach to instructing mothers about newborn care. From a psychoanalytic perspective, "regression in the service of the other"—that is, reverting to a prior state when one did not so much "know" as "feel," or when one is in touch with earlier ways of being and ways of relating—is a part of clinical work that establishes the "precondition for empathy" (Olinick, 1969; Balint, 1968; Cooper, 1989). Similarly, mothers of newborns may engage in "regression in the service of the baby" (Bergman, 1999; also see Mahler et al., 1999; Winnicott, 1960), a process in which the mother may "move in and out of states of loss of interest in other relationships so that she can lose herself in empathy and intimacy with her infant" (Bergman, 1999, p. 165; Odent, 1984). Lest regression become gender stereotyped, Odent (1999a) has noted that fathers who support their partners in birth often regress after the baby is born, coming down with nameless aches, flu, or "feeling drained." In this extension of professional empathy for the emotionally demanding states that mother and baby are experiencing, developmental care providers aim to "hold" and serve as guardians of the developmental environment of mother and newborn and their family.

This shared developmental environment is understood as a space in which emotion, sensory experience, and the mutual awareness of mother and newborn are continually communicated, thanks to the newborn's capacity for "affect sharing" and "emotional contagion." Newborns evidence an awareness of the difference between their own cry and the cries of other newborns, and newborns find the cries of other newborns to be compelling. Neurologic research has demonstrated that "affect sharing [and] emotional contagion [are] already developed in the newborn. Emotion recognition and sharing emerge in the newborn much earlier than 'theory of mind' [i.e., thinking]" (Lagercrantz & Changeux, 2009, p. 258).

This body of research about newborns has transformed our understanding of the emotional dimension of what previously has been defined as exclusively instinctual behavior in the newborn. The hunger for air that emerges at birth can be called a primordial emotion (Denton, 2005). This first arousal drives the newborn to spontaneously explore the world, particularly to search for food in the mother's breast (Lagercrantz & Changeux, 2009). No longer seen only as a physiological state, newborn crying has "neural correlates for a 'conscious' social communication of the newborn with his/her caretaker" (Lagercrantz & Changeux, 2009, p. 258).

Research with infants and mothers has further shown that newborns register maternal emotion through a multiplicity of avenues, including maternal facial expression, physiological indicators of maternal distress, maternal voice, and maternal handling of the newborn (Markova & Legerstee, 2006). As one large study of depressed mothers concluded:

> Not every baby is [severely] affected by a depressed mother who perhaps cries when she meets his gaze. Others, however, react by rejecting the mother's attempts to make contact and start whining. (Karolinska Institutet, 2010 citing Salomonsson, 2010)

Studies of pregnant women who lost their partners on September 11, 2001, provide a poignant window into their newborns' frustrated efforts to soothe their bereaved mothers (Moscowitz, 2012).

It is precisely this bidirectional communication of emotion between mother and newborn, newborn and mother, which developmental care providers can help to "hold" or contain. Within this developmental environment occur the many "hidden co-regulators" (Hofer, 1994; also see Hofer, 1984):

> "The seemingly minor aspects of social interaction . . . the non-verbal signals, mannerisms, tones of voices, gestures, facial expressions, brief touches, and even the timing of events and pauses between words . . . which have physiologic consequences—often outside the awareness of the participants. (Hofer, 1984, p. 194)

Given the impossibility and undesirability of trying to educate mothers to mechanically orchestrate co-regulation with their newborn, developmental care might adopt an approach in the spirit of "biological nurturing," which promotes "nurturing and enjoyment" (Batacan, 2010) of not just newborn caregiving but also maternal–newborn intimacy and communication. This approach shares the central aim of psychoanalytic mother–infant observation (Miller, 1997) and mother–infant psychoanalytic treatment—namely, to enable mother and baby "to find each other in a calm, safe environment" (Karolinska Institutet, 2010; Salomonsson, 2014) and attune to each other (Markova & Legerstee, 2006). As we will see in the next sections, newborn development in the first 28 days is characterized by sequences of organized and seemingly disorganized behavior. By "seeing" these sequences, the developmental processes they contain, and the challenges that newborn and mother encounter in sustaining their teamwork, developmental care providers can facilitate empathy and contain the mother and newborn while attending to the successful completion of essential developmental processes.

Developmental Care and Neonatal Behavioral Transition

At birth, the newborn engages her senses and capacities for expression in the air and light of the extrauterine world. The dramatic increase in oxygenation, withdrawal of intrauterine neurosteriods, catecholamine rush, and presence of peaked and pulsatile oxytocin "turn up" the senses in the baby's first moments of life. The baby enters her new human environment engulfed in a flood of sensory neural impulses that ushers in postnatal neural network formation, which will shape the infant's brain (Lagercrantz & Changeux, 2009).

During fetal life, gamma-aminobutyric acid (GABA) is the dominant excitatory neurotransmitter; in extrauterine life, however, GABA becomes an inhibitory neurotransmitter and glutamate and aspartate serve as the dominant excitatory hormones (Lagercrantz, Hanson, Evrard, & Rodeck, 2002; Letinic, Zoncu, & Rakic, 2002). The fetus is comparatively sedated by the low oxygen tension of fetal blood and neurosteroid suppressors of neuronal activity (pregnanolone and prostaglandin D_2) (Mellor, Diesch, Gunn, & Bennett, 2005). One viewpoint considers the fetus "unconscious," with birth arousing the newborn to wakefulness and conscious experience (Lagercrantz & Changeux, 2009). Interestingly, at the time of transition from fetal to newborn life, the functions of the primary neurotransmitter chemicals change, triggered by altered intracellular ion concentrations and oxytocin release that occur around the time of birth (Tyzio et al., 2006).

The baby's brain at birth has an almost adult number of neurons, albeit with immature connections among them. Overproduction of synapses accompanied by a process of synaptic elimination and stabilization in the earliest months of life is a "pruning" process guided by interactions with the environment (Lagercrantz & Changeux, 2009; Monk & Hane, 2014; Nelson & Bosquet, 2000). This brain-shaping process begins in the first moments of life and continues into adolescence.

The presence and maturing functionality of brain structures and early connections among them provide the potential for conscious content in the newborn period, according to brain researchers. Starting at about 34 weeks' gestational age, a synchrony of EEG impulses across the two hemispheres of the fetus's brain and the formation of long-range colossal connections provides neurobiological evidence of a global neural workspace (GNW) (Changeux & Dehaene, 2008; Vanhatalo & Kaila, 2006). The vertical brain stem, diencephalic, and thalamo-cortical pathways that regulate states of consciousness become established; once these pathways connect with the GNW, the hard-wiring necessary for newborn consciousness is present.

In summarizing the research on newborn consciousness, Lagercrantz and Changeux (2009, p. 259) detail the newborn's considerable capacity for awareness and emotion:

[T]he newborn infant can be awake, exhibit sensory awareness, and process memorized mental representations. It is also able to differentiate between self and non-self touch, express emotions, and show signs of shared feelings. Yet, it is unreflective, present oriented, and makes little reference to a concept of him/herself. *Newborn infants display features characteristic of what may be referred to as basic consciousness* and they still have to undergo considerable maturation to reach the level of adult consciousness.

The baby's birth and earliest experiences release biological substrates that are known to accompany "positive emotion" (Dixon, Skinner, & Foureur, 2013; Nissen, Lilja, Widström, & Uvnäs-Moberg, 1995; Odent, 1999b). Specifically, high levels of oxytocin and the physiology of transition start up the nerve connections between the brain stem and the right prefrontal cortex (Lipton, 2005), a collection called the reticular activating system (RAS). The RAS links somatic (bodily) and neural function and is fully activated by the end of the first period of reactivity of the transition to extrauterine life: Put simply, the mind–body connection is established.

These awakenings of consciousness in the birthing newborn co-occur with maternal consciousness alterations that facilitate birth. The baby experiences a *birth of consciousness*, whereas the mother experiences a *consciousness of birth*—the first experience of dyadic consciousness in the early moments of newborn life and newborn–parental acquaintance. Primal states of awareness (Odent, 1986) predominate for mother and baby and facilitate the newborn's transition to extrauterine life, completing the first process of neonatal behavioral development and ushering in what Winnicott calls the "holding phase," which may last beyond the first 28 days. It is a time when developmental care calls for "holding" the dyad, by providing emotional containment and ethical guardianship as mother and baby begin to recover from the birth experience.

The Predictable Behavioral Sequence

The behavioral and psychological aspects of transition in the well newborn include the initial state changes, readiness for interactions, and accompanying behaviors involved in recovery from birth and neonatal emergence. Within each of the three periods of transition, optimal developmental care for the dyad maintains the goal of facilitating and fostering healthy *process completion* (Winnicott, 1960).

The first period of reactivity is primarily influenced by high levels of catecholamine, the hormone of the sympathetic nervous system. Concurrently, neurosuppressor hormone levels decrease as oxytocin and oxygen levels increase (Lagercrantz & Changeux, 2009).

The first period of wakefulness including active and quiet alert states can last as long as 2 hours (Graves & Haley, 2013).

Newborns supported prone on the mother's abdomen and chest demonstrate exploratory behaviors as they touch their mother's skin for the first time. Skin-to-skin contact with the mother keeps the newborn warm and supports the pre-latch sequence of neonatal behaviors. The newborn is drawn to the aroma of components in the mother's breastmilk, which resembles the aroma of the amniotic fluid on the baby's hands. Guided by touch and smell, the newborn's process of "crawling" along the mother's body in the direction of the breast activates neurologic connections that support development of pre-latch, latch, and feeding behavior. Baby behavior includes the anti-gravity movement of head righting and lifting, which progresses and supports successful root, gape, latch, and suck (Colson, Meek, & Hawdon, 2008; Righard & Alade, 1990).

The newborn gut is activated by mechanical ingestion of air and hormonal changes that activate gut maturation (Van Woudenberg, Wills, & Rubarth, 2012). The baby's successful first experience on the mother's body, including salivation, latching, sucking, and ingesting the first drops of colostrum, stimulates postnatal gastrointestinal startup. Peristalsis begins and post-birth immunologic, digestive, and excretory processes are initiated.

Developmental care guides providers to foster newborn–maternal exploration and the completion of the first feeding without undue interruption (Widströmet et al., 2011; Widström & Thingström Paulsson, 1993; Winnicott, 1960). Affective (rather than cognitive) approaches to communication are optimal during this time period. Rather than an occasion for providing information-driven patient education, this is the time to facilitate mother and newborn in exploring and becoming acquainted in "the self-attach space" of the maternal abdomen (Cadwell, 2007). Developmental care respects the newborn's process of breastfeeding in the initial hours and days after birth (Cadwell, 2007; Righard & Alade, 1990). At birth, hand-drying of the newborn is minimized to preserve the olfactory cue of amniotic fluid that stimulates suckling first on the neonate's hands and then on the maternal nipple. The most important role of professional providers is to maintain patience, empathy, and noninterference in "holding" the mother's and baby's efforts.

Developmental care engages with parents in interpreting newborn behavior and its relational qualities. Even for mothers with older children, each baby presents something new and different in terms of the infant's needs and experience of development, which must be learned firsthand. Providers can foster tactful observation of moments of each newborn's response to the mother, noting the many ways that the mother is co-regulating the newborn through touch, heartbeat, voice, warmth, smell, feeding, and holding.

The post-birth sleep period is characterized by a drowsy to deep sleep state that commonly lasts approximately 1 to 4 hours. The baby is usually difficult to rouse or wake during this time, and bowel sounds are usually present (Graves & Haley, 2013; Van Woudenberg et al.,

2012). Developmental care includes interpreting the baby's cues of state change toward sleep (i.e., disengagement or eye rubbing) and helping parents understand this state as restorative rest from the exertion of birth and activity of the first period of reactivity.

Developmental care aims to avoid interrupting the first period of sleep. With potential new visitors arriving and eager to "meet the baby" and medical administrative staff eager to conduct their procedures, ethical guardianship of this period of first sleep is warranted. There is no need for separation, as care can be provided while the newborn is being held by parents. If both mother and newborn are recovering normally from birth, the baby can remain prone on the mother's abdomen. If the mother needs a time of separation to restore herself through food, sleep, and bathing, the newborn can remain skin-to-skin with the mother's partner.

The behaviors of the second period of reactivity may look disorganized and distressing to parents, who commonly interpret them as illness or difficulty breathing. Attending to parents' interpretations can assist parents to appreciate these behaviors as protective strengths related to adjusting to extrauterine life. Providers should support the mother in holding the baby in prone position, patting the neonate's back to facilitate secretion drainage, and massaging the back to support normal process. After several hours of the second period of reactivity, the baby is calm, with stable vital signs, and feeds again, signaling the end of transition.

Newborn States: Co-regulation for Process Completion

Behavioral states are the foundation for understanding the newborn and her capacity for organized behavior. Defined as "recurrent ensembles of behavior that have similar characteristics" (Nugent, Keefer, Minear, Johnson, & Blanchard, 2007, p. 9), states are an innate organizing structure. This "structure" of different newborn behavior states, their distinctiveness in the individual, and the quality (speed, ease, and reliability) of passage among states all factor into early newborn behavioral patterns. Newborn behavior includes the qualities of the baby's states and the ease of passage among them. The baby's first extrauterine experience of states is biologically informed by the hormonal environment of birth during transition.

An example of state maintenance variation can be seen in the quality of newborn sleep. Some newborns sleep soundly and quietly for extended periods without rousing to stimulation in the environment. Other newborns sleep fitfully, rousing at intervals to cry out during sleep, and are easily disturbed by activities in the environment. State change variation is evident in an infant who rouses slowly from sleep through drowsy, then quiet alert, to active alert, and then to crying. Another infant might pass rapidly (or even imperceptibly) through state changes and wake into a full-blown, lusty cry. After birth for days or even months, some infants are unable to transition smoothly from state to state. In an over-stimulating environment, some babies remain in light sleep to protect their central nervous system, whereas other babies have difficulty achieving any restful sleep (Appleton, 2011, p. 206).

Regulation—a critical concept in newborn behavior—refers to the baby's state maintenance and change capabilities in the face of both internal and external stimuli (VandenBerg, 2007). As an internal characteristic, regulation varies from baby to baby. Ongoing closeness of baby and mother (i.e., smell, skin, touch, voice, heartbeat, and handling/caretaking behavior) assists in co-regulation (Beebe & Lachmann, 1998). During co-regulation, a mother's affect assists the neonate in tolerating and communicating emotions such as hunger and fear. Through sensual, emotional, "body language" and rhythms shared between mother and newborn, the relational basis for the newborn's "self-regulation" through parent–infant synchrony becomes evident (Feldman, 2007).

The ability to regulate his or her own states is often called the "first developmental task of the newborn" (Nugent et al., 2007 p. 37). However, newborn regulation of states also depends on maternal provision of "hidden regulators" that may calm, support, or complicate newborn state transition and maintenance (Hofer, 1994). Regulation and co-regulation begin with parents' sensitive recognition and timely responsiveness to cues and newborn states. Providers' sensitive recognition of and ability to "hold" the emotional dimensions of mother and baby states is a critical component of supporting healthy dyadic co-regulation.

Parents' and providers' interactions with newborns facilitates state regulation when such interactions are attuned to the newborn's state and cues (Nugent et al., 2007, p. 37). Parents' and providers' empathetic responses enable babies to organize and establish predictable patterns of state maintenance and change. Consistent responsiveness assists the baby in moving from profound uncertainty about survival in the world to trusting and anticipating predictable parental response for survival (Winnicott, 1960).

Providers can assist parents by providing concrete examples of behavioral strategies to help their newborn modulate and regulate his or her states. For babies who exhibit subtle states, for parents who are very concrete or externally directed, and for parents struggling with or who are unaware of the need for co-regulation, concrete examples are very helpful. Nursing Child Assessment Satellite Training's (NCAST) *Keys to Caregiving* program is a well-documented instructional resource for behavioral strategies that may be shared and demonstrated to regulate infants (NCAST, 1990).

Working together, providers and parents should observe the newborn's states, ability to self-regulate, and opportunities for co-regulation. For example, the newborn's physical examination is an ideal opportunity for teaching and learning (Appleton, 2011, p. 207). Co-regulation strategies used by healthcare providers may be discussed and practiced with parents throughout the teaching opportunity of the physical exam.

For instance, when the neonate cries during the physical assessment, the provider has an opportunity to present strategies and skills for consoling (co-regulating) a crying baby to the parents. Staged interventions include observing (for 15 seconds) for self-consoling such as hand-to-mouth behaviors (Appleton, 2011, p. 208). While such self-regulation is appreciated by healthcare providers, hand-to-mouth behaviors may be interpreted by parents as a precursor to thumb sucking or face scratching. An interpretive opportunity between provider and parent can be realized as self-soothing hand-to-mouth behaviors are presented as a strength and an innate capacity of the baby to manage his own states, and an early effort to develop awareness of his own body (Hoffer, 1949).

Developmental care providers can facilitate and support parents in recognizing behavioral "cues" as signals for readiness to change states. Feeding readiness cues of salivation, lip smacking, and rooting are among the first behavioral cues that parents will likely see in the early hours of transition (Widström et al., 2011). Eye rubbing is an expression of sleep readiness in many babies from the beginning of neonatal life. Engagement and disengagement cues are listed in **Table 6-1**. Learning to identify and read an infant's cues supports the parents' abilities to modify their interactions before the baby becomes distressed. Prompt and consistent response to the baby's cues affords newborns the benefit of receiving immediate fulfillment of their needs, similar to the intrauterine experience (Winnicott, 1960). Such consistency also facilitates an emerging sense of efficacy, as the infant experiences her own important contribution to needs satisfaction.

From a behavioral perspective, co-regulation comprises the newborn and parental processes of cue recognition, responsiveness, and action leading to satisfaction and relaxation of parent and baby. The reward of successful co-regulation is the mutual experience of satisfied needs and relaxation for both members of the dyad. Co-regulation through social interaction continues well beyond one sequence or process and well beyond the neonatal period.

Ideally, co-regulation will begin in the parental–newborn embrace at birth. Skin-to-skin care provides warmth, audible and familiar maternal heartbeat and voice, and olfactory recognition of the mother's smell. Prone positioning of the infant on the maternal abdomen regulates the micro-reflexes necessary for exploration of the maternal abdomen and breast. In response to the newborn's exploration, maternal hormone release occurs. Another example of co-regulation is the supply-and-demand nature of maternal milk. In these interactions, emotional experience is being shaped, communicated, and learned as parent and newborn engage in signaling and communication that bring satisfaction, acquaintance, and attunement.

The Neonatal Behavioral Assessment Scale (NBAS; also called the Brazelton Examination) measures the individuality of a newborn's neurobehavioral state (Als, Tronick, Lester, & Brazelton, 1977). The NBAS demonstrates to parents their neonate's inborn capacities, including the ability to change or maintain state when disruptive stimuli are introduced (Nugent et al., 2007, p. 2). While performing the examination, the advanced practice provider teaches parents about their newborn's competencies for state regulation, modeling strategies for maintaining a supportive environment for the individual infant. For example, sequential methods

Table 6-1: Self-Regulatory Versus Stress Behaviors

Organization (Ready for Engagement)	Disorganization (Ready for Disengagement)
Physiologic	
Cardiorespiratory: stable heart and/or respiratory rate; regular, slow respirations	Cardiorespiratory: increase or decrease in respiratory rate; irregular respirations; apnea; gasping; bradycardia; blood pressure instability; sneezing, hiccoughs, coughing, sighing
Color: pink, stable	Color: mottling, duskiness; cyanosis—central or generalized; pallor or plethora
Gastrointestinal: tolerates feedings	Gastrointestinal: abdominal distention; spitting up; vomiting; gagging; stooling
Behavioral	
Body movements smooth and synchronous: consistent tone of all body parts; arms and legs flexed with smooth movements	Tremors, jittery and jerking movements; hypotonia or hypertonia (flaccid trunk, extremities; movements arching, flailing, extended extremities; finger splays, fisting)
States: well-defined sleep–wake	Unable to modulate states: sudden state changes; more active than quiet sleep; awake states with gaze aversion, frowning, grimacing, staring, irritability, wide-eyed "help me" look
Self-quieting behaviors: hand-to-mouth, hand or foot clasping, finger folding or grasping, sucking, foot or leg bracing	Limited use of self-quieting behaviors (may need assistance from caregiver)
Attentive behaviors: alert gaze; fixes and follows visual stimuli; ceases to suck or slows suck rate; turns toward auditory stimuli; smiles; imitates; opens mouth, extends tongue; vocalizes: coos, babbles, habituates to stimuli	May demonstrate any of above stress signals when attempting to interact with one or more modes of stimuli (e.g., rocking, talking) simultaneously in environment (either animate or inanimate)

Reproduced from Gardner, S. L., Goldson, E., & Hernandez, J. A. (2016). The neonate and the environment: Impact on development. In S. L. Gardner, B. S. Carter, M. Enzman-Hines, & J. A. Hernandez (Eds.), *Merenstein and Gardner's handbook of neonatal intensive care* (8th ed., pp. 262–314). St. Louis, MO: Mosby-Elsevier.

for consoling a fussing baby are presented: (1) talking with a soothing voice with repetitive rhythmic content, (2) placement of the parental hand to contain limbs, and (3) picking up, cuddling, and rocking the newborn. Using aspects of the NBAS, parents can learn which strategies and types of regulatory interactions are needed to assist this particular newborn to transition from fussy to quiet or active alert.

"Co-regulation Boot Camp": Bringing in the Milk

Once transition is completed, mother and newborn enter a period when the baby's states are not yet stabilized and prefeeding, feeding, and postfeeding behaviors may vary. Parents may now struggle to interpret the newborn's needs in the context of the unpredictability in this period. The breastfeeding dyad is working on their "fit" as the newborn seeks to master the root, gape, latch, and effective sucking tasks and as the mother experiments with positioning and guiding the baby (Walker, 2014, p. 259). During this period, the newborn is truly dependent on the mother to provide basic needs according to the baby's as yet unpatterned cues. This co-regulation "boot camp" period occurs from 3 to 5 days after birth for the breastfeeding dyad and over a shorter period for the formula-feeding dyad. After the initial sleep period, feeding sessions may not be followed by the deep relaxation and sleep that occur after the feeding of the more mature infant. Alternatively, feeding sessions may be characterized by the newborn falling asleep before feeding seems complete. Because this period requires moment-to-moment maternal attention, mothers may worry that breastfeeding will consume all of their time, because in these first days, it often does.

During the colostral phase of breastfeeding, the baby is learning to refine prelatch behaviors and working toward mastering the gape, latch, suck, and swallow skills of breastfeeding. The colostral phase of breastfeeding is characterized by a small volume (2 to 20 mL/breast for the first feeding) of breastmilk (Lawrence & Lawrence, 2011), which is compatible with the newborn's stomach capacity of approximately 20 mL (Bergman, 2013). Frequent feedings are physiologic and facilitate a co-regulated process to establish a mature milk supply by the end of the first 2 weeks of life (Lawrence & Lawrence, 2011). Frequent feedings activate the neonatal gut's functionality in terms of hunger, satiety, and digestion, as well as evacuation of bilirubin-laden meconium. These necessary co-regulated frequent feedings, if not understood by the mother and her family, may result in worry about the success of breastfeeding. Mothers (and family members) may worry about milk supply ("I don't have enough milk; my baby is hungry") and the success of breastfeeding ("Breastfeeding is not working"). Mothers may be hyperalert to their baby's behavior and hypervigilant to any indication that something may be wrong with the baby or themselves.

Newborns are explicitly or implicitly compared by their mothers to older infants who eat, sleep, and wake in predictable three-hour cycles. While acknowledging the meaning a mother attributes to her baby's behavior, the developmental care provider can help parents identify and attend to the moment-to-moment needs of this particular baby during this unique phase. Breastfeeding boot camp can represent a "touchpoint" for the dyad, when it seems that newborn development and maternal care are not moving forward. By acknowledging the newborn's role in co-regulating milk production (i.e., "My baby is doing exactly what it takes on her part to bring in the milk so she will be satisfied"), mothers may relax and be comforted by the normalcy of the baby's behavior. Fears that parents begin to form around early breastfeeding challenges may be eased by acknowledging that baby's behavior in the early days predicts neither later baby behavior nor long-term breastfeeding success.

At this time, the dyad is vulnerable to maternal-, family-, and provider-driven interventions targeted at eating and satiety. Giving formula and forced placement of the newborn at the breast are common interventions that alter the natural process. Well-intentioned relatives and friends often advocate interventions to alleviate the stress of this time, such as introducing formula and/or cereal. Providers typically intervene with instructions on prescriptive latch methods, undermining maternal confidence and the baby's skill development and interrupting the dyad's evolving co-regulation skills. Developmental care providers need to effectively "hold" the emotional turbulence of the dyad during this period and refrain from excessive intervention or instruction as a means to soothe their own anxieties. At the same time, providers need to remain aware of the emergence of symptoms of maternal anxiety or depression, particularly at moments when breastfeeding becomes challenging (Ystrom, 2012).

As lactogenesis progresses and small amounts of colostrum are replaced by transitional milk in larger volumes, the newborn initiates audible swallowing behaviors and expresses satiety after a feed. The baby's hands relax, the baby falls into a deep, calm sleep, and the infant has a satisfied facial expression after feeding. This is the process-completion moment everyone has been waiting and working for!

As soon as the newborn becomes familiar with the mother's breast and nipple and coordinates his breastfeeding skills, the breast becomes fuller and harder while the nipple changes texture, form, and consistency. Newborns often respond to the unfamiliarity of a now more difficult-to-grasp nipple with side-to-side head shaking, crying, and pulling away. These behaviors occur just when the mother may be experiencing breast pain from fullness and needs the newborn to effectively suck to reduce edema and pressure. Because side-to-side adult head movements signal refusal ("No"), parents may interpret the newborn's reactions to the changed nipple as refusal. Providers can reinterpret neonatal behaviors as an attempt to get reoriented at the breast. Demonstrating hand expression as a method of softening the areola and reassuring the mother that breast edema is temporary are strategies to assist the nursing dyad in managing this distressing new circumstance. If new mothers interpret "breasts full of milk" as their condition for the duration of breastfeeding, they are likely to abandon breastfeeding.

Stools become "transitional" as milk replaces colostrum and the gut finally evacuates all meconium. At this point, the stools are the result of what is ingested during extrauterine life. Mature stooling patterns correspond to the volume and content of milk; neonates often stool with every feeding. Although a wide range of normal frequency and volume exist, a pattern becomes apparent for the specific infant. Frequent stooling evacuates meconium from the neonatal gut, thereby decreasing reabsorption of bilirubin from the intestines and contributing to the resolution of physiologic jaundice and the management of hyperbilirubinemia (Walker, 2014, p. 346).

Together, the mother and newborn co-regulate multiple, interrelated developmental processes. The mother's breasts empty, soften, and increase in weight, filling predictably with the baby's feeding cycle throughout the day. The newborn's now predictable wake, eat, satiety, and sleep cycles complement the feedings. In addition, there may be at least one quiet alert state conducive to face-to-face socialization daily. While each mother–newborn pair may still face some challenges at this time, they enjoy the comfort of predictability in breastfeeding and the proof that breastfeeding is successful.

Newborn Growth Spurt: Expanding and Maturing the Milk

After weeks of predictable sleep–wake–feed–satiety cycles, the neonate begins to "eat all the time." The baby feeds well, then wants to feed again in a matter of minutes. This healthy pattern, called "cluster feeding," may occur at any time, but is associated with increasing the milk supply and assuring adequate intake during growth spurts (Lawrence & Lawrence, 2011, p. 250). If cluster feeding has not been part of this dyad's feeding pattern, mothers may experience it as a frustrating disorganization and regression in feeding success.

Mothers, and others, may conclude from the baby's demand for frequent feeding during this period that "there is not enough milk" when, in fact, the mother's breastmilk is maturing. Cessation of breastfeeding and/or introduction of formula supplementation may occur if breastmilk is thought to be insufficient. Providers can "hold" the frustration of this phase, assuring mothers and concerned family members that the neonate's increased appetite is a normal and healthy development. Reassurance of an adequate milk supply can be demonstrated by adequate neonatal weight gain. Strategies to facilitate the innate capacity to increase maternal milk supply include (1) physical holding (perhaps skin-to-skin in the supported prone position on the maternal abdomen), (2) increasing maternal relaxation and rest, (3) facilitating opportunities for infant feeding, and (4) ensuring maternal nutrition and hydration.

Co-regulation for Conformity: Days, Nights, and Elimination

The next developmental phase focuses on the family's need to socialize their new member to a standard wake–sleep cycle that conforms to the family's and society's norm (i.e., wakefulness in the daytime and uninterrupted sleep at night) (Lancy, 2015). At the 10-day to 2-week visit, the newborn's physical growth is assessed with an expectation of weight gain of ½ to 1 ounce per day beginning at the second week of life. If satisfactory weight gain is achieved, the concept of "socializing" newborn sleep is typically a topic of interest to parents because of their sleep deprivation, care of other children, and working in and/or outside the home. Many parents view their need to reorganize neonatal sleep behavior as not only part of socialization, but also an economic necessity.

Using a developmental care approach, professional care providers "hold" and address parental anxieties and exhaustion while promoting empathy for the baby. At least half of all babies experience their longer period of wakefulness and crying during the night. This night-waking pattern often follows the same circadian cycle of the fetus in utero. Many mothers will remember that their neonate, as a fetus, had a consistent and predictable intrauterine active period in the middle of the night. Parental strategies to reorganize neonatal sleep–wake cycles need to be the least disruptive for the infant. When active and quiet alert stages with the infant occur during daylight hours, whereas calming, less stimulating interactions are promoted during the nighttime hours, the infant's circadian rhythm will begin to reorganize (Hagan, Shaw, & Duncan, 2008, p. 311). To extend nighttime sleeping intervals, providers may encourage parents to interact with their infant during the evening, thereby prolonging evening wakefulness and offering a later nighttime feeding. Using quieting music, calming massage, low lights, and minimal vocalizations should gradually shorten nighttime alert phases.

Strategies to change an infant's sleep pattern must avoid interrupting states that are not accompanied by state-change cues. For example, daytime waking of an infant after 2 hours of sleep is state interruption rather than completion. Few infants tolerate this approach, which may herald further disruption in self-regulation and overall behavior predictability. Because substantial infant learning occurs during sleep, strategies of sleep-state interruption should not be encouraged (Monk & Hane, 2014, p. 15).

Premature or adult-driven reorganization of infant sleep–wake cycles is not a simple, quick, or easy process. Infants do not normally "sleep through the night" or for periods that exceed 5 hours until they are at least 3 months of age (Monk & Hane, 2014). Parental fatigue and frustration can increase the risk of depression during this period, while the newborn is at higher risk for shaking or other harm (Oldbury & Adams, 2015). Developmental care providers can talk openly with parents about their feelings and frustrations, assess for maternal depression (referring for treatment if indicated), suggest or recruit support for respite and rest, and suggest childcare arrangements for parents returning to work.

During this time, parental concerns about changing elimination patterns may also arise. As the infant's gastrointestinal tract matures, stooling frequency changes from every feeding to stooling several times per day. Coupled with the sometimes "red-faced" efforts to stool, these changes may cause parents to interpret their baby as being "constipated." Formula-fed infants often experience a parent-induced formula change in response to such concerns, while breastfeeding mothers may worry that their dietary habits are causing gastrointestinal distress in their infant. Parents may use home-created solutions, over-the-counter remedies, and/or nutritional supplements in an attempt to "calm" the baby.

A developmental care approach explores parents' anxieties and identifies neonatal symptoms, behavior, stool consistency, and type of feeding. Developmental changes in stool patterns and a definition of constipation should be explained to parents. Breastfed babies are rarely constipated and (contrary to popular belief) formula-fed infants are *not* constipated by the iron in term formula. Parental advice to relieve the baby's symptoms includes using warm baths and bicycling leg exercises to relieve gas.

Saying Goodbye to the Neonatal Period: Colic, Fatigue, and Mother/Baby Blues

The majority of neonates develop a period of crying during the day. This late afternoon and evening crying begins at about 3 weeks of age and peaks between 4 to 6 weeks of age. If the crying period exceeds 3 hours, occurs at least 3 times per week, lasts at least 3 weeks, and has no discernible cause, it is termed "colic" (Kurth, Kennedy, Spichiger, Hösli, & Stutz, 2011, p. 188). Disquieting infant crying is most commonly cited reason for parents consulting health professionals (Long, 2001).

Although there is no universally accepted understanding of the origins of this "crying period," developmental changes in the infant's gastrointestinal and central nervous system, as well as the circadian rhythm of human milk production, may contribute to late afternoon "fussiness." Because the circadian rhythm of human milk production is lowest in volume, fat, and calories in the early evening, infants become hungry sooner after their previous feeding. During this time of day, the mother may be fatigued, the baby wants to nurse continuously, and the household may be busy with meal preparation and socializing. In the face of these challenges, after having achieved a predictable feeding pattern, the dyad once again experiences disorganization that can be interpreted as "taking one step back." As parents and family members seek strategies to console the infant, their coping mechanisms and capacity for empathy may be taxed to the limit.

While crying periods are viewed as part of individual variation and due to developmental processes (Nugent et al., 2007, p. 108), some theorists hypothesize that crying can best be understood in the interactional context. Evidence supports the premise that if parents respond immediately to infant crying, the infant will cry less compared to an infant whose crying is ignored (Nugent et al., 2007, p. 110). In addition, newborn crying is no longer seen as exclusively a physiologic state. Rather, infant crying has neural correlates to social communication between baby and caretaker. Lagercrantz and Changeux (2009) describe crying in newborns as producing "[c]haracteristic sounds and grimaces with vigorous body movements to the extent that crying may be viewed as a distinct state of consciousness interpreted as [the newborn's] 'honest signaling of need or vigor' (Soltis, 2004, p. 444)."

After birth, the amount of newborn crying is associated with maternal fatigue and tiredness: as newborn crying increases, so does maternal fatigue (Kurth et al., 2011). Extreme parental fatigue and sleep deprivation may contribute to the development of postpartum depression. Marked fatigue in mothers has the potential to decrease empathetic responsiveness to unrelenting newborn crying—what one qualitative study calls "parental colic" (Thompson, Harris, & Bitowski, 2001).

The onset of newborn crying periods also overlaps and follows the time when mothers may be experiencing "baby blues." Baby blues may be associated with the dramatic hormonal adjustments that occur during the postpartum period. Clinically, women report feeling emotional and teary. What does it mean when mother and baby both experience intense crying at the close of the neonatal period? As the family adjusts to life with the newborn, the newborn may be spending more time in a crib, carrier, car seat, or being held by others. Increased separation from the mother can be experienced as a loss for the baby. Loss of shared physical proximity with mother also includes loss of access to maternal "hidden regulators" of infant states, emotions, and behavior (Hofer, 1994).

Like the mother, the newborn may be experiencing distress and fatigue during this period. Becoming part of a household and experiencing the family cycle of activity during the day and calm and sleep at night are experiences that may overwhelm a newborn who is not ready for "living with" (Winnicott, 1986) the whole family. Even though the baby may nap, ongoing fatigue may trigger distress and disorganization. Afternoon attention from siblings arriving home from school and adults arriving home from work may be overwhelming to a fatigued newborn or a fatigued parent just emerging from the "boot camp" experience.

Infant research has documented newborn crying in relation to unspoken maternal distress, what Fraiberg, Adelson, and Shapiro (1975) call "ghosts in the nursery." A mother–infant psychoanalytic approach addresses the mother's sources of distress with the infant present, even "talking to the baby" and putting words to a newborn's acute emotional states (Salomonsson, 2014). Providers using this approach can open new avenues for soothing and supporting the mother and newborn as a dyad.

During this period of inconsolable crying, infants are vulnerable to abuse and shaken-baby syndrome (Carbaugh, 2004). For the depressed mother, it is a time of increased risk for self-harm (Ystrom, 2012). Parents can be supported through the provision of information about these feelings and by referrals to sources of support. Developmental care providers can help parents understand that these intense and distressing emotions may be, in part, their own experience of "holding" the distress of their baby's development (Winnicott, 1960), particularly as the newborn emerges from the neonatal period into his or her "birth" as an infant (Mahler et al., 1999). This is another remarkable process-completion step—the successful developmental journey of the neonate through the challenging first month of life, with its foundation in the mother–infant relationship.

Sharing strategies for dealing with infant crying periods reassures parents that crying episodes are commonplace and gives them tools to cope with the stress created by this behavior. First, parents should be sure that the baby's physical needs are met: baby is fed, diaper is changed, and baby is in a soothing and safe environment. Use of a soothing sequence of behaviors and cues such as holding securely, swaddling, soft music, rocking, and a quiet environment are conducive to quieting an infant. Parental consideration of using a more highly structured daily routine as well as decreasing overall stimulation assists some babies to quiet themselves (Hagan et al., 2008). This strategy is particularly helpful for a "rapid-state-change baby," who typically does best with predictability and calm in the environment. Help parents examine family routines and consider ways to change afternoon and evening activities to expose the infant to less stimulation. Additionally, reducing maternal–infant separation and providing co-regulation via bodily closeness may quiet the infant. Parents can consider wearing the baby in a soft carrier or in skin-to-skin nurturing positions so that heartbeat, warmth, movement, and mutual frontal position may calm the infant. With these supports, the newborn may be able to better tolerate the challenges of development.

Without clinical supervision support, the emotional demands of providing "holding" for a newborn and family may contribute to provider burnout and the mechanistic delivery of care. For these reasons, emerging models of developmental care may include mother–baby psychotherapists partnering with home-visiting nurses, midwives, and pediatric providers. These partnerships can help hone providers' developmental care skills and deepen their clinical observations with the goal of bringing a dyadic approach to mother–infant care.

Conclusion

Caring practice must be reevaluated to ensure that all members of the team are able to provide adequate holding for the infant's development (Regis, Kakehashhi, & Pinheiro, 2005, p. 43). We invite providers to engage in developmental care that "holds" the shared psychological field of mother and newborn, containing both the joys and the terrors of newborn development and parenting. With that invitation comes the responsibility to empower developmental care providers with the education and professional supports to practice "holding" and sustain the demands of this approach. Ineffective strategies employed by systems to manage emotionality in health care have included "processes of psychosocial distancing, task allocation, and the depersonalization of patients" (Menzies, 1959, cited in Rafferty, 2010, p. 247). A more viable alternative is to provide developmental education and workplace supports, including clinical supervision that "attends to the emotional world" of the care provider and helps providers to "develop ways of learning emotionally" from their experiences of care provision (Rafferty, 2010, p. 247). Extending Winnicott's theory to clinical supervision, Rafferty sees

> holding as active, empathic concern for the professional health and welfare of one's colleagues, which leads to a defined relationship based on mutual trust. Holding extends into the concept of handling, through its requirement to identify the necessary conditions for professional development, and provide opportunities for finding useful meaning in the challenges of change and loss. (Rafferty, 2010, p. 245)

In this sense, developmental care is aspirational, containing a vision of a transformed professional environment that could translate to improved family and newborn health and well-being.

Developmental care may also have a role in promoting health equity. How might the practice of holding the developmental space of the mother and newborn help support women who experience a hostile "outside world" or troubled family members intruding into their internal world, impinging upon their resilience, and affecting their newborn's chance to thrive? How might this relational approach to developmental care help increase food security in a community, facilitating newborn access to optimal nutrition through breastfeeding and families' access to healthy food in their neighborhoods? For developmental care to have these impacts, advocacy is needed on behalf of public policies that will assure access to essential resources such as maternal nutrition, postpartum depression prevention (Werner et al., 2015), and mental health services and that will establish the community-level conditions for empowered and meaningful motherhood, fatherhood, and child development. Policy makers, the health professions, and communities together can help "hold" and enrich the social-structural space for newborn development.

Even in an ideally supported environment, however, developmental care is needed to cushion families and providers as they become attuned to the intimate psychological space of the mother and newborn. We know that strengthening parents' capacity for empathy strengthens sensitivity to infant cues for both mothers and fathers (Graham, 1993). Through creative interprofessional collaborations, providers can cultivate their "holding skills," integrating holding into dyad-focused developmental care, and bringing this approach into families' homes and hearts.

Student Practice Activities

The following questions are intended for reflection and discussion on features of "developmental care" of the mother–infant dyad. There are no correct or incorrect answers for these questions.

1. What is involved in "holding the space for birth"?

2. How is "holding the space for mother and newborn" both similar to and different from "holding the space for birth"?

3. Why does a developmental care approach favor affective over didactic approaches to the mother in the first moments and day of life? Develop your own explanation of why this strategy is unrelated to mothers' intelligence.

4. How is breastfeeding a process of co-regulation involving *actions* and *processes* on the part of the mother and on the part of the infant?

5. What does it mean for mother and infant to "discover each other" in the first month of life?

Multiple Choice

1. During the second period of reactivity the infant's behavior is often affected by which condition?
    A) Clearing the airway and intestines
    B) Hyperbilirubinemia
    C) Prolonged sleep
    D) Very high levels of catecholamines and oxytocin

2. The phrase "co-regulation boot camp," as used in this chapter, describes which period of time for the mother–infant dyad?
    A) Birth and initial feeding
    B) Completion of the second period of reactivity and milk "coming in"
    C) Milk coming in and 28 days post birth
    D) The initial feeding and the second period of reactivity

3. Which aspects of newborn state regulation are likely to be observable during the newborn physical assessment?
    A) Maternal co-regulation
    B) Quality of active sleep
    C) Self-quieting behaviors
    D) Transition from active to deep sleep

4. Which criteria must newborn behavior meet to be defined as colic?
    A) Evening crying episodes where infant is inconsolable
    B) Infant drawing knees to abdomen during crying episodes
    C) Three-hour crying periods at least three times a week for three weeks
    D) Three-hour crying periods with no identifiable cause daily for a week

5. What does the practice of "holding" the mother–newborn pair require?
    A) A thermoneutral environment
    B) Empathy and awareness of the emotional experience of the dyad
    C) Extensive interviews with a mother about parenting philosophy
    D) Provision of advice and education about newborn care

References

Als, H., Tronick, E., Lester, B., & Brazelton, T. (1977). The Brazelton Neonatal Behavioral Assessment Scale (BNBAS). *Journal of Abnormal Child Psychiatry, 5,* 3.

Appleton, J. (2011). Newborn behavioural aspects. In A. Lomax (Ed.), *Examination of the newborn* (pp. 201–217). Chichester, UK: John Wiley & Sons.

Balint, M. (1968). *The basic fault: Therapeutic aspects of regression.* London, UK: Tavistock.

Batacan, J. (2010). A new approach: Biological nurturing and laid-back breastfeeding. *International Journal of Childbirth Education, 25*(2), 7–9.

Beebe, B., & Lachmann, F. M. (1998). Co-constructing inner and relational processes: Self- and mutual regulation in infant research and adult treatment. *Psychoanalytic Psychology, 15,* 480–516.

Bergman, A. (1999). *Ours, yours, mine: Mutuality and the emergence of the separate self.* North vale, NJ: Jason Aronson.

Bergman, N. J. (2013). Neonatal stomach volume and physiology suggest feeding at 1-h intervals. *Acta Paediatrica, 102*(8), 773–770.

Blonsky, P. P. (1930). *Reflexive psychology.* Moscow/Leningrad, Russia.

Brazelton, T. (1992). *On becoming a family: The growth of attachment before and after birth.* New York, NY: Delacorte.

Brazelton, T. B., & Sparrow, J. D. (2001). *Touchpoints: 3–6.* Cambridge, MA: Perseus.

Brazelton, T. B., & Sparrow, J. (2003). *The touchpoints model of development.* Boston, MA: Brazelton Touchpoints Center.

Cadwell, K. (2007). Latching-on and suckling of the healthy term neonate: Breastfeeding assessment. *Journal of Midwifery and Women's Health, 52,* 638.

Carbaugh, S. F. (2004). Understanding shaken baby syndrome. *Advances in Neonatal Care, 4,* 105–114.

Changeux, J.-P., & Dehaene, S. (2008). The neuronal workspace model: Conscious processing and learning. In R. Menzel (Ed.), *Learning theory and behavior* (Vol. 1, pp. 729–758). Oxford, UK: Elsevier.

Colson, S., Meek, J., & Hawdon, J. (2008). Optimal positions for the release of primitive neonatal reflexes stimulating breastfeeding. *Early Human Development, 84,* 441–449.

Cooper, A. M. (1989). Concepts of therapeutic effectiveness in psychoanalysis: A historical review. *Psychoanalytic Inquiry, 9,* 4–25.

Denton, D. (2005). *The primordial emotions.* Oxford, UK: Oxford University Press.

Dixon, L., Skinner, J., & Foureur, M. (2013). The emotional and hormonal pathways of labour and birth: Integrating mind, body and behaviour. *New Zealand College of Midwives Journal, 48,* 15–23.

Eldredge, N. (1985). *Time frames: The evolution of punctuated equilibria.* Princeton, NJ: Princeton University Press.

Fahey, K., Foureur, M., & Hastie, C. (Eds.). (2008). *Birth territory and midwifery guardianship: Theory for practice, education and research.* New York, NY: Books for Midwives.

Fahey, K., & Hastie, C. (2008). Midwifery guardianship: Reclaiming the sacred in birth. In K. Fahey, M. Foureur, & C. Hastie (Eds.), *Birth territory and midwifery guardianship: Theory for practice education and research* (pp. 21–37). Edinburgh, UK: Elsevier.

Fahey, K. A., & Parratt, J. M. (2006). Birth territory: A theory for midwifery practice. *Women and Birth, 19*(2), 45–50.

Feldman, R. (2007). Parent–infant synchrony: Biological foundations and developmental outcomes. *Current Directions in Psychological Science, 16,* 340.

Fogel, A., & Garvey, A. (2007). Alive communication. *Infant Behavior and Development, 30*(2), 251–257.

Fraiberg, S., Adelson, E., & Shapiro, V. (1975). Ghosts in the nursery: A psychoanalytic approach to the problems of impaired infant–mother relationships. *Child and Adolescent Psychiatry, 14*(3), 387–421.

Gersick, C. J. G. (1988). Time and transition in work teams: Toward a new model of group development. *Academy of Management Journal, 31*(1), 9–41.

Gersick, C. J. G. (1989). Marking time: Predictable transitions in task groups. *Academy of Management Journal, 32*(2), 274–309.

Gersick, C. J. G. (1991). Revolutionary change theories: A multilevel exploration of the punctuated equilibrium paradigm. *Academy of Management Review, 16*(1), 10–36.

Gould, S. J., & Eldredge, N. (1977). Punctuated equilibria: The tempo and mode of evolution reconsidered. *Paleobiology, 3,* 115–151.

Graham, M. (1993). Parental sensitivity to infant cues: Similarities and differences between mothers and fathers. *Journal of Pediatric Nursing, 8*(6), 376–384.

Graves, B., & Haley, M. (2013). Newborn transition. *Journal of Midwifery and Women's Health, 58,* 662–670.

Hagan, J. F., Shaw, J. S., & Duncan, P. M. (Eds.). (2008). *Bright futures: Guidelines for health supervision of infants, children and adolescents* (3rd ed.). Elk Grove Village, IL: American Academy of Pediatrics.

Hastie, C. (2008). The spiritual and emotional territory of the unborn and the newborn baby. In K. Fahey, M. Foureur, & C. Hastie (Eds.), *Birth territory and midwifery guardianship: Theory for practice education and research* (pp. 79–93). Edinburgh, UK: Elsevier.

Hofer, M. A. (1984). Relationships as regulators: A psychobiologic perspective on bereavement. *Psychosomatic Medicine, 46*(3), 183–197.

Hofer, M. (1994). Hidden regulators in attachment, separation, and loss. *Monographs of the Society for Research in Child Development, 59*, 192–207.

Hoffer, W. (1949). Mouth, hand, and ego-integration. *Psychoanalytic Study of the Child, 3–4*, 49–56.

Kamel, H., & Dockrell, J. E. (2000). Divergent perspectives, multiple meanings: A comparison of caregivers' and observers' interpretations of infant behavior. *Journal of Reproductive and Infant Psychology, 18*(1), 41–60.

Karolinska Institutet. (April 19, 2010). Mother-infant psychoanalysis may create a beneficial circle in the event of poor bonding. Retrieved from https://www.sciencedaily.com/releases/2010/04/100413072042.htm

Klaus, M. H., & Kennell, J. H. (1976). *Maternal–infant bonding: The impact of early separation or loss on family development.* St. Louis, MO: CV Mosby.

Kurth, E., Kennedy, H., Spichiger, E., Hösli, I., & Stutz, E. (2011). Crying babies, tired mothers: What do we know? A systematic review. *Midwifery, 27*(2), 187–194.

Lagercrantz, H., & Changeux, J. (2009). The emergence of human consciousness: From fetal to neonatal life. *Pediatric Research, 6*(3), 255–260.

Lagercrantz, H., Hanson, M., Evrard, P., & Rodeck, C. (2002). *The newborn brain.* Cambridge, UK: Cambridge University Press.

Lancy, D. (2015). *The anthropology of childhood: Cherubs, chattel, changelings.* Cambridge, UK: Cambridge University Press.

Lawrence, R., & Lawrence, M. (2011). *Breastfeeding: A guide for the medical profession* (7th ed.). St. Louis, MO: Mosby.

Letinic, K., Zoncu, R., & Rakic, P. (2002). Origin of GABAergic neurons in the human neocortex. *Nature, 417*, 645–649.

Lipton, B. H. (2005). *The biology of belief.* Santa Rosa Mountain, CA: Elite Books.

Long, T. (2001). Excessive infantile crying: A review of the literature. *Journal of Child Health Care, 5*(3), 111–116.

Mahler, S., Pine, F., & Bergman, A. (1999). *The psychological birth of the human infant: Symbiosis and individuation.* New York, NY: Basic Books.

Markova, G., & Legerstee, M. (2006). Contingency, imitation, and affect sharing: Foundations of infants' social awareness. *Developmental Psychology, 42*(1), 132–141.

Mellor, D., Diesch, T., Gunn, A., & Bennet, L. (2005). The importance of "awareness" for understanding fetal pain. *Brain Research Reviews, 49*, 455–471.

Menzies, I. (1959). A case study in the functioning of social systems as a defense against anxiety: A report on a study of the nursing service of a general hospital. *Human Relations, 13*, 119–121.

Mercer, R. T. (1995). *Becoming a mother: Research on maternal identity from Rubin to the present.* New York, NY: Springer.

Miller, L. (Ed.). (1997). *Closely observed infants.* London, UK: Bristol Classical Press.

Monk, C., & Hane, A. (2014). Fetal and infant neurobehavioral development: Basic processes and environmental influences. In A. Wenzel (Ed.), *The Oxford handbook of perinatal psychology.* Retrieved from http://psychology.williams.edu/files/Fetal_and_Infant_Neurobehavioral_Development.pdf doi:10.1093/oxfordhb/9780199778072.013.20

Moskowitz, S. (2012). Primary maternal preoccupation disrupted by trauma and loss: Early years of the project. *Journal of Infant, Child, and Adolescent Psychotherapy: Special Issue on Mothers, Infants and Young Children of September 11, 2001, 10*(2–3), 229–237.

Nelson, C., & Bosquet, M. (2000). Neurobiology of fetal and infant development: Implications for infant mental health. In C. H. Zeanah, Jr. (Ed.), *Handbook of infant mental health* (2nd ed., pp. 37–59). New York, NY: Guilford Press.

Nissen, E., Lilja, G., Widström, A., & Uvnäs-Moberg, K. (1995). Elevation of oxytocin levels in early postpartum women. *Acta Obstetrica Gynecologica, 74,* 530–533.

Nugent, J., Keefer, C., Minear, S., Johnson, L., & Blanchard, Y. (2007). *Understanding newborn behavior and early relationships: The newborn behavioral observations system handbook.* Baltimore, MD: Paul H. Brookes Publishing.

Nursing Child Assessment Satellite Training (NCAST). (1990). *Keys to caregiving study guide.* Seattle, WA: NCAST Publications.

Odent, M. (1983). Birth under water. *Lancet, 2,* 1476–1477.

Odent, M. (1984). *Birth reborn.* New York, NY: Pantheon.

Odent, M. (1986). *Primal health.* London, UK: Century Hutchinson.

Odent, M. (1999a). Is the participation of the father at birth dangerous? *Midwifery Today, 51,* 23–24.

Odent, M. (1999b). *The scientification of love.* London, UK: Free Association Books.

Oldbury, S., & Adams, K. (2015). The impact of infant crying on the parent–infant relationship. *Community Practitioner, 88*(3), 29–34.

Olinick, S. L. (1969). On empathy, and regression in service of the other. *British Journal of Medical Psychiatry, 42*(1), 41–49.

Pancheri, L. (1997). Interpretation and change in psychoanalysis: What is left of classical interpretation. *Journal of European Psychoanalysis, 5.* Retrieved from http://www.psychomedia.it/jep/number5/pancheri.htm

Rafferty, M. (2010). Using Winnicott (1960) to create a model for clinical supervision. In L. de Raeve, M. Rafferty, & M. Paget (Eds.), *Nurses and their patients: Informing practice through psychodynamic insights.* Keswick, UK: M&K Publishing,

Regis, F., Kakehashi, T., & Pinheiro, E. (2005). Analysis of the care given to hospitalized newborns according to the Winnicottian perspective. *Revista Brazileida Enfermagen, 56*(1), 39–43.

Righard, L., & Alade, M. (1990). Effect of delivery room routine on success of first breastfeed. *Lancet, 336,* 1105–1107.

Rubin, R. (1967). Attainment of the maternal role: Part I: Processes. *Nursing Research, 16*(3), 237–245.

Salomonsson, B. (2010). *"Baby worries": A randomized control trial of mother–infant psychoanalytic treatment.* Stockholm, Sweden: Karolinska Institutet.

Salomonsson, B. (2014). *Psychoanalytic therapy with infants and their parents: Practice, theory and results.* New York, NY: Routledge.

Soltis, J. (2004). The signal functions of early infant crying. *Behavior and Brain Science, 27,* 443–458.

Sparrow, J., & Brazelton, T. B. (2009). A developmental approach to the prevention of common behavioral problems. In T. K. McInerny, H. M. Adam, D. Campbell, D. K. Kamat, & K. J. Kelleher (Eds.), *Textbook of pediatric care* (pp. 1163–1167). Elk Grove Village, IL: American Academy of Pediatrics.

Thompson, P., Harris, C., & Bitowski, B. (2001). Effects of infant colic on the family: Implications for practice. *Issues in Comprehensive Pediatric Nursing, 9*(4), 273–285.

Trevarthen, C. (2011). What is it like to be a person who knows nothing? Defining the active intersubjective mind of a newborn human being. *Infant and Child Development, 20*(1), 119–135.

Trevarthen, C., & Aiken, K. J. (2001). Infant intersubjectivity: Research, theory and clinical applications. *Journal of Child Psychology and Psychiatry, 1*, 3–48.

Tyzio, R., Cossart, R., Khalilov, I., Minlebaev, M., Hubner, C. A., Represa, A., . . . Khazipov, R. (2006). Maternal oxytocin triggers a transient inhibitory switch in GABA signaling in the fetal brain during delivery. *Science, 314,* 1788–1792.

VandenBerg, K. (2007). State systems development in high-risk newborns in the neonatal intensive care unit: Identification and management of sleep, alertness, and crying. *Journal of Perinatal & Neonatal Nursing, 21*(2), 130–139.

Vanhatalo, S., & Kaila, K. (2006). Development of neonatal EEG activity: From phenomenology to physiology. *Seminars in Fetal and Neonatal Medicine, 11,* 471– 478.

Van Woudenberg, C., Wills, C., & Rubarth, L. (2012). Newborn transition to extrauterine life. *Neonatal Network, 31*(5), 319.

Vygotsky, L. S. (1998). Part 2: Problems of the child. In R. Rieber (Ed.), *The collected works of L. S. Vygotsky* (Vol. 5, pp. 187–205). Berlin, Germany: Springer.

Walker, M. (2014). *Breastfeeding management for the clinician: Using the evidence.* Burlington, MA: Jones & Bartlett Learning.

Werner, E. A., Gustafsson, H. C., Lee, S., Feng, T., Jiang, N., Desai, P., & Monk, C. (2015, August 2). PREPP: Postpartum depression prevention through the mother–infant dyad. *Archives of Women's Mental Health.* [Epub ahead of print]. doi: 10.1007/s00737-015-0549-5

Widström, A. M., Lilja, G., Aaltomaa-Michalias, P., Dahllöf, A., Lintula, M., & Nissen, E. (2011). Newborn behaviour to locate the breast when skin-to-skin: A possible method for enabling early self-regulation. *Acta Paediatrica, 100*(1), 79–85.

Widström, A. M., & Thingström-Paulsson, J. (1993). The position of the tongue during rooting reflexes elicited in newborn infants before the first suckle. *Acta Paediatrica, 82*(3), 281–283.

Winnicott, D. W. (1960). The theory of the parent–infant relationship. *International Journal of Psychoanalysis, 41,* 585–595.

Winnicott, D. W. (1965). *The maturational processes and the facilitating environment.* London, UK: Hogarth Press & Institute of Psychoanalysis.

Winnicott, D. W. (1986). *Holding and interpretation: Fragment of an analysis.* London, UK: Hogarth Press & Institute of Psychoanalysis.

Ystrom, E. (2012). Breastfeeding cessation and symptoms of anxiety and depression: A longitudinal cohort study. *BMC Pregnancy and Childbirth, 12,* 36.

CHAPTER 7

NEWBORN DISCHARGE TIMING

Katrina Wu and Rachel Stapleton

Introduction

Natalie peers down at her little baby boy, Charlie, as his nurse takes his temperature for the last time before heading home. While she is looking forward to taking Charlie home to join his three older siblings, she has been grateful for her 2-day hospital stay. This time away from the busyness that comes with raising her family has given her a chance to bond with Charlie.

Down the street at a free-standing birth center, Monica feels empowered. Breastfeeding her 4-hour-old newborn could not feel more peaceful, considering her long and trying labor. As her husband brings in the car seat in preparation for heading home, Monica exclaims, "This is exactly why we chose to come here! We were able to have the birth experience we wanted, and now I can't believe we get to go home and snuggle into our own beds."

Both Natalie and Monica felt supported and pleased with their immediate postpartum experiences. Though the length of their postpartum stays varied greatly, both mothers left their birth sites prepared to care for their newborns. The timing of newborn discharge varies across institutions and birth settings, and many factors need to be considered in determining an appropriate length of stay. This chapter explores the dynamics involved in the decision making around newborn discharge timing.

Historical Perspective

Home was the most common birth site in the United States until about the 1940s and 1950s. Nearly all women were giving birth in the hospital by the 1960s, which led to much longer hospital stays postpartum, averaging about 4 to 5 days by 1970 (Kuper, 1997). As a countercultural swing began drawing women back to the home setting for birth, families began to request shorter hospitals stays. Hospitals responded by offering educational programs that resulted in postpartum stays of approximately 12 hours as an alternative to home birth (Kuper, 1997). Soon after, shorter hospital stays were implemented with all mothers and newborns, and by the 1990s insurance companies would often deny reimbursement for postpartum stays beyond 24 hours following vaginal births (American Academy of Pediatrics [AAP], 2004). In an effort to ensure adequate postpartum health promotion, many states began passing bills safeguarding minimum postpartum stays. This led Congress to pass the Newborns' and Mothers' Health Protection Act of 1996, which required that insurance companies cover a minimum of 48 hours' postpartum care following vaginal births and 96 hours' postpartum care following cesarean births (Bradley, 1996). Of note, this act does not require this full length of stay, should families and providers consider an earlier discharge time appropriate.

Ethical Considerations

The bioethical principles of nonmaleficence, beneficence, autonomy, and justice should all be considered when determining appropriate discharge timing. First, a newborn's safety must be a high priority. The principle of nonmaleficence urges providers to consider whether early discharge might either lead to harm or increase a newborn's chance of being readmitted. If staying longer at a birth site would provide specific benefits to the family, such as having additional lactation support, then the principle of beneficence may encourage a longer stay. Because newborns are unable to exercise their autonomy, parents should be included as decision-making partners in determining readiness for discharge. Justice should also be considered amidst the landscape of rising healthcare costs and families who are either uninsured or underinsured. Appropriate length of stay and the use of outpatient services can help to mitigate the cost of hospital admission.

Data Collection

Determining the timing of newborn discharge is a complex, clinical decision made jointly by the newborn's family, maternal, and pediatric providers, and any other team members who have been involved in the newborn's care, such as nursing staff and social workers. Given that the goal is simultaneous discharge of mother and baby to their home, communication among providers and an awareness of the mother's postpartum recovery can also influence when a newborn is discharged.

History

The first step in evaluating newborns' readiness for discharge is considering their history prenatally, their labor and birth experience, and their transition following the birth. The practitioner should review the prenatal history for any concerns, such as abnormal ultrasound findings. The mother's prenatal course can also affect the newborn's transition during the postnatal period. For instance, if the mother had gestational diabetes or substance abuse issues, more time may be needed to ensure a healthy transition.

Assessing the labor for factors that could potentially affect a newborn's discharge timing is also necessary. If the mother was positive for group B *Streptococcus*, the provider should determine if adequate antibiotic prophylaxis occurred during labor and ensure no infection signs have appeared since the woman gave birth. Providers should also assess for adequate treatment of any other infections that may have surfaced, such as chorioamnionitis.

Reviewing fetal heart rate patterns during labor and Apgar scores following the birth provides insight into the newborn's stability in the immediate postpartum period and possibly beyond. Providers must also take into account the gestational age and weight at birth and consider whether these factors affected the newborn's transition to extrauterine life. As mothers and some newborns require more recovery time following cesarean births, the route of birth will have an impact on discharge timing.

Evaluating the newborn's postpartum history also includes ensuring culturally appropriate bonding as the newborn integrates into his or her family, successful feeding, appropriate weight loss, consistently normal vital signs, and absence or appropriate recovery from hyperbilirubinemia and hypoglycemia.

Physical Examination

Once the history has been completed, the newborn must be personally observed and assessed by an appropriate healthcare provider to determine the infant's readiness for discharge. The physical exam should not reveal any concerns that would warrant a longer admission, such as major congenital defects, concerning heart murmurs, signs of infection, or significant jaundice. Aside from the absence of concerning pathology, healthy vital signs and other indicators of successful physiologic transition following the birth should be noted. A healthcare provider should note successful physiologic transition following the birth and currently stable vital signs. According to the American Academy of Pediatrics (AAP, 2015), these criteria include no signs of respiratory distress and a respiratory rate less than 60 breaths per minute. The newborn's axillary temperature should be in the range of 36.5°C to 37.4°C (97.7°F to 99.3°F). The newborn's heart rate may range from 70 to 190 beats per minute depending on whether the newborn is awake or asleep. If the heart rate remains in the lower or upper end for an extended period of time or if the heart rate is accompanied by signs of circulatory compromise, more evaluation may be needed (AAP, 2015).

Prior to going home, the newborn should have established successful feeding. Best practice advocates that a healthcare team member be available for breastfeeding support postpartum, and observe an effective latch during a feeding session. The newborn's intake and output should both be appropriate for his or her age, taking into account the expected irregularity of feedings within the first 24 hours. Parents should continue to record both feeding frequency and duration as well as urination and stooling following discharge, making an earlier discharge possible even if a newborn has not yet urinated, for example.

Routine Newborn Medications and Newborn Screening

The newborn provider should ensure that erythromycin eye ointment, vitamin K injection, and hepatitis B vaccine have all been offered and administered according to parents' consent.

Several routine screens are conducted on healthy newborns either prior to hospital discharge or shortly after discharge in a home or outpatient setting—namely, a blood test, a hearing screen, and a critical congenital heart disease screen (CCHD). Since 2005, the U.S. Department of Health has recommended that the newborn blood sample, which tests for a number of health conditions that ultimately vary by state, be collected between 24 and 48 hours following the birth, arriving at the laboratory no more than 24 hours after collection (AAP, Newborn Screening Authoring Committee, 2008; Baby's First Test, 2015; Health Resources and Services Association [HRSA] & American College of Medical Genetics [ACMG], 2005). The Centers for Disease Control and Prevention (CDC, 2015) recommends hearing screening be conducted within the first month of life, but ideally prior to a hospital discharge. While such screening has not yet been implemented in all states, the CDC (2014a) recommends CCHD screening with a pulse oximeter for newborns between 24 and 48 hours of life. In hospital settings, accomplishing these screening tests prior to discharge is reasonable. For births that take place at home or in birth centers, the tests are typically conducted during home visits 1 to 2 days following the birth.

Teaching and Counseling

The healthcare provider not only needs to assess the newborn physically, but must also determine the family's readiness to care for their newborn once they leave their birth setting. Providers can best assess readiness while providing this education and observing care firsthand.

The family should have the knowledge and skills to appropriately care for their newborn at home. Providing training during pregnancy and in the immediate postpartum period can improve families' confidence and preparedness to go home. Ideally, many of these topics will have been addressed during the pregnancy, and then are simply reviewed prior to discharge. These topics include, but are not limited to, infant safety, such as car seat use and sleeping positions; logging newborn feeding and output with an understanding of normalcy; signs of distress or illness; and umbilical cord care.

Healthcare providers should also ensure the safety of the newborn's potential home environment. Risk factors that may need to be assessed include mental illness, history of child abuse, and substance abuse. Families should also have a support network in place upon going home or have adequate social resources available in case additional help is needed.

Standards of Care

Hospital Setting

According to the AAP (2015), the time spent in the hospital before discharge needs to be long enough to ensure that the most common complications would have already occurred while the mother and baby are in the care of a health provider and that the newborn and mother have ample time to rest and recover. Most newborn and maternal complications happen within 12 hours after birth; however, some complications, such as hyperbilirubinemia and delayed postpartum hemorrhage, can arise later in the postpartum period. Ultimately, stability of the mother and newborn is the primary factor in determining discharge timing. Physiologic stability of the newborn includes having vital signs within normal parameters for at least 12 hours prior to discharge (**Box 7-1**) (AAP, 2015). In the hospital setting, the decision of stability is made by a team of healthcare providers, which is most often led by pediatric care providers. If applicable, identification and management of complications, such as sepsis and high-risk jaundice, also need to be resolved before the newborn leaves the hospital (AAP, 2015).

The newborn should have a minimum of two successful feeding sessions prior to leaving the hospital (AAP, 2015). A healthcare team member should observe and document the feeding sessions, making specific note of the latch and the newborn's ability to suck and swallow (Hagan, Shaw, & Duncan, 2008). If the newborn is having trouble with feedings, a referral to lactation services should be made. In regard to output, the newborn should have urinated and stooled at least one time before discharge (AAP, 2015).

Ideally, the mother will be discharged home with her newborn. In addition to her physiologic stability, providers should evaluate the family's social stability. The family's readiness to care for their newborn's needs and their ability to access support and further healthcare

Box 7-1: General Criteria for Newborn Discharge

- Breastfeeding established (2+ feedings in hospital)
- 1 stool and 1 void (if > 24-hour admission)
- Newborn screenings complete or planned for follow-up visit
- Newborn medications administered (erythromycin eye ointment, vitamin K injection, hepatitis B vaccine)
- Mother receives tetanus–diphtheria–pertussis (Tdap) vaccine if not previously vaccinated
- Physical examination and labs essentially normal
- Stable vital signs (for 12 hours in hospital)
- Axillary temperature 36.5–37.4°C (97.7–99.3°F)
- Respiratory rate < 60 breaths/min, no signs of distress
- Heart rate 70–190 beats/min
- Adequate social support
- Car seat installation
- Discharge teaching on newborn care and warning signs

Data from American Academy of Pediatrics. (2015). Hospital stay for healthy term newborn infants. *Pediatrics, 135*(5). 949–953. doi: 10.1542/peds.2015-0699

resources are critical to determining discharge timing. For example, if parents are required to be away from home due to extenuating circumstances, an appropriate caretaker needs to be established prior to discharge.

When indicated, laboratory results should also be reviewed prior to discharge. These results may include cord blood and direct Coombs testing, toxicology results, and results of sexually transmitted infection testing in the mother (AAP, 2015). Immunizations for the mother, such as Tdap (tetanus, diphtheria, and acellular pertussis) for protection against pertussis in the newborn, and the hepatitis B vaccine for the newborn may also be given prior to leaving the hospital (CDC, 2014b).

If the family requested a male newborn circumcision, ensure this procedure has taken place or is coordinated in the outpatient setting. If the circumcision is performed, assess the site for any excessive bleeding or signs of infection, and teach parents how to care for the circumcision prior to discharge (AAP, 2015).

The decision of discharge timing should be individualized to each mother–infant dyad; in light of this need for tailoring, early discharge should not be considered for all families. If an infant is to be discharged from the hospital prior to 48 hours after the birth, the AAP (2015) recommends a follow-up visit be scheduled within the next 48 hours (Escobar et al., 2001; Escobar et al., 2005; Kotagal, Atherton, Eshett, Schoettker, & Perlstein, 1999; Meara, Kotagal,

Atherton, & Lieu, 2004; Nelson, 1999). This visit should be conducted by a provider skilled in newborn examination and could take place in an outpatient setting or at home. Although outcomes are comparable, home visits have been found to be more costly, yet yield greater patient satisfaction (Escobar et al., 2001). The focus of the visit is to evaluate for appropriate care of the newborn and the expected physiologic transition from birth. Holistic care of the entire family should be provided at this visit as well, including assessment for maternal postpartum depression (AAP, 2015).

Birth Center and Home Settings

In the United States, the vast majority of home and birth center births are attended by certified professional midwives (CPMs), certified nurse–midwives (CNMs)/certified midwives (CMs), and traditional midwives (Stapleton, Osborne, & Illuzzi, 2013). CPMs are trained to oversee normal newborn care until approximately 6 weeks postpartum, while CNMs and CMs can manage well-newborn care until 28 days of life (American College of Nurse–Midwives [ACNM], 2012; National Association of Certified Professional Midwives [NACPM], 2004). While it is common to transfer the newborn's primary care to the ongoing pediatric providers prior to these time limits, midwives are the discharging providers following home and birth center births. The primary difference in discharge timing from these sites in comparison to timing at the hospital is that postpartum admissions are significantly shorter in the former, typically averaging 3 to 6 hours. Clinical decision making around discharge can be more complex in birth centers and homes, as midwives are continually assessing both for the potential need to transfer to the hospital and for the newborn's readiness for discharge.

Newborn activities that take place in the home or birth center prior to discharge include establishing breastfeeding; conducting a full newborn physical examination, including weight and measurements; and administering erythromycin eye ointment and vitamin K injection. By the time the newborn is 3 to 6 hours of age, midwives will have assisted in these activities and can assess if the newborn's vital signs and general stability are appropriate for discharge. Birth records with the newborn's history are then transmitted to the ongoing pediatric provider. Depending on the midwife practice's postpartum visit schedule, there may be an overlap in newborn care with the pediatric care provider over the first few weeks of life.

The American Association of Birth Centers (AABC, 1995) stresses that early discharge is offered in a maternity healthcare context that uniquely prepares women to identify normal findings in their newborns, while also empowering parents to recognize abnormal findings that warrant contacting their midwife or pediatric provider. This system incorporates rigorous prenatal education for parents in preparation for early newborn assessment and care, ultimately instilling confidence in parenting. While newborn care basics are certainly covered, education also includes extensive breastfeeding preparedness; identifying signs of respiratory distress, such as nasal flaring, retractions, tachypnea with attempted feedings, and central cyanosis; and identifying signs of infection, with instructions on taking the newborn's temperature following discharge. In addition to reviewing these instructions prior to discharge, plans are scheduled for a follow-up within the first 2 days.

Prenatally, providers assist families in identifying postpartum resources and preparing for interdependence postpartum (AABC, 1995). These resources range from friends and family who can help provide postpartum meals and household maintenance to community healthcare resources available for lactation and mental health support.

In addition to maternal assessment, the home visit should include the newborn blood screen, CCHD screen, and possibly the hearing screen. The nurse or midwife would also review the newborn's breastfeeding and output log and provide breastfeeding support as needed. Finally, this visit would include an assessment of the newborn's weight, vital signs, and risk for jaundice. The immediate postpartum period together with the home visit comprise the same activities accomplished during the immediate postpartum period during hospital stays.

Risk of Readmission

The risk of readmission is a primary factor in considering when to discharge the mother and baby. Fortunately, the vast majority of newborns who are born term or close to term do not develop problems after birth. Therefore, the risk of readmission in healthy infants is low. One study found that in 7021 term or near-term newborns born in the hospital, 8% were identified as having complications after birth (Jackson et al., 2000). The most commonly reported problems involved tachypnea and temperature abnormalities for the infant. Of the problems identified, 69% were diagnosed by the practitioner while performing the first examination on the newborn during the immediate postpartum period. As some of these complications occur further from birth, this possibility stresses the need for follow-up within days after discharge (Jackson et al., 2000).

Increasing length of hospital stays has shown mixed results in terms of whether they decrease readmission rates (AAP, Subcommittee on Hyperbilirubinemia, 2004; Gentile et al., 1981; Maisels et al., 2009). Confounding variables make it difficult to draw consistent conclusions across all studies (Datar & Sood, 2006; Grupp-Phelan, Taylor, Liu, & Davis, 1999; Kotagal et al., 1999; Paul, Lehman, Hollenbeak, & Maisels, 2006; Watt, Sword, & Krueger, 2005). The majority of readmissions are related to feeding difficulties, including jaundice and dehydration (Danielsen, Castles, Damberg, & Gould, 2000; Escobar et al., 2005). Whether newborns are discharged early or not, this finding highlights the need for strong breastfeeding support for all mothers during and after admission. **Box 7-2** presents an evidence-based list of risk factors for readmission.

Box 7-2: Risk Factors for Readmission

- Small for gestational age
- Low birth weight
- Shorter gestation (late-preterm infants)
- Feeding difficulties
- Primiparity
- White or Asian race
- Instrumental deliveries

Data from Bernstein, H. H., Spino, C., Finch, S., Wasserman, R., Slora, E., Lalama, C., . . . McCormick, M. C. (2007). Decision-making for postpartum discharge of 4300 mothers and their healthy infants: The life around newborn discharge study. *Pediatrics, 120*(2), 391–400; Danielsen, B., Castles, A. G., Damberg, C. L., & Gould, J. B. (2000). Newborn discharge timing and readmissions: California, 1992–1995. *Pediatrics, 106*, 31–39; Escobar, G. J., Greene, J. D., Hulac, P., Kincannon, E., Bischoff, K., Gardner, M., . . . France, E. (2005). Rehospitalisation after birth hospitalisation: Patterns among infants of all gestations. *Archives of Disease in Childhood, 90*(2), 125–131. doi: 10.1136/adc.2003.039974; Paul, I. M., Lehman, E. B., Hollenbeak, C. S., & Maisels, M. J. (2006). Preventable newborn readmissions since passage of the Newborns' and Mothers' Health Protection Act. *Pediatrics, 118*(6), 2349–2358; Watt, S., Sword, W., & Krueger, P. (2005). Longer postpartum hospitalization options: Who stays, who leaves, what changes? *BMC Pregnancy Childbirth, 5*(13). doi: 10:1186/1471-2393-5-13.

In regard to midwife-attended home and birth center births, two large studies have evaluated newborn outcomes in the United States. In 2013, the National Birth Center Study II released its prospective findings on birth center outcomes from 2007 to 2010, which included birth data from 15,574 women planning birth center births (Stapleton et al., 2013). The newborn transfer rate in the immediate postpartum period prior to discharge was 2.6%, with the most common reason for transfer being respiratory issues such as transient tachypnea of the newborn. The urgent newborn transfer rate was 0.7%, with the most common reason for such transfer being an Apgar score less than 7 at 5 minutes postpartum.

In 2014, the Midwives' Alliance of North America published data on 16,924 midwife-attended home births (Cheyney et al., 2014). This prospective study revealed a 0.9% newborn transfer rate in the immediate postpartum period and a 2.8% admission rate to the neonatal intensive care unit (NICU) in the first 6 weeks of life, which included the immediate postpartum period prior to discharge.

The model of care for home and birth center settings provides additional preparedness to improve parenting competence, and also incorporates the use of home visits in the first few days following discharge to ensure appropriate physiologic and social transitions. The findings from the National Birth Center Study II and the Midwives' Alliance of North America indicate that the vast majority of newborns are discharged from home and birth center settings without immediate or delayed complications that could require hospitalization.

Cultural Considerations

In light of the United States' increasing cultural, ethnic, religious, and racial diversity, it is more important now than ever that providers exercise cultural humility. The concept of cultural humility involves keeping a continually open mind, committing to reflective lifelong learning, and realizing that full cultural competence is an unattainable goal (Tervalon & Murray-Garcia, 1998). It also acknowledges the power differential that inherently accompanies a provider–patient relationship and seeks to humbly keep patients with their values and goals at the center of their care.

In considering newborn discharge, cultural humility is particularly necessary in assessing how and when families bond with their newborns, realizing that the amount and timing of eye contact and displays of physical and verbal affection vary across families and cultures. The degree to which parents desire to provide all newborn care as opposed to having extended family or hospital staff assist them during admission can also vary and cannot be consistently used to gauge parents' desire or readiness for independence. Providers must graciously exercise humility in considering a family's ability to safely care for their newborn at home.

Leininger's culture care diversity and universality theory provides a helpful framework for considering newborn care customs (McQuiston & Webb, 1995). Leininger explains that all cultures have practices and remedies that have been passed down for centuries. Providers can accommodate these instinctive and familiar culturally based caring practices alongside the professional knowledge they received from training and evidence-based practice to provide the most appropriate care for any given family or community (McQuiston & Webb, 1995). If certain practices are known to cause harm, however, providers should address these concerns with thorough counseling and informed consent. Honoring families and communities as they seek to gently care for and raise up their next generation through the heartbeat of time-honored traditions greatly enhances the healthcare experience of all families.

Examples of common practices in certain cultures include some Asian women desiring to keep their rooms and all liquids and foods warm in the postpartum period; women from several cultures including Hispanic, Native American, Asian, and Somali refraining from breastfeeding until their milk has fully come in; and differences in newborn bathing and swaddling practices (Dixon, 1992; Steinman et al., 2010; Weibert, 2002). Cultural humility does not assume that every family will make decisions consistent with cultural generalizations. Nevertheless, having at least a basic understanding of the beliefs and practices of the patient population assists in providing more meaningful and competent care. It fosters healthier and more respectful client–provider relationships by giving providers insight that aids them in asking pertinent questions and better anticipating families' needs. As an example, if a provider is discharging a newborn whose parents are religious Jews on the Sabbath, it would be culturally sensitive to ask if they would like assistance with carrying their belongings to their transportation. While not all religious Jews adhere to the same work restrictions on the Sabbath, being aware that some would not be able to carry their belongings to their car, wash their newborns, write down discharge instructions, or drive their cars can help providers better anticipate potential needs their clients may have in preparing for discharge.

Conclusion

Clinical decision making in determining discharge timing for newborns essentially centers on stability. This complex decision must take many factors into account, including the newborn's history, physiologic stability, and social environment. In addition to evaluating these components, providers seek to assess parental readiness and include families as shared decision makers when determining the most appropriate discharge time for individualized care. Ultimately, providers aim to promote a safe and nurturing transition for families to welcome their newborns into their homes.

Student Practice Activities

Multiple Choice

1. When should the newborn screening blood sample be collected following the birth?
    A) Less than 12 hours
    B) 12–24 hours
    C) 24–48 hours
    D) 48–72 hours

2. In what year did Congress pass the Newborns' and Mothers' Health Protection Act, ensuring insurance coverage for adequate hospital stays postpartum?
    A) 1960
    B) 1972
    C) 1985
    D) 1996

3. According to the American Academy of Pediatrics, which of the following sets of vital signs would indicate a newborn is ready for discharge?
    A) HR: 158, RR: 42, T: 96.5
    B) HR: 122, RR: 58, T: 99.0
    C) HR: 120, RR: 72, T: 97.8
    D) HR: 136, RR: 56, T: 99.5

4. When does the majority of early home care education occur for families planning a home birth?
    A) Prenatally
    B) In labor
    C) Immediate postpartum, prior to discharge
    D) At a postpartum home visit within 2 days of the birth

5. The American Academy of Pediatrics recommends newborn vital signs be stable for ____ hours prior to hospital discharge.
    A) 2
    B) 6
    C) 12
    D) 24

6. The Newborns' and Mothers' Health Protection Act ensures insurance coverage for at least ____ hours following cesarean births.
    A) 24 hours
    B) 48 hours
    C) 72 hours
    D) 96 hours

Hospital Birth Case Study

Courtney gave birth to Jasmine 2 days ago following an essentially healthy pregnancy. On the day of the birth, Courtney had a difficult time latching Jasmine, and was experiencing some nipple pain. A lactation consultant has been working with the mother and baby, and breastfeeding has since improved. Jasmine's weight loss is at 7% today, and a bilirubin level was collected at 40 hours of age because of mild jaundice on examination. The results came back as lower risk at 8 mg/dL. Jasmine has passed her CCHD and hearing screen, and her metabolic screen has been sent to the lab.

1. Which additional information would you want to glean from Jasmine's chart?
2. Which questions do you still have for the family?
3. Which questions do you have for additional healthcare staff?
4. Are there any additional laboratory tests or physical assessments that you feel are necessary?
5. Based on the information provided, would you consider Jasmine appropriate for discharge today?

Home Birth Case Study

Marquisia is now 1 hour old. Her fetal heart tones were stable throughout labor and pushing, and her Apgar scores were 7 at 1 minute and 8 at 5 minutes. Since birth, her respiratory rate has been in the 60s to 80s. On physical exam, you hear clearing lung sounds in all fields and do not see nasal flaring or retractions. You note acrocyanosis. Twenty minutes following the birth, Marquisia began to nurse. She had a strong latch and successfully nursed for 15 minutes on each side.

1. Which additional information would you like to know, either from her history or exam findings?
2. Would you consider Marquisia stable currently? Why or why not?
3. Discuss possible indications for a hospital transfer. Discuss criteria that would still need to be met, should the midwife consider discharging her rather than transferring.
4. How would you make a plan for Marquisia?

References

American Academy of Pediatrics (AAP). (2004). Hospital stays for healthy term newborns. *Pediatrics, 113*(5), 1434–1436.

American Academy of Pediatrics (AAP). (2015). Hospital stay for healthy term newborn infants. *Pediatrics, 135*(5), 949–953. doi: 10.1542/peds.2015-0699

American Academy of Pediatrics (AAP), Newborn Screening Authoring Committee. (2008). Newborn screening expands: Recommendations for pediatricians and medical homes: Implications for the system. *Pediatrics, 121*(1), 192–217.

American Academy of Pediatrics (AAP), Subcommittee on Hyperbilirubinemia. (2004). Management of hyperbilirubinemia in the newborn infant 35 or more weeks of gestation. *Pediatrics, 114*(1), 297–316.

American Association of Birth Centers (AABC). (1995). Position statement: Early discharge. Retrieved from http:// c.ymcdn.com/sites/www.birthcenters.org/resource/collection/46992E86-D0A4-476E-8B09-F5ECE203B16E/ EARLYDC.pdf

American College of Nurse–Midwives (ACNM). (2012). ACNM core competencies for midwifery practice. Retrieved from http://www.midwife.org/ACNM/files/ACNMLibraryData/UPLOADFILENAME/000000000050/ Core%20Comptencies%20Dec%202012.pdf

Baby's First Test. (2015). The recommended uniform screening panel. Retrieved from http://www.babysfirsttest.org/

Bradley, W. (1996). Newborns' and Mothers' Health Protection Act of 1996, Public Law No. 104–204.

Centers for Disease Control and Prevention (CDC). (2014a). Pulse oximetry screening for critical congenital heart defects. Retrieved from http://www.cdc.gov/features/congenitalheartdefects/

Centers for Disease Control and Prevention (CDC). (2014b). Recommended immunization schedule for persons aged 0 through 18 years: United States. Retrieved from http://www.cdc.gov/vaccines/schedules/downloads/ child/0-18yrs-schedule.pdf

Centers for Disease Control and Prevention (CDC). (2015). Hearing loss in children: Screening and diagnosis. Retrieved from http://www.cdc.gov/ncbddd/hearingloss/screening.html

Cheyney, M., Bovbjerg, M., Everson, C., Gordon, W., Hannibal, D., & Vedam, S. (2014). Outcomes of care for 16,924 planned home births in the United States: The Midwives Alliance of North America Statistics Project, 2004 to 2009. *Journal of Midwifery and Women's Health, 59*(1), 17–27. doi: 10.1111/jmwh.12172

Danielsen, B., Castles, A. G., Damberg, C. L., & Gould, J. B. (2000). Newborn discharge timing and readmissions: California, 1992–1995. *Pediatrics, 106*, 31–39.

Datar, A., & Sood, N. (2006). Impact of postpartum hospital-stay legislation on newborn length of stay, readmission, and mortality in California. *Pediatrics, 118*(1), 63–72.

Dixon, G. (1992). Colostrum avoidance and early infant feeding in Asian societies. *Asia Pacific Journal of Clinical Nutrition, 1*(4), 225–229.

Escobar, G. J., Braveman, P. A., Ackerson, L., Odouli, R., Coleman-Phox, K., Capra, A. M., . . . Lieu, T. A. (2001). A randomized comparison of home visits and hospital-based group follow-up visits after early postpartum discharge. *Pediatrics, 108*(3), 719–727.

Escobar, G. J., Greene, J. D., Hulac, P., Kincannon, E., Bischoff, K., Gardner, M., . . . France, E. (2005). Rehospitalisation after birth hospitalisation: Patterns among infants of all gestations. *Archives of Disease in Childhood, 90*(2), 125–131. doi: 10.1136/adc.2003.039974

Gentile, R., Stevenson, G., Dooley, T., Franklin, D., Kawabori, I., & Pearlman, A. (1981). Pulsed Doppler echocardiographic determination of time of ductal closure in normal newborn infants. *Journal of Pediatrics, 98*(3), 443–448.

Grupp-Phelan, J., Taylor, J. A., Liu, L. L., & Davis, R. L. (1999). Early newborn hospital discharge and readmission for mild and severe jaundice. *Archives of Pediatric and Adolescent Medicine, 153*(12), 1283–1288.

Hagan, J. F., Shaw, J. S., & Duncan, P. M. (2008). *Bright futures: Guidelines for health supervision of infants, children, and adolescents* (3rd ed.). Elk Grove Village, IL: American Academy of Pediatrics.

Health Resources and Services Association (HRSA) & American College of Medical Genetics (ACMG). (2005). Newborn screening: Toward a uniform panel and system. Retrieved from http://mchb.hrsa.gov/programs/newbornscreening/ screeningreportpdf.pdf

Jackson, G., Kennedy, K., Sendelbach, D., Talley, D., Aldridge, C., Vedro, D., & Laptook, A. (2000). Problem identification in apparently well neonates: Implications for early discharge. *Clinical Pediatrics, 39*(10), 581–590.

Kotagal, U. R., Atherton, H. D., Eshett, R., Schoettker, P. J., & Perlstein, P. H. (1999). Safety of early discharge for Medicaid newborns. *Journal of the American Medical Association, 282*(12), 1150–1156.

Kuper, D (1997). Newborns' and mothers' health protection act: Putting the brakes on drive-through deliveries. *Marquette Law Review, 80*(2), 668–689.

Maisels, M. J., Bhutani, V. K., Bogen, D., Newman, T. B., Stark, A. R., & Watchko, J. F. (2009). Hyperbilirubinemia in the newborn infant < or = 35 weeks' gestation: An update with clarifications. *Pediatrics, 124*(4), 1193–1198.

McQuiston, C. M., & Webb, A. A. (1995). *Foundations of nursing theory: Contributions of 12 key theorists.* Thousand Oaks, CA: Sage.

Meara, E., Kotagal, U. R., Atherton, H. D., & Lieu, T. A. (2004). Impact of early newborn discharge legislation and early follow-up visits on infant outcomes in a state Medicaid population. *Pediatrics, 113*(6), 1619–1627.

National Association of Certified Professional Midwives (NACPM). (2004). Essential documents of the National Association of Certified Professional Midwives. Retrieved from http://www.nacpm.org/Resources/nacpm-standards.pdf

Nelson, V. R. (1999). The effect of newborn early discharge follow-up program on pediatric urgent care utilization. *Journal of Pediatric Health Care, 13*(2), 58–61.

Paul, I. M., Lehman, E. B., Hollenbeak, C. S., & Maisels, M. J. (2006). Preventable newborn readmissions since passage of the Newborns' and Mothers' Health Protection Act. *Pediatrics, 118*(6), 2349–2358.

Stapleton, S. R., Osborne, C., & Illuzzi, J. (2013). Outcomes of care in birth centers: Demonstration of a durable model. *Journal of Midwifery & Women's Health, 58*(1), 3–14. doi: 10.1111/jmwh.12003

Steinman, L., Doescher, M., Keppel, G., Pak-Gorstein, S., Graham, E., Haq, A., . . . Spicer, P. (2010). Understanding infant feeding beliefs, practices and preferred nutrition education and health provider approaches: An exploratory study with Somali mothers in the USA. *Maternal& Child Nutrition, 6*(1), 67–88.

Tervalon, M., & Murray-Garcia, J. (1998). Cultural humility versus cultural competence: A critical distinction in defining physician training outcomes in multicultural education. *Journal of Health Care for the Poor and Underserved, 9*(2), 117–125.

Watt, S., Sword, W., & Krueger, P. (2005). Longer postpartum hospitalization options: Who stays, who leaves, what changes? *BMC Pregnancy Childbirth, 5*(13). doi: 10:1186/1471-2393-5-13

Weibert, S. (2002). Cultural diversity and breastfeeding. *San Diego County Breastfeeding Coalition, 2*(3), 1–8.

CHAPTER 8

DISCHARGE TEACHING

Cara Busenhart

A recent survey of new mothers found that a significant amount of teaching must be performed before discharge of a newborn infant from the hospital or birth center. Even when the newborn is born at home, the parents must be provided with education about normal newborn care and follow-up, despite the fact that the newborn will not be "discharged" from a healthcare facility.

Ideally, teaching and preparation for care of the newborn should begin during the pregnancy and continue through the birth and into the well-child care environments. Teaching and instruction should be individualized for each infant and family, after carefully assessing the family's educational preparation, language and cultural needs, health literacy, and physical capabilities.

Timing of Discharge

The decision to discharge the infant and mother from the birth facility is often a joint decision between the family, obstetric provider, and neonatal/pediatric provider (if they are different individuals). The length of stay should be long enough to assess for newborn problems and to ensure the family is prepared to care for the newborn at home (McKee-Garrett, 2015).

A routine stay of 24 to 48 hours in the hospital or 12 hours (or less) in a free-standing birth center is typical after a normal vaginal birth. The hospital stay may be longer for cesarean delivery or a pregnancy with complications. The American Academy of Pediatrics (AAP)

Box 8-1: American Academy of Pediatrics Recommendations for Discharge of Healthy Term Newborns

- No neonatal abnormality requiring hospitalization
- Vital signs are normal for at least 12 hours
- Has urinated and stooled at least once spontaneously
- Completed at least two successful feedings
- If circumcised, the infant has no evidence of excessive bleeding at the circumcision site for at least 2 hours
- Does not have significant jaundice
- Screened and monitored for sepsis
- Maternal laboratory testing results have been reviewed (including HIV, syphilis, and hepatitis B surface antigen)
- Initial hepatitis B vaccine given
- Screening tests completed (hearing, metabolic, and critical congenital heart disease)
- Mother/family has received training on care of the infant and has demonstrated competency
- Confirmation of an appropriate car seat for travel received
- Family, environmental, and social risk factors assessed and addressed
- Appropriate follow-up care identified and communicated to the mother/family

Data from Benitz, W. E. (2015). Hospital stay for healthy term newborn infants. *Pediatrics, 135*(5), 948–953.

has recommended minimum criteria and conditions for newborn discharge (**Box 8-1**). For late-preterm newborns, 18 discharge criteria must be (**Box 8-2**) met prior to discharge (Engle, Tomashek, Wallman, & Committee on Fetus and Newborn, 2007). The AAP also recommends a follow-up visit, in the office or the family home, within 48 hours for all newborns who are discharged from a delivery facility prior to 72 hours (Rosenberg & Grover, 2013). An early visit is particularly important for infants who are born late preterm, are small for gestational age, have difficulty breastfeeding, or have medical, social, or financial risk factors.

Standard of Care/National Guidelines for Care

There are no national guidelines for a standardized discharge teaching curriculum from nursing or medical professional organizations. The American Academy of Family Physicians does recommend key areas that should be addressed as the basis of a hospital discharge list: (1) feeding, (2) urination patterns, (3) bowel movements, (4) umbilical cord care, (5) skin care, (6) genital care, (7) signs of illness, (8) prevention of sudden infant death syndrome, (9) car seat selection and proper use, and (10) follow-up appointment made at discharge (Langan, 2006).

Box 8-2: American Academy of Pediatrics Discharge Criteria for Late-Preterm Infants

- Accurate gestational aging done
- Timing of discharge individualized—the late-preterm infant may not be able to be discharged or ready for discharge before 48 hours
- Follow-up care within 24 to 48 hours of discharge has been arranged
- Vital signs (heart/respiratory rates, axillary temperature) within normal range
- Stooled at least once
- Successfully fed by breast/bottle for 24 hours prior to discharge; weight loss greater than 2% to 3% of birth weight per day or a maximum of 7% of birth weight after birth should be assessed for dehydration (and jaundice) before discharge
- Breastfeeding ability/success evaluated and documented at least twice daily after birth
- Feeding plan developed and taught to parents, who understand how to carry it out and why the feeding plan is important
- Risk of developing severe hyperbilirubinemia is assessed using nomograms, with follow-up plans determined
- Physical examination totally normal with no abnormality
- Circumcision site with no active bleeding for at least 2 hours before discharge
- Evaluation of maternal/neonatal laboratory work complete
- Hepatitis B vaccine given or plans for outpatient administration made
- Initial newborn genetic screen drawn; repeat follow-up screen scheduled
- Passes car seat test/challenge
- Hearing screen done
- Critical congenital cardiac disease screening done
- Social, environmental, and familial risk factors assessed and, if necessary, discharge delayed until plans for interventions have been developed
- Parents are able through education and demonstration to provide care for their newborn after discharge

Data from Engle, W. A., Tomashek, K. M., Wallman, C., & Committee on Fetus and Newborn. (2007). "Late-preterm" infants: A population at risk. *Pediatrics, 120,* 1390–1401.

Without published guidelines, care providers are left to create and design a curriculum that is appropriate for their patient population. This chapter presents key concepts that are important to include in discharge teaching for newborn infants and their families.

Parental perceptions of the discharge process often differ from provider perceptions of this process. The mother and family should be offered an opportunity to ask questions and to have all questions answered. Unfortunately, many parents are often left with unanswered questions (Sneath, 2009). Additionally, the mother and family should be given instruction on how to reach a care provider with any concerns after discharge, including how to seek emergency care for serious concerns (Langan, 2006).

Preparation for Discharge

Newborn Screens

Screening of newborns is conducted to detect life-threatening disorders or conditions that may cause lifelong health implications before the disorder becomes symptomatic (Kemper, 2015). Screening tests that are available for newborns include metabolic disorders, hearing, hyperbilirubinemia (jaundice), and critical congenital heart defects.

In the United States, screening programs are managed at the state level and include screening procedures, diagnosis, treatment of disease, follow-up, and tracking of outcomes (Kemper, 2015). While there is variability between state screening programs, the U.S. Secretary of Health and Human Services has established a recommended list of conditions that should be included in all screening programs. The Recommended Uniform Screening Panel (RUSP) includes such conditions as (1) primary congenital hypothyroidism, (2) congenital adrenal hyperplasia, (3) hemoglobinopathies, (4) critical congenital heart disease, (5) cystic fibrosis, (6) classic galactosemia, (7) hearing loss, (8) severe combined immunodeficiencies, (9) phenylketonuria, and (10) maple syrup urine disease (Kemper, 2015).

Metabolic Screening   Metabolic screening should be performed as close to hospital discharge as possible to permit the most accurate results (Kemper, 2015). If the infant is not born in a hospital, the parents should arrange for screening with their healthcare provider when the child is 1 to 2 days of age (March of Dimes, 2015; Newborn Screening Clearinghouse [NSC], 2015). Some states require that screening occurs again around 2 weeks of age (March of Dimes, 2015).

Metabolic screening is completed with a blood test, requiring a heel lance to collect blood on a special type of paper, which is then sent to a lab for analysis (NSC, 2015). Results of the test are typically available within a week and are communicated to the healthcare provider of record for the infant (March of Dimes, 2015). This relatively rapid turnaround time allows for early identification and treatment of disorders.

State screening programs vary in terms of the number of conditions included in their screening panel. A panel of 32 specific conditions is encouraged in the RUSP; however, states are not legally required to include all disorders or conditions in their screening program (NSC, 2015). All states include sickle cell disease, phenylketonuria, and hypothyroidism in their screening panel, and nearly all states include cystic fibrosis screening (Shapira, 2010). Expanded newborn screening, also referred to as supplemental screening (NSC, 2015), includes additional screening beyond the basics covered in state screening and aids in the diagnosis of inborn errors of metabolism (Rosenberg & Grover, 2013), such as organic acid metabolism disorders, fatty acid oxidation disorders, and amino acid metabolism disorders, as well as hemoglobin disorders and other disorders (March of Dimes, 2015). These rare disorders prevent the human body from turning food into energy (Patel, 2013), block processing of amino acids to make protein, impact oxygen delivery to the body (March of Dimes, 2015), and may lead to varying degrees of developmental delay (Patel, 2013).

Baby's First Test is an educational website for parents and healthcare professionals regarding newborn screening. On this site, parents can find information about screening specific to their state of residence or the location of their birthing facility (Kemper, 2015).

Hearing Screening Significant hearing loss is the most common disorder at birth (Adcock & Freysdottir, 2015). Hearing loss may lead to delays in language development, behavioral and psychosocial difficulties, and poor academic achievement. To prevent these complications, universal hearing screening—that is, screening of all newborns—is recommended in the United States to detect hearing loss (McKee-Garrett, 2015). Although not all states have laws mandating such screening, all states have implemented universal newborn hearing screening (Adcock & Freysdottir, 2015). Early diagnosis and intervention can improve speech, development of language, and educational attainment in affected individuals (Adcock & Freysdottir, 2015; Rosenberg & Grover, 2013). Similar to metabolic screening, hearing screening is performed prior to discharge from the hospital or around 1 to 2 days of age (March of Dimes, 2015).

Two types of hearing screen techniques are approved by the AAP's Task Force on Newborn and Infant Hearing: auditory brain stem responses (ABR) and otoacoustic emissions (OAE). Both of these techniques are inexpensive, portable, reproducible, and automated (Adcock & Freysdottir, 2015). **Table 8-1** compares the two screening techniques.

Infants who are referred for audiologic assessment after failing the hearing screen should be evaluated by 3 months of age (Adcock & Freysdottir, 2015). If intervention is necessary, it should be implemented by 6 months of age and should be individualized to the infant and family (Adcock & Freysdottir, 2015).

Hyperbilirubinemia/Jaundice Screening All infants should be screened every 8 to 12 hours after birth for the presence of jaundice (McKee-Garrett, 2015). If jaundice is present prior to 24 hours of age or appears excessive for the age, a bilirubin measurement should be performed. The AAP (2015e) suggests that all newborns should be screened for jaundice and hyperbilirubinemia before discharge from the hospital or the birth center.

Screening for hyperbilirubinemia, either with total serum bilirubin or transcutaneous bilirubin levels, has become common practice in the United States. Such screening is suggested to prevent chronic bilirubin encephalopathy. Despite this common practice, the U.S.

Table 8-1: Comparison of Auditory Brain Stem Responses and Otoacoustic Emissions Hearing Screening Techniques

	Auditory Brain Stem Responses	Otoacoustic Emissions
Testing time	• Infants must be asleep for testing, with delays noted with any infant movement	• Less patient preparation time • Shorter testing time (5 minutes versus 13 minutes) • Infant may be awake, feeding, or sucking on pacifier
Interference	• Subject to movement artifact from the infant	• Not subject to movement artifact from the infant • Sensitive to background noise
False-positive results	• Lower incidence of false-positive test results • Referral rate of 4%	• More infants falsely appear to have hearing loss in first 3 days of life with otoacoustic emissions (likely due to occlusion of ear canal with vernix) • Referral rate of 15%
Tympanic membrane mobility	• Does not require normal middle ear	• Requires a normal middle ear • Reduced tympanic membrane mobility can reduce screening pass rates
Auditory neuropathy	• Can detect hearing loss in infants with auditory neuropathy • Appropriate screening test for infants at risk for auditory neuropathy (preterm, hypoxia, hyperbilirubinemia, neurologic impairment)	• Cannot detect hearing loss in infants with auditory neuropathy, which may cause a false-negative result
Relative costs	• Total cost of screening and evaluation may be lower due to lower referral rate	• Lower actual screening cost

Modified from Adcock, L. M., & Freysdottir, D. (2015). Screening the newborn for hearing loss. In T. W. Post (Ed), *UpToDate*, Waltham, MA: UpToDate. Accessed on June 24, 2016.

Preventive Services Task Force (2015) has concluded that there is insufficient evidence to recommend screening all infants for hyperbilirubinemia.

Critical Congenital Heart Disease Screening   Congenital heart disease is the most common congenital disorder in newborns (Altman, 2015). Critical cardiac lesions—referring to those lesions requiring surgery or other invasive intervention in the first year of life—carry an increased risk of morbidity and mortality when there is a delay in diagnosis or referral to a tertiary center. Critical congenital heart disease (CCHD) includes (1) hypoplastic left heart syndrome, (2) pulmonary atresia, (3) tetralogy of Fallot, (4) total anomalous pulmonary venous return, (5) transposition of the great arteries, (6) tricuspid atresia, and (7) truncus arteriosus (Altman, 2015).

In 2011, the U.S. Health and Human Services Secretary's Advisory Committee on Heritable Disorders in Newborns and Children recommended that all infants be screened for CCHD with pulse oximetry (McKee-Garrett, 2015), as physical examination alone is often insufficient to detect critical lesions (Altman, 2015). The AAP, American Heart Association, and American College of Cardiology Foundation have all endorsed this recommendation. Most states now require pulse oximetry screening for CCHD as part of the panel of newborn screening (McKee-Garrett, 2015).

Like other screening tests, pulse oximetry screening for CCHD should be done as close to the infant's discharge from the hospital as possible (Altman, 2015). If the infant is not born in the hospital, parents should be advised to follow up with their pediatric care provider within 1 to 2 days of birth so that the screening can be done at the pediatric office. To perform this test, a motion-tolerant pulse oximeter is placed on the right hand and either foot, with screening occurring simultaneously or in direct sequence (Altman, 2015). Screening results for CCHD are positive when they meet one of the following criteria: (1) SpO_2 measurements less than 90%; (2) SpO_2 measurement less than 95% in both upper and lower extremities on three measurements (separated by at least an hour); or (3) differences in SpO_2 of more than 3% between the upper and lower extremities (Altman, 2015).

If screening is positive for CCHD, the infant should be referred to a healthcare team (i.e., neonatology and pediatric cardiology) who can appropriately manage the condition. Parents and clinicians should also be aware of and look for nonspecific symptoms of undiagnosed CCHD, including poor feeding, poor weight gain, cyanosis, respiratory difficulties, decreased activity, irritability, and excessive sweating (Altman, 2015).

Feeding

Regardless of how the infant is fed, either with breastmilk or formula, parents should be encouraged to record the feeding time and amount, in either minutes (breast) or ounces (formula). Infants should be fed frequently in the first few days of life to avoid hypoglycemia (McKee-Garrett, 2015).

Breastfeeding Breastfeeding is encouraged because of its benefits to both mother and infant. Breastfed infants should be fed at least 8 to 12 times within 24 hours during hospitalization and until the mother's milk supply is established. Skin-to-skin contact, on-demand feedings, support with lactation resources, and infrequent separation of the mother and infant are all measures that contribute to lactation success (McKee-Garrett, 2015).

Formula Feeding Healthy newborns who are fed formula should be offered the standard 19–20 cal/oz formula. On-demand feedings are encouraged, with no breaks longer than 4 to 5 hours. In the first few days of life, 0.5 to 1 ounce per feed is appropriate (McKee-Garrett, 2015).

Elimination

Urination Patterns Frequency of urination varies greatly between infants (AAP, 2015a). In the first week of life, an infant will generally have one void, or urination, for the number of days of age. After day 6, an infant may void as often as once every hour to as few times as 6 voids in 24 hours (AAP, 2015a). The color of urination should be light to dark yellow.

Bowel Movements Infants' bowel movements vary in their frequency, consistency, and color (AAP, 2015a). All infants should have their first bowel movement within the first 24 hours. Meconium is black, tarry, and without odor because newborns do not have bacterial colonization of their gut until after the first feeding (Hill, 2015). Over the next few days, the stools will transition from dark to dark green to yellow in color. Breastfed infants will often have stools that are watery with seedy-appearing consistency. Formula-fed infants may have less watery stools that are pasty in consistency (Hill, 2015). Stools should not be clay colored or bloody; these findings should be reported and investigated immediately.

Infection Control

The most effective way to prevent infections in newborns is good hand washing or hand hygiene (Centers for Disease Control and Prevention [CDC], 2015). Parents and caregivers should be instructed to wash their hands before touching the infant, after touching a child's urine or saliva, after wiping a child's nose, and after changing diapers. If soap and water are unavailable, an alcohol-based hand sanitizer should be used (CDC, 2015). In addition to hand washing, caregivers should be instructed *not* to put any infant care items in their mouth. When kissing an infant, they should also be encouraged to avoid contact with saliva (kiss on forehead or cheek).

Immunizations

Immunizations also prevent the spread of infections to newborns. Maternal immunization with the influenza vaccine and tetanus–diphtheria–pertussis (Tdap) vaccine is recommended during pregnancy to protect the unimmunized newborn/neonate from infection. All pregnant women should receive the inactivated flu vaccine during flu season (CDC, 2014b). Infants cannot receive the flu vaccine until they have reached 6 months of age, so all caregivers and family members should be vaccinated to reduce the risk of the infant coming in contact with an infected individual.

Between 27 and 36 weeks' gestation, Tdap vaccine should be given to pregnant women during each pregnancy. Additionally, all caregivers and close family members should be vaccinated against pertussis (CDC, 2014b). Pertussis (whooping cough) may be very serious for infants who cannot protect themselves. Vaccination of close contacts conveys protection for the infant.

Hepatitis B vaccine is typically given in three doses, with the first dose being administered at birth (CDC, 2014a). The second dose is given between 1 and 2 months of age, and the third dose between 6 and 18 months of age. All babies should begin the hepatitis B vaccine series prior to leaving the hospital or birth center (CDC, 2014a; McKee-Garrett, 2015).

Infant Care

Parenting and infant care are learned behaviors. They are not a "spectator sport"; rather, parents learn infant care by doing infant care. Parents need to be taught about normal newborn physical findings as well as how to care for their care newborn. Practice and caring for their own baby is the best teacher as the healthcare professional supervises, instructs, and supports their efforts.

Bathing   Bathing an infant approximately three times per week is adequate to keep the infant clean. Bathing more frequently may dry out the infant's skin. Until the umbilical cord falls off (at about 1 to 2 weeks), a sponge bath should be used. After the umbilical cord falls off, the infant may be placed directly into the bath, with approximately 2 inches of water in the tub. Warm (100°F)—not hot—water and a mild soap should be used. Supplies should be kept within arm's reach, and parents should be taught to never leave the infant. Parents should be instructed to avoid drafty areas and to dry the infant thoroughly after completing the bath (AAP, 2015b).

Diapering   Parents should be changing their baby's diapers prior to discharge. They should be instructed on diaper-changing technique and safety measures. During diapering, an infant should never be left unattended or on a high surface without a safety strap. An easily remembered rule is "Always have one hand on your baby." Encourage parents and caregivers to keep all supplies within arm's reach (Jana, 2015).

Instruct parents to clean their infant, particularly girls, by gently wiping from front to back (Jana, 2015). Diaper dermatitis occurs when newborn skin is exposed to urine, feces, enzymes, bile salts, and microorganisms (Lund & Durand, 2016).To prevent diaper rash, parents should change the diaper as soon as possible after a bowel movement and change wet diapers frequently (AAP, 2015d). Additionally, the infant's bottom should be exposed to air as often as feasible. If diaper rash occurs, diaper wipes should be avoided, as they irritate the skin further (AAP, 2015d).

Diaper rash occurs more frequently under certain conditions: (1) when babies are not kept clean and dry, (2) when babies have diarrhea, (3) when babies begin to eat solid food, and (4) when babies take antibiotics (AAP, 2015d). If diaper rash occurs, parents should be instructed to use an oil-based barrier ointment.

Cord Care The only care necessary for the umbilical cord stump is to keep it clean and dry (AAP, 2015f). Alcohol cleansing and triple dye are no longer necessary in developed countries (McKee-Garrett, 2015). The cord will eventually shrivel and fall off around 2 weeks of age. As the cord separates, some blood may be seen on the top of the baby's diaper that is near the cord—this is normal and heralds the separation process. Parents should be instructed to watch for signs of omphalitis, an infection of the cord stump. Signs of omphalitis include a foul-smelling yellowish discharge from the cord, red skin around the base of the cord, and crying when the cord is touched (AAP, 2015f).

Skin Care Infant skin is delicate and needs special care. In general, if skin care items are necessary, it is best to use products that are designed for babies and to avoid use on the infant's hands or face (Stanford Children's Health, 2015). Lotions are rarely necessary, although parents enjoy the smell; use products with no additives or fragrance. If powders are used, parents should be instructed to put the powder in their hand and then apply the hand to the baby's skin. Talc can be breathed into and has been seen in infants' lungs. Infant clothes should be washed in a mild soap and rinsed twice, and no dryer sheets should be used.

Circumcision

The decision to have a male infant circumcised is personal and may be influenced by geographic area, socioeconomic status, religious affiliation, insurance coverage, birth facility, and race or ethnic group (Baskin, 2015). Circumcision has been associated with some medical benefits, including reduced rates of urinary tract infection, penile cancer, and sexually transmitted infections. Risks of complications should be discussed with parents, including inadequate skin removal, bleeding, infection, urethral complications, glans injury, removal of excessive skin, adhesions, and anesthetic complications. The AAP's Task Force on Circumcision (2012) has concluded that the benefits to health for male circumcision justify access to the circumcision procedure for any families that choose it.

The circumcision procedure may be performed with various techniques, including use of the Gomco clamp, Plastibell device, or Mogen clamp (Weismiller, 2015). Provider choice often determines the modality of the technique. Parents should be instructed on post-circumcision care appropriate to the technique used by their healthcare provider. Regardless of technique, the infant should void within 12 hours of the procedure. Some blood may be noticed in the diaper, but if the blood spotting is greater than a quarter size, the surgical provider should be notified (Weismiller, 2015). Normal healing will include slight swelling and the formation of a crust on the glans (AAP, 2015c). Cleansing gently with water (and soap, if soiled) is all that is necessary to keep the penis clean. Petroleum ointment or a water-based lubricant is placed over the wound for 3 to 5 days to avoid adhesion of the glans to the infant diaper (Weismiller, 2015).

Safety

A culture of safety in the home where infants and young children live prevents injury or death. Parents must be taught how to baby-proof their home. As advocates for their baby, parents must also instruct others (i.e., grandparents, babysitters, family, friends) and make sure that their homes are safe. **Table 8-2** provides a review of key concepts for newborn safety recommendations.

Table 8-2: Newborn Safety Recommendations

Babywearing	• Make sure the infant's airway is open at all times. • Keep the infant in an upright position. • Provide support for the infant's developing neck and back. • Inspect the carrier for wear or damage, including weak spots, loose stitching, or worn fabric. • Baby carriers should not be used in motor vehicles (Babywearing International, 2015).
Car seats	• The car seat should meet national safety standards. • Installation should be according to the manufacturer's instructions. • The infant should be placed in an appropriate-size car seat and rear-facing until 2 years of age (or longer if the child is able to tolerate it). • Car seats should not be used for infant sleeping. • Never leave the baby unattended in a car seat (AboutKidsHealth, 2015).
Cribs	• Place the crib away from window blinds or curtains. • Do not use window coverings with cords. • Do not place any items in the crib with the infant, including toys, bumper pads, or blankets. • Use a firm mattress that fits snugly in the crib. • Slats should be spaced no more than 6 cm apart (James, 2009).
Other infant equipment	• Be sure that all swings, cribs, strollers, carriers, bassinets, changing tables, playpens, and toys meet national safety standards. • Used equipment should meet current safety standards. • Do not use infant seats or swings for sleeping babies (AboutKidsHealth, 2015).

(Continued)

Table 8-2: Newborn Safety Recommendations (*Continued*)

Fall prevention	• Never place the infant on a raised surface without keeping a hand on the child. • Do not place an infant seat on a raised surface. • Keep care items within reach if the infant is on a raised surface (AboutKidsHealth, 2015).
Infant cardiopulmonary resuscitation (CPR)	• Take an infant CPR course prior to birth. • Encourage all family and caregivers to take a CPR and first aid course (AboutKidsHealth, 2015).
Nose suctioning	• Suction the nose before a feeding or before bedtime. • Avoid suctioning after a feeding. • If the baby vomits and milk is coming from nose and mouth, suction the *nose first* and then the mouth. • Clean the bulb suction well between uses (Cincinnati Children's Hospital, 2015).
Pets	• Do not leave the newborn alone with a pet (AboutKidsHealth, 2015).
Taking temperature	• Rectal temperatures are contraindicated in the newborn because of the risk for perforation. Teach parents to take axillary temperatures.
Heating formula or breastmilk	• Never heat liquids in a microwave because "hot spots" in the liquid can burn an infant's mouth.
Vaporizer	• Use cool mist—never a warm mist vaporizer—to prevent accidental burns.
Siblings	• Never leave the baby alone with young sibling(s). • Supervise siblings and ensure they hold the baby *only* when they are seated.

Sleep Environment An appropriate sleep environment is encouraged to prevent sudden infant death syndrome (SIDS) or sudden unexplained infant death (SUID). A sudden infant death in an infant younger than 1 year of age that is unexplained after thorough investigation is classified as SIDS (Corwin, 2015).

Infant and environmental factors that increase risk for SIDS include (1) preterm birth or low birth weight, (2) prone sleeping position (not on back), (3) sleeping on a soft surface or with bedding accessories, (4) bed-sharing, (5) overheating, and (6) parental smoking (Corwin, 2015). To reduce an infant's risk of SIDS and other sleep-related causes of infant death, the National Institute of Child Health and Human Development developed the Safe to Sleep public education campaign (U.S. Department of Health and Human Services, 2014). Its recommendations for parents and caregivers to reduce the incidence of SIDS and sleep accidents are listed in **Box 8-3**.

Some infant care practices have been associated with a decreased incidence of SIDS and sleep-related causes of death. Use of an oscillating fan in the infant's room, swaddling in the

Box 8-3: Recommendations for a Safe Sleep Environment

- Use a firm sleep surface covered by a snug fitted sheet.
- Do *not* use pillows, blankets, sheepskins, or crib bumpers in any baby sleep area.
- Keep soft objects, toys, loose bedding and sleep positioners (Corwin, 2015) out of the baby's sleep area.
- Do *not* smoke or let anyone smoke around the baby.
- Make sure nothing covers the baby's head.
- *Always* place the baby on his or her back for sleep, for naps and at night.
- Dress the baby in sleep clothing, such as a one-piece sleeper, and do not use a blanket.
- The baby's sleep area should be near where the parents sleep.
- The baby should not sleep in an adult bed, on a couch, or on a chair alone, with parents, or with any other persons.
- Instruct all of the baby's care providers—babysitters, grandparents, family, friends, and childcare facilities—to follow these recommendations every time the baby is put to sleep.

Modified from U.S. Department of Health and Human Services. (2014). What does a safe sleep environment look like? Safe to Sleep® public education campaign. Retrieved from http://www.nichd.nih.gov/sts/about/environment/Pages/look.aspx

supine position, room-sharing, breastfeeding, and use of a pacifier have all reduced the risk of SIDS (Corwin, 2015).

How to Recognize a Sick Baby Every parent needs to be taught the signs and symptoms of a septic/infected baby. A teaching sheet, written in their primary language, should also be given to them at discharge, especially for first-time parents. All parents—but especially parents with older children—need to be instructed that a newborn is *never* to be given medicine, even acetaminophen, without consulting with the baby's healthcare provider. Newborns whom parents think are "sick enough" to medicate are sick enough to be seen by a provider.

Follow-Up Care

Follow-up care for the newborn should be arranged prior to discharge. The follow-up visit may take place in the office/clinic or the home. The timing of the visit should be based on the characteristics of the birth, length of stay after birth, and any issues that arose in the immediate newborn transition (McKee-Garrett, 2015). For a stay of less than 48 hours, a well-child visit is recommended within 48 hours of discharge. For a typical stay longer than 48 hours, a well-child visit within 3 to 5 days after discharge is appropriate. Early, comprehensive

Box 8-4: Components of Follow-Up Newborn Visit

- Assessment of the general health of the newborn
- Assessment of the mother–infant–family interaction
- Assessment of infant behavior
- Reinforcement of maternal and family education for infant care, including feeding, supine sleep position, child safety seats, and encouragement of breastfeeding
- Review of results of outstanding laboratory tests, including the newborn screen
- Performance of any necessary tests, such as a bilirubin check for jaundice
- Establishment of the relationship with a medical home for the newborn
- Assessment of parental well-being, including assessment of fatigue and postpartum depression in the mother

Modified from McKee-Garrett, T. M. (2016). Overview of the routine management of the healthy newborn infant. In T. W. Post (Ed.), *UpToDate*. Waltham, MA: UpToDate. Accessed on June 24, 2016.

follow-up visits decrease rates of rehospitalization for infants. Important components of a follow-up visit are listed in **Box 8-4**.

Student Practice Activities

Learning Activities

1. For each of the discussion/reflection prompts below, outline key concepts and teaching points that you will review with parents and caregivers. Address any controversies and/or care options that may be present.
   A) Parents of a 6-hour-old newborn desire discharge from the hospital due to their lack of health insurance payment for an extended stay. The infant was born without incident to a healthy 26-year-old mother with no known risk factors.
   B) A new mother asks why she should not place her infant to sleep "on her tummy." She is concerned about her new infant spitting up/choking and requests reassurance that her baby will "be okay on her back."
   c) Parents of a 48-hour-old infant who is being discharged do not have a pediatric healthcare provider selected to care for their infant after discharge.

2. Develop a teaching plan for each of the following scenarios:
   A) A father of a 36-hour-old newborn requests information on available screening tests for his child. He has not had any prior education about screening for conditions/disorders, screening process, diagnosis, or follow-up of abnormal results.

B) An infant is being discharged from the free-standing birth center where the child was born 6 hours ago. The parents are requesting follow-up in their home. Discuss timing of the follow-up visit and components of that visit.

C) An infant is being discharged from the birth facility at 48 hours of age. The baby boy did not pass his hearing screen in the right ear using the OAE testing modality. Discuss the necessity of any follow-up testing and the timeline for follow-up.

3. Design a one-page teaching sheet on infant care that parents may take home after discharge. Consider ease of use, clarity of language, and use of space within your document. How would this teaching sheet look different based on location of birth or length of stay prior to discharge?

Multiple Choice

1. Which of the following newborns is not ready for discharge at this time?
   A) Infant birth weight 2750 g; gestational age exam indicates term infant
   B) Infant requires phototherapy; home health referral and phototherapy arranged
   C) Male infant, circumcision 1 hour ago; no void since procedure
   D) Metabolic screening is complete; baby has appointment with pediatrician in 48 hours

2. The National Institute for Child Health and Development has recommended which of the following positions for sleeping newborns? (Choose all that apply.)
   A) Lateral
   B) Prone
   C) Semi-recumbent
   D) Supine

3. Which of the following bathing techniques is appropriate for a newborn at 3 weeks of age?
   A) Place infant in approximately 2 inches of water.
   B) Bathe the infant every day.
   C) Use a bath ring to support the infant.
   D) Water temperature should be cool to the touch on inside of wrist.

References

AboutKidsHealth. (2015). Newborn baby safety. Retrieved from http://www.aboutkidshealth.ca/en/resourcecentres/pregnancybabies/newbornbabies/newbornbabysafety/pages/default.aspx

Adcock, L. M., & Freysdottir, D. (2015). Screening the newborn for hearing loss. In M. S. Kim (Ed.), *UpToDate*. Retrieved from http://www.uptodate.com/contents/screening-the-newborn-for-hearing-loss

Altman, C. A. (2015). Congenital heart disease in the newborn: Presentation and screening for critical CHD. In D. R. Fulton & L. E. Weisman (Eds.), *UpToDate*. Retrieved from http://www.uptodate.com/home/index.html

American Academy of Pediatrics (AAP). (2012). Circumcision policy statement. *Pediatrics, 130*(3), 585–586.

American Academy of Pediatrics (AAP). (2015a). Baby's first days: Bowel movements & urination. Retrieved from https://www.healthychildren.org/English/ages-stages/baby/Pages/Babys-First-Days-Bowel-Movements-and-Urination.aspx

American Academy of Pediatrics (AAP). (2015b). Bathing your newborn. Retrieved from https://www.healthychildren.org/English/ages-stages/baby/bathing-skin-care/Pages/Bathing-Your-Newborn.aspx

American Academy of Pediatrics (AAP). (2015c). Caring for your son's penis. Retrieved from https://www.healthychildren.org/English/ages-stages/baby/bathing-skin-care/Pages/Caring-For-Your-Sons-Penis.aspx

American Academy of Pediatrics (AAP). (2015d). Diaper rash. Retrieved from https://www.healthychildren.org/English/ages-stages/baby/diapers-clothing/Pages/Diaper-Rash.aspx

American Academy of Pediatrics (AAP). (2015e). Newborn jaundice screening. Retrieved from https://www.healthychildren.org/English/ages-stages/baby/Pages/Newborn-Jaundice-Screening.aspx

American Academy of Pediatrics (AAP). (2015f). Umbilical cord care. Retrieved from https://www.healthychildren.org/English/ages-stages/baby/bathing-skin-care/Pages/Umbilical-Cord-Care.aspx

Babywearing International. (2015). Safety. Retrieved from http://babywearinginternational.org/what-is-babywearing/safety/

Baskin, L. S. (2015). Neonatal circumcision: Risks and benefits. In K. Eckler (Ed.), *UpToDate*. Retrieved from http://www.uptodate.com/contents/neonatal-circumcision-risks-and-benefits

Centers for Disease Control and Prevention (CDC). (2014a). Hepatitis B and the vaccine to prevent it: Fact sheet for parents. Retrieved from http://www.cdc.gov/vaccines/vpd-vac/hepb/fs-parents.html

Centers for Disease Control and Prevention (CDC). (2014b). Vaccines for pregnant women. Retrieved from http://www.cdc.gov/vaccines/adults/rec-vac/pregnant.html

Centers for Disease Control and Prevention (CDC). (2015). Protect your unborn baby or newborn from infections. Retrieved from http://www.cdc.gov/features/prenatalinfections/

Cincinnati Children's Hospital. (2015). Suctioning the nose with a bulb syringe. Retrieved from http://www.cincinnatichildrens.org/health/s/suction/

Corwin, M. J. (2015). Sudden infant death syndrome: Risk factors and risk reduction strategies. In G. B. Mallory & T. K. Duryea (Eds.), *UpToDate*. Retrieved from http://www.uptodate.com/home/index.html

Engle, W. A., Tomashek, K. M., Wallman, C., & Committee on Fetus and Newborn. (2007). "Late-preterm" infants: A population at risk. *Pediatrics, 120*, 1390–1401.

Hill, D. L. (2015). Baby's first bowel movements. American Academy of Pediatrics. Retrieved from https://www.healthychildren.org/English/ages-stages/baby/diapers-clothing/Pages/Babys-First-Bowel-Movements.aspx

James, A. (2009). Nursery equipment safety for newborn babies. AboutKidsHealth. Retrieved from http://www
.aboutkidshealth.ca/En/ResourceCentres/PregnancyBabies/NewbornBabies/NewbornBabySafety/Pages/
Nursery-Equipment-Safety-for-Newborn-Babies.aspx

Jana, L. A. (2015). Changing diapers. American Academy of Pediatrics. Retrieved from https://www.healthychildren
.org/English/ages-stages/baby/diapers-clothing/Pages/Changing-Diapers.aspx

Kemper, A. R. (2015). Newborn screening. In M. S. Kim (Ed.), *UpToDate.* Retrieved from http://www.uptodate.com/
contents/newborn-screening?source=search_result

Langan, R. C. (2006). Discharge procedures for healthy newborns. *American Family Physician, 73*(5), 849–852.

Lund, C., & Durand, D. J. (2016). Skin and skin care. In S. L. Gardner, B. S. Carter, M. Enzman-Hines, & J. A. Hernandez
(Eds.), *Merenstein and Gardner's handbook of neonatal intensive care* (8th ed., pp. 464–478). St. Louis, MO:
Elsevier-Mosby.

March of Dimes. (2015). Newborn screening tests for your baby. Retrieved from http://www.marchofdimes.org/baby/
newborn-screening-tests-for-your-baby.aspx

McKee-Garrett, T. M. (2015). Overview of the routine management of the healthy newborn infant. In L. E. Weisman
(Ed.), *UpToDate.* Retrieved from http://www.uptodate.com/home/index.html

Newborn Screening Clearinghouse (NSC). (2015). Baby's first test. Retrieved from http://www.babysfirsttest.org/
newborn-screening/states

Patel, S. (2013). Inborn errors of metabolism. *MedlinePlus.* U.S. National Library of Medicine. Retrieved from
https://www.nlm.nih.gov/medlineplus/ency/article/002438.htm

Rosenberg, A. A., & Grover, T. (2013). The newborn infant. In W. W. Hay, M. J. Levin, R. R. Deterding, & M. J. Abzug
(Eds.), *Current diagnosis & treatment: Pediatrics* (22nd ed.). Retrieved from http://accessmedicine.mhmedical
.com.proxy.kumc.edu:2048/content.aspx?bookid=1016

Shapira, S. K. (2010). CDC commentary: The critical importance of newborn screening and follow-up. *Medscape.*
Retrieved from http://www.medscape.com/viewarticle/725824

Sneath, N. (2009). Discharge teaching in the NICU: Are parents prepared? An integrative review of parents' perceptions. *Neonatal Network, 4,* 237–246.

Stanford Children's Health. (2015). Bathing and skin care. Retrieved from http://www.stanfordchildrens.org/en/topic/
default?id=bathing-and-skin-care-90-P02628

U.S. Department of Health and Human Services. (2014). What does a safe sleep environment look like? Safe to Sleep®
public education campaign. Retrieved from http://www.nichd.nih.gov/sts/about/environment/Pages/look.aspx

U.S. Preventive Services Task Force (USPSTF). (2015). Hyperbilirubinemia: Screening infants. Final update summary. Retrieved from http://www.uspreventiveservicestaskforce.org/Page/Document/UpdateSummaryFinal/
hyperbilirubinemia-screening-infants

Weismiller, D. G. (2015). Techniques for neonatal circumcision. In K. Eckler (Ed.), *UpToDate.* Retrieved from http://
www.uptodate.com/contents/techniques-for-neonatal-circumcision?source=search_result

CHAPTER 9

HYPERBILIRUBINEMIA OF THE NEWBORN BORN AFTER 35 WEEKS' GESTATION

Susan Dragoo

Jaundice is the most common transitional finding in the newborn period, appreciable in more than 80% of all newborns in the United States. In the healthy newborn, jaundice progresses in a predictable pattern with a clinical presentation that includes yellow skin, conjunctiva, and mucous membranes. It initially becomes visually apparent on the face and is followed by caudal progression to the trunk and extremities.

At low levels, bilirubin—a weak acid—has antioxidant properties that make it capable of binding to membrane lipids and limiting damage created by peroxidation. At elevated levels, bilirubin is toxic, having the ability to create neuronal damage and neurologic dysfunction. In the newborn, the clinical significance of bilirubin is the propensity for its disposition in the skin and mucous membranes, which produces the characteristic yellow color associated with jaundice. Hyperbilirubinemia progresses through predictable stages, with physical findings beginning with visible jaundice and progressing to acute bilirubin encephalopathy (ABE) with sleeping difficulty, feeding difficulty, and lethargy (**Figure 9-1**). If untreated, the newborn may progress from ABE to chronic bilirubin encephalopathy (CBE) with athetoid cerebral palsy, hearing loss, and dental hyperplasia (Kaplan, Wong, Sibley, & Stevenson, 2015).

Box 9-1 lists terminology related to hyperbilirubinemia. This chapter reviews the pathophysiology of bilirubin, differentiates physiologic jaundice from pathologic jaundice, reviews current treatment options for hyperbilirubinemia, and describes an appropriate follow-up plan for the newborn with hyperbilirubinemia.

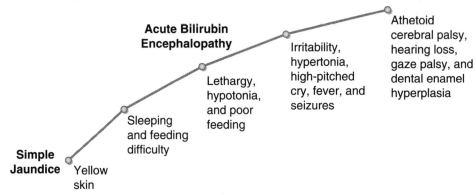

Figure 9-1: Predictable trajectory of hyperbilirubinemia through common stages.

Box 9-1: Terminology

Bilirubin	A biologically active end product of heme catabolism. A weak acid with a pH of 7.4 (see conjugated and unconjugated bilirubin).
Conjugated bilirubin	Bilirubin that is bound to glucuronic acid by uridine diphosphate (UDP). Conjugated bilirubin is water soluble, more easily excreted into bile, and eliminated from the body through the bowel.
Unconjugated bilirubin	Bilirubin that is not bound. Unconjugated bilirubin is not water soluble, making it more difficult to excrete from the body.
Jaundice	The easily identifiable yellow color that occurs as a result of bilirubin deposits in the skin and mucous membranes. The name comes from the French *jaune*, meaning "yellow."
Physiologic jaundice	Jaundice that is characterized by a gradual rise in total bilirubin that occurs between 48 and 120 hours of age. It is usually benign, is self-limiting, and requires only surveillance from the healthcare team.
Pathologic jaundice	Defined by timing of jaundice or by the rate of rise of total serum bilirubin (TSB). Jaundice is pathologic when it occurs within the first 24 hours of life, when it occurs after the first week of life, or when it lasts longer than 2 weeks. Pathologic jaundice is also defined as a TSB rise of 5 mg/dL or greater per day of life or a TSB greater than 18 mg/dL.
Severe hyperbilirubinemia	TSB greater than the 95th percentile for age, which requires phototherapy.
Kernicterus	A pathologic diagnosis characterized by bilirubin staining of the brain stem nuclei and cerebellum. This term is derived from the German *kern*, meaning "kernel or nucleus," and the Greek *ikteros*, meaning "jaundice."

Bilirubin encephalopathy	Clinical central nervous system findings caused by bilirubin toxicity to the basal ganglia and brain stem nuclei. Without intervention, bilirubin encephalopathy has the potential to progress from an acute to chronic state.

- Acute bilirubin encephalopathy (ABE): Early bilirubin toxicity that may be transient and reversible. ABE has two phases: early and intermediate. The early phase is characterized by lethargy, hypotonia, and poor suck. The intermediate phase is characterized by moderate stupor, irritability, and hypertonia. Hypertonia is manifested by a backward arching of the neck (retrocollis) and trunk (opisthotonos). The infant may also develop a fever and high-pitched cry that alternates with drowsiness and hypotonia.
- Chronic bilirubin encephalopathy (CBE): Chronic and permanent clinical sequelae of bilirubin toxicity. Clinical manifestations include pronounced retrocollis, opisthotonos, shrill cry, absent feeding, apnea, fever, deep stupor/coma, seizures, and possibly death.

Reproduced from Kaplan, M., Wong, R., Sibley, E., & Stevenson, D. (2015). Neonatal jaundice and liver diseases. In R. J. Martin, A. A. Fanaroff, & M. C. Walsh (Eds.). *Fanaroff & Martin's neonatal–perinatal medicine* (pp. 1618–1673). Philadelphia, PA: Elsevier.

Incidence

In late-preterm and full-term infants, bilirubin levels increase soon after birth. Normally, bilirubin levels increase following an hour-specific percentile track and decline by the end of the first week. For most newborns, bilirubin reaches its peak of approximately 6 mg/dL between the second and fourth days of life. Late-preterm infants reach their peak bilirubin levels later (5 to 7 days of life), demonstrate a higher peak than full-term infants, and are 2.4 times more likely to develop significant hyperbilirubinemia than neonates born at 38 to 40 weeks' gestation (Bhutani & Johnson, 2006; Wallenstein & Bhutani, 2013). In approximately 6.1% of healthy newborns, bilirubin levels increase to 12 mg/dL; in another 3% of healthy newborns, bilirubin levels increase to 15 mg/dL. Bilirubin generally returns to a normal level (less than 1 mg/dL) by the time the infant reaches 12 days of age, in what is a self-limiting process for most newborns. In some newborns, however, the rate of rise accelerates, such that they are vulnerable to severe hyperbilirubinemia and bilirubin neurotoxicity, if left untreated.

Bilirubin Metabolism

Adult Metabolism of Bilirubin

Throughout the life span, bilirubin production and elimination from the body is an ongoing process. Approximately 75% of bilirubin is derived from the lysis of red blood cells (RBCs). Hemolysis releases iron protoporphyrin (heme), which is then catalyzed by heme oxygenase and converted to biliverdin and subsequently into bilirubin (unconjugated). Unconjugated bilirubin becomes bound to albumin and is transported to the liver. In the hepatocytes, bilirubin comes under the influence of the hepatic enzyme isozyme uridine diphosphate (UDP) glucurononosyl transferase 1A1 (UGT1A1). The UDP UGT1A1 works to bind the bilirubin to glucuronic acid. In this conjugated (water-soluble) form, bilirubin can be excreted into bile and eliminated from the body through the bowel (**Figure 9-2**).

Homeostasis depends on the body's ability to conjugate and excrete bilirubin at a rate that is in balance with the rate of hemolysis. Any process that increases hemolysis, increases intestinal uptake of bilirubin, or slows the ability to excrete bilirubin jeopardizes this balancing act. Homeostasis is challenged at birth as the newborn transitions from intrauterine to extrauterine life.

Newborn Metabolism of Bilirubin

Hematologic Metabolism On the first day of life, bilirubin production in the normal newborn occurs at approximately 2 to 3 times the rate of production in adults, averaging approximately 8 to 10 mg/kg of the newborn's body weight per day. Hematologic factors that contribute to the development of rapid increases in bilirubin levels include relative polycythemia at birth and increased heme degradation incidental to the shortened erythrocyte life span of the neonate. The RBC life span is 70 to 90 days in newborns, as compared to the considerably longer 120 days in older children and adults.

On the first day of life, the high hemoglobin and hematocrit levels required for survival of the fetus in the low-oxygen environment of the uterus are no longer necessary, and degradation of the extraneous red blood cells begins. The increased rate of hemolysis and subsequent release of heme drives rapid production of bilirubin and increases the risk of hyperbilirubinemia. During the next two postnatal days, however, bilirubin production decreases rapidly.

Enterohepatic Factors Conditions that are associated with slow intestinal transit time and increased enterohepatic circulation increase the incidence of hyperbilirubinemia. Conjugation of bilirubin takes place in the hepatocytes, with the conjugated bilirubin being excreted into bile and subsequently into the intestines. Bilirubin is absorbed in small amounts from the bowel and returned to the liver as part of the enterohepatic circulation. Intestinal slowing increases

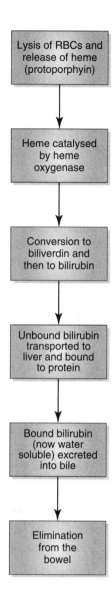

Figure 9-2: Metabolism of bilirubin.

the propensity for fragile conjugation bonds to be broken, causing bilirubin to be returned to the unconjugated state. Unconjugated bilirubin is easily absorbed from the intestinal tract and is once again returned to liver, thereby repeating the cycle (**Figure 9-3**).

In the newborn, hepatic uptake of bilirubin is slower than that in an older child or adult. This delay in uptake can be traced to decreased levels of hepatic proteins as well as decreased

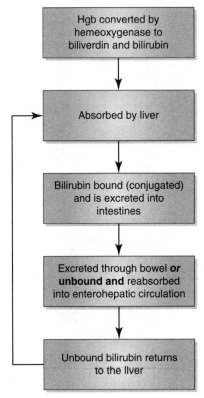

Figure 9-3: Pathway of bilirubin synthesis, transport, and metabolism.

hepatic blood flow. Intestinal transit is also slowed owing to the low feeding volume and low bulk. This combination perpetuates the enterohepatic cycle of increased bilirubin uptake in the intestine and slow hepatic uptake. Together, the increased uptake and slowed excretion of bilirubin place the newborn at increased risk for hyperbilirubinemia.

Intestinal Flora An estimated 25% of the bilirubin excreted into the intestine is reabsorbed as unconjugated bilirubin, and approximately 10% of the bilirubin excreted into the intestine is excreted in stool as unaltered bilirubin. The remaining bilirubin is converted to urobilinoids, most of which are excreted in stool. Small amounts of these urobilinoids are reabsorbed in the colon and returned to the enterohepatic circulation or excreted through the kidneys. The diminished bacterial flora in the newborn bowel decreases the ability of the newborn gut to reduce bilirubin to urobilinogen. As a consequence, the bilirubin pool in the newborn intestine is increased in comparison to the pool in an older child, which further increases uptake of bilirubin into the enterohepatic circulation.

Current Guidelines for Management

In an effort to reduce the frequency of severe neonatal hyperbilirubinemia and bilirubin encephalopathy, the American Academy of Pediatrics' (AAP) Subcommittee on Hyperbilirubinemia has developed a set of guidelines for identification and management of hyperbilirubinemia
in the newborn infant born at 35 weeks' gestation or later; **Box 9-2** describes key concepts
underlying these guidelines. The AAP guidelines are in alignment with the Institute of Medicine's (IOM) position statement on patient safety and timeliness of interventions, and include
primary and secondary prevention mechanisms as well as recommendations for laboratory
evaluation, risk assessment, follow-up, and treatment.

Promote and Support Successful Breastfeeding

Physiologic jaundice is associated with hepatic immaturity, decreased ability to conjugate bilirubin, decreased rate of excretion, and mild dehydration. Poor caloric intake and/or dehydration associated with inadequate breastfeeding may contribute to higher levels of unconjugated

---

Box 9-2: Clinician Guidelines for Management of Hyperbilirubinemia: Key Concepts

- Promote and support successful breastfeeding.
- Establish nursery protocols for identification and evaluation of hyperbilirubinemia.
- Measure the total serum bilirubin (TSB) or transcutaneous bilirubin (TcB) level of infants who are jaundiced in the first 24 hours of life.
- Recognize that visual estimation of the degree of jaundice can lead to errors, particularly in darkly pigmented infants.
- Interpret all bilirubin levels according to the infant's age in hours.
- Recognize that infants at less than 38 weeks' gestation, and particularly those who are breast-fed, are at higher risk of developing hyperbilirubinemia and require closer surveillance and monitoring.
- Perform a systematic assessment on all infants before discharge for the risk of severe hyperbilirubinemia.
- Provide parents with written and verbal information about newborn jaundice.
- Provide appropriate follow-up based on the time of discharge and the risk assessment.
- Treat newborns, when indicated, with phototherapy or exchange transfusion.

bilirubin and the subsequent development of hyperbilirubinemia. Increased feeding will frequently resolve the problem as hydration status improves and frequency of stooling increases.

Promotion of successful breastfeeding is a primary prevention mechanism for hyperbilirubinemia. The AAP and World Health Organization (WHO) recommend breastfeeding for all healthy term and late-preterm newborns. All breastfeeding mothers must be assessed for adequacy of breastfeeding. Simplified, successful breastfeeding requires adequate milk production and the ability of the baby to initiate a latch and to coordinate sucking and swallowing. The mother should be assisted in increasing her milk supply by ensuring a minimum of 8 to 12 feedings per day. Using a breast pump after or between feedings can be an additional strategy to improve milk production, as increasing the milk demand increases the milk supply. If the newborn is not latching well, the mother should receive education and assistance to resolve the problem.

While supplementation with formula is not optimal, it may be considered if the infant has excessive weight loss (more than 10% of birth weight), exhibits signs of dehydration, or becomes severely jaundiced. Signs of adequate intake include transition to seedy, mustard-colored stools by the third or fourth day of life, and 3 to 4 stools and 4 to 6 wet diapers per day by the fourth day of life.

Establish Nursery Protocols for Identification and Evaluation of Hyperbilirubinemia

The overriding goal for nursery protocols is to reduce the preventable causes of ABE. The IOM recommends establishing institutional systems and cultures that empower all members of the healthcare team to work toward the common goal of patient safety. Studies demonstrate that standard work and a systems approach provide consistent means for early identification and intervention for the newborn at risk for ABE. Protocols should include use of checklists and reminders that decrease the need for clinician memory of care to be provided or that has been provided, as this reduces the risk of human error and increases overall patient safety. Circumstances in which nurses can request a bilirubin level without a physician order should be clearly identified, as this promotes timely identification and prevents delay in treatment.

Perform a Systematic Assessment of All Infants Before Discharge for the Risk of Severe Hyperbilirubinemia

Systematic assessment for hyperbilirubinemia includes clinical risk assessment, visual inspection, bilirubin measurements (direct plasma, transcutaneous estimation, or a combination of methods), and use of tools (such as nomograms) to interpret the results (Bhutani et al., 2013; Bhutani, Vilms, & Hamerman-Johnson, 2010).

Risk Factor Screening Screening begins with identification of risk factors that can be categorized by prenatal history, familial history, intrapartum events, and postnatal circumstances (such as feeding methods). The Centers for Disease Control and Prevention (CDC) has suggested a mnemonic, JAUNDICE, as a way to easily recall the most common risk factors for hyperbilirubinemia (**Box 9-3**).

Prenatal Risk Factors Prenatal risk factors for hyperbilirubinemia include advanced maternal age, maternal diabetes, and first-trimester bleeding during the current pregnancy. Maternal blood type and Rh factor may direct early laboratory studies to determine risk for hemolysis or hemolytic disease and may include neonatal ABO typing, Rh type, and Coombs screening (AAP, 2004). Familial risk factors include a sibling with a history of neonatal jaundice, and Asian, American Indian, or Greek ethnicity. An O or Rh-negative maternal blood type places the newborn at risk for ABO or Rh incompatibility and hemolytic anemia.

Neonatal, Intrapartum, and Postnatal Risk Factors Male gender and gestational age less than 38 weeks (i.e., late-preterm infant) increase the risk of hyperbilirubinemia. Intrapartum events that place the newborn at greater risk for jaundice include operative vaginal delivery, Pitocin augmentation or induction, cephalohematoma, and significant bruising, as reabsorption of the hemolyzed blood products increases the release of heme and leads to subsequent elevation of bilirubin.

Box 9-3: Major Risk Factors for Hyperbilirubinemia in Full-Term Newborns: JAUNDICE Mnemonic

- **J**aundice within first 24 hours after birth
- **A** sibling who was jaundiced as a neonate
- **U**nrecognized hemolysis, such as ABO blood type incompatibility or Rh incompatibility
- **N**onoptimal sucking/nursing
- **D**eficiency in glucose-6-phosphate dehydrogenase, a genetic disorder
- **I**nfection
- **C**ephalohematomas/bruising
- **E**ast Asian or Mediterranean descent

Reproduced from Centers for Disease Control and Prevention. (2015). Jaundice & kernicterus. Guidelines and tools for health professionals. Retrieved from http://www.cdc.gov/ncbddd/jaundice/hcp.html

Breastfeeding Breastfed infants are 3 times more likely to have a total serum bilirubin (TSB) level greater than 12 mg/dL, and 6 times more likely to have a level greater than 15 mg/dL. Bilirubin levels in breastfed infant may reach as high as 25 to 30 mg/dL. The exact mechanism for breastfeeding-related jaundice is unclear, but may be related to poor caloric or fluid intake and/or increased weight loss. Infants who lose more than 7% of their birth weight are at increased risk for becoming significantly dehydrated and have a higher likelihood of significant jaundice. Additional mechanisms that increase likelihood of breastfeeding jaundice may include slow passage of meconium and the type or number of bacteria in the intestine, as this adds to enterohepatic bilirubin circulation. Breastmilk jaundice differs from physiologic jaundice in that the bilirubin levels rise during the second week of life—a time when physiological jaundice is improving. Breastmilk jaundice may be prolonged, peaking at 4 weeks of age and lasting up to 12 weeks.

Identification of risk factors should prompt clinicians to heighten surveillance for hyperbilirubinemia. Risk-scoring tools are available to aid in differentiating high-risk newborns from low-risk newborns (**Table 9-1**). In the risk-scoring tool in Table 9-1, all risk factor scores

Table 9-1: Risk Score for Neonatal Hyperbilirubinemia

Variable	Score
Birth weight:	
• 2000–2500 g (4 lb, 7 oz–5 lb, 8 oz)	0
• 2501–3000 g (5 lb, 8 oz–6 lb, 10 oz)	3
• 3001–3500 g (6 lb, 10 oz–7 lb, 11 oz)	6
• 3501–4000 g (7 lb, 11 oz–8 lb, 13 oz)	9
• 4001–4500 g (8 lb, 13 oz–9 lb, 15 oz)	12
• 4501–5000 g (9 lb, 15 oz–11 lb, 1 oz)	15
Oxytocin (Pitocin) used during delivery	4
Vacuum-assisted delivery	4
Breastfeeding and bottle-feeding	4
Exclusive breastfeeding	5
Gestational age < 38 weeks	5

Note: A total score of 8 or more suggests an increased risk of hyperbilirubinemia. A total serum or transcutaneous bilirubin level should be obtained.
Data from Bhutani, K. R., Nihtianova, L. X., & Schwartz, C. A. (2005). Identifying newborns at risk of significant hyperbilirubinemia: A comparison of two recommended approaches. *Archives of Disease in Childhood*, 90(4), 417.

are added to give a total score; a score greater than 8 would prompt early bilirubin measurement by transcutaneous bilirubinometry (TcB) or serum testing.

Visual Inspection A TSB greater than 2 mg/dL is appreciable in virtually all newborns in the first several days of life, gradually rising to a peak of 5 to 6 mg/dL on the third to fourth days of life. Jaundice is visually apparent when the TSB is 5 mg/dL or greater (Kaplan, et al., 2015). Visual inspection for jaundice should be performed along with vital signs measurement, and should occur no less than every 8 hours when hyperbilirubinemia is suspected. This is accomplished by blanching the skin with digital pressure on the forehead, sternum, or knee to reveal the underlying color or tone. Assessment of jaundice must be performed in a well-lit room, and natural lighting or daylight is preferred.

Inspection is useful for identifying jaundice, but it is not an accurate method to determine bilirubin levels. Its degree of accuracy varies with the clinician's experience level and the newborn skin differences that come with ethnic variation. For this reason, it is important to obtain bilirubin levels for all newborns who appear jaundiced with a TSB/TcB measurement regardless of age in hours.

Bilirubin Measurement Bilirubin measurement can be obtained by transcutaneous or serum means. The specimen for TSB measurement is most commonly obtained from a heel puncture or by intravenous draw. While the TSB is the most accurate measurement, obtaining the blood sample is invasive and painful for the newborn. The specimen must be obtained from a free-flowing blood source, as a difficult draw may result in a hemolyzed specimen that can be incorrectly interpreted as elevated.

Transcutaneous bilirubinometry is a noninvasive means of objectively measuring skin color and estimating TSB levels. Multiple studies have demonstrated that handheld TcB devices can accurately estimate TSB in term and late-preterm infants of varying races and ethnicities to within 2 to 3 mg/dL of the TSB when the TSB is less than 15 mg/dL (Maisels & Kring, 2006; Muchowski, 2014; Taylor et al., 2015). A limitation of the TcB technology is that it tends to underestimate the bilirubin level with TSB levels greater than 15 mg/dL. It is recommended that all TcB levels greater than 15 mg/dL and above the 75th percentile be confirmed with TSB measurements.

Clinical Application The AAP (2004) has developed an algorithm for bilirubin assessment that incorporates both assessment of risk factors and visual assessment. Its recommendations state that evaluation of bilirubin should be performed by TSB or TcB on every newborn who appears to be jaundiced in the first 24 hours after birth, on every newborn with jaundice that appears excessive for age, or if there is any doubt about the degree of jaundice. The AAP also recommends that all newborns be screened prior to discharge by a TSB or TcB measurement.

While this measurement may occur when the newborn is between 18 and 48 hours of life, a standardized approach suggests that it be paired with another consistently occurring task (i.e., concurrent to the routine metabolic screening test) to create consistency and ownership for all members of the team. TcB and TSB results should be plotted on a nomogram (**Figure 9-4**) and interpreted based on the infant's age in hours to appreciate the newborn's risk for subsequent severe hyperbilirubinemia (Bhutani et al., 2010). In the case of home or birth center care with discharge between 6–2 hours of life, the bilirubin screening will be performed by the follow-up care provider at the 24–48 hour visit.

There is no global recommendation for single versus serial bilirubin assessment. While a single bilirubin measurement can alert the clinician to infants with bilirubin levels greater than the 75th percentile for age in hours, serial bilirubin measurements (i.e., daily noninvasive

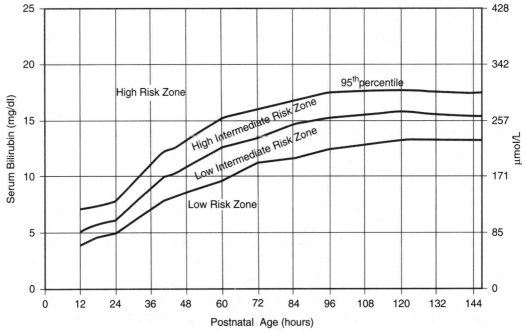

Figure 9-4: Nomogram for designation of risk in 2840 well newborns at 36 or more weeks' gestation with birth weight of 2000 grams or more or 35 or more weeks' gestation with birth weight of 2500 grams or more based on the hour-specific total serum bilirubin levels. Before discharge the serum bilirubin level was obtained, and the zone in which the value fell predicted the likelihood of a subsequent bilirubin level exceeding the 95th percentile (high-risk zone).

Reproduced from Bhutani R. K., Johnson, L., & Sivieri, E. M. (1999). Predictive ability of predischarge hour-specific serum bilirubin for subsequent significant hyperbilirubinemia in healthy term and near-term newborns. Reproduced with permission from *Journal of Pediatrics, 103*(1), 6–14. Copyright (c) 1999 by the AAP.

TcB determinations) can track rapid rates of bilirubin rise (more than 0.2 mg per 100 mL per hour), which enhances their predictive value for hyperbilirubinemia.

Treat Newborns, When Indicated, with Phototherapy or Exchange Transfusion

Historically, and prior to the use of phototherapy, the only treatment option for hyperbilirubinemia was an exchange transfusion. The use of phototherapy as an early intervention has curtailed, though not eliminated, the need for exchange transfusions.

Phototherapy

Technical Features of Phototherapy The visible light spectrum ranges from approximately 350 to 800 nm. Bilirubin absorbs visible light in the blue region of the spectrum, which is found at wavelengths of ± 460 nm. Phototherapy takes advantage of this property by creating a photochemical reaction that transforms the unconjugated bilirubin molecules that are bound to human serum albumin into photoproducts that can then be excreted from the body. Current phototherapy devices employ either a fluorescent-tube or light-emitting diode (LED) lights that emit light within the 460 to 490 nm range, which is within the blue–green spectrum (Bhutani and the Committee on Fetus and Newborn of the AAP, 2011).

Indications for Phototherapy The AAP has issued comprehensive guidelines based on limited evidence for the initiation of phototherapy in infants greater than 35 weeks' gestation. There is no single TSB concentration at which phototherapy should be initiated; rather, the infant's gestational age, postnatal age, and risk factors must be taken into consideration. Tools are available to aid in the decision-making process for treatment of hyperbilirubinemia. Online applications are increasingly popular for this purpose; the BiliTool, for example, is recognized and recommended by the AAP as an aid to decision making for the jaundiced newborn. Case studies at the end of the chapter will give the reader the opportunity to use this online tool.

The nomogram is another tool that is recognized by the AAP for its ability to aid decision making about initiation of phototherapy in newborns greater than 35 weeks' gestation (**Figure 9-5**). Recommendations related to nomograms are based on limited evidence, and the levels for initiation of treatment are estimates.

Regardless of the tool used, the bilirubin level itself does not dictate initiation of phototherapy; rather, the clinician must establish the infant's risk level and consider this along with the bilirubin level to make a clinical decision (Bhutani et al., 2013). As the nomogram in Figure 9-5 suggests, a newborn at 48 hours with a TSB of 13 should be started on phototherapy if at high risk for hyperbilirubinemia, may be started on phototherapy if at medium risk, and should continue with surveillance if at low risk (Bromiker, Bin-Nun, Schimmel, Hammerman & Kaplan, 2012).

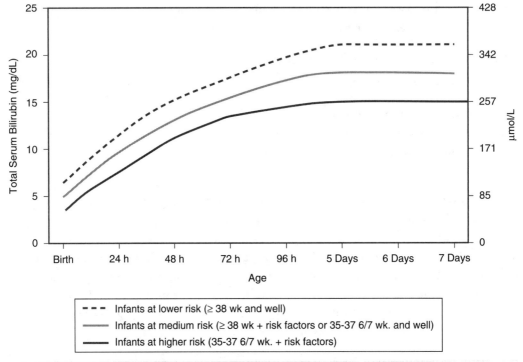

• Use total bilirubin. Do not subtract direct reacting or conjugated bilirubin.
• Risk factors = isoimmune hemolytic disease, G6PD deficiency, asphyxia, significant lethargy, temperature instability, sepsis, acidosis, or albumin < 3.0g/dL (if measured)
• For well infants 35-37 6/7 wk can adjust TSB levels for intervention around the medium risk line. It is an option to intervene at lower TSB levels for infants closer to 35 wks and at higher TSB levels for those closer to 37 6/7 wk.
• It is an option to provide conventional phototherapy in hospital or at home at TSB levels 2-3 mg/dL (35-50mmol/L) below those shown but home phototherapy should not be used in any infant with risk factors.

Figure 9-5: Nomogram showing management of hyperbilirubinemia in newborn infants.
Reproduced from American Academy of Pediatrics, Subcommittee on Hyperbilirubinemia: Clinical Practice Guideline. (2004). Management of hyperbilirubinemia in the newborn infant 35 or more weeks of gestation. Reproduced with permission from *Pediatrics, 114*(1), 297–316, Copyright (c) 2004 by the AAP.

Discontinuation of Phototherapy The decision to discontinue phototherapy should be based on the overall clinical presentation of the newborn. Clinical response in the form of decreasing TSB levels should be evident within 4 to 6 hours, in the form of a decrease of more than 2 mg/dL in serum concentration. This decrease is variable, however; its precise magnitude depends on the infant's rate of bilirubin production, enterohepatic circulation, bilirubin elimination, and degree of tissue bilirubin deposition. It is reasonable to discontinue phototherapy once the TSB has fallen below the 75th percentile for hours-of-life age and below the 40th percentile in newborns with risk factors or a lower (less than 38 weeks) gestational age.

Illumination   The distance of the light should be such that maximum illumination for optimal body exposure can be achieved. Maximum body exposure to illumination is paramount for efficient reduction in TSB, as the effectiveness of phototherapy is dose dependent (Bhutani and the Committee on Fetus and Newborn of the AAP, 2011). Although complete exposure is impossible due to use of eye masks and diapers, it is possible with the use of overhead light sources and lighted mattresses to achieve approximately 80% body exposure.

Safety and Protective Measures   The newborn must be evaluated for response to therapy as evidenced by improvement and resolution of bilirubin, or alternatively, by deterioration and progression of jaundice (Bhutani and the Committee on Fetus and Newborn of the AAP, 2011). The newborn must be assessed frequently for adequate hydration and nutrition. Phototherapy should be interrupted for breastfeeding unless the newborn's bilirubin levels are approaching those that require exchange transfusion. The newborn temperature must be monitored frequently. Temperature control must be maintained, with attention being paid to prevention of iatrogenic hyperthermia. The caregiving team must stay alert to signs suggestive of early bilirubin encephalopathy, such as altered sleeping patterns, deteriorating feeding patterns, or irritability and crying with inability to be consoled.

The current literature suggests that placing the newborn in a supine position during phototherapy does not compromise illumination coverage, delay bilirubin response, or increase the length of treatment time (Lee Wan Fei & Abdullah, 2015) Placing the baby in a supine position provides a consistent message to parents that is in alignment with "back to sleep" policies for safe sleep practices.

Eye masks are routinely used during phototherapy, as retinal damage has been documented in the unpatched eyes of newborn monkeys. Purulent eye discharge and conjunctivitis have been reported with prolonged use of eye patches.

Although concerns have been raised regarding phototherapy exposure of the genitalia and reproductive system, such worries are unsubstantiated. Diapering should be minimized, as it is not required for protection from exposure harms; rather, diapers are used for hygiene purposes only.

Adverse Effects of Phototherapy   Short-term effects of phototherapy include maternal separation with potential for interference with maternal bonding, intestinal hypermotility with diarrhea, and temperature instability. Long-term effects may include increased risk for childhood asthma.

Exchange Transfusion   Although phototherapy is effective in the treatment of hyperbilirubinemia, exchange transfusion is occasionally indicated. A nomogram for exchange transfusion based on TSB levels is available. Exchange transfusion should be performed in infants with TSB levels in the range indicated by the nomogram, with TSB levels of 25 mg/dL or greater, and with jaundice and signs of acute bilirubin encephalopathy. Approximately 85% of blood is replaced during an exchange transfusion, resulting in an approximately 50% reduction in bilirubin.

Although mortality rates from this procedure are low (approximately 2%), as many as 74% of newborns experience some form of adverse events from exchange transfusion, including thrombocytopenia or metabolic acidosis. The AAP recommends that exchange transfusion be performed by trained personnel in a neonatal intensive care unit (NICU).

Provide Parents with Written and Verbal Information About Newborn Jaundice; Provide Appropriate Follow-Up Based on the Time of Discharge and the Risk Assessment

Prior to discharge, parents of the newborn should receive clear verbal and written instructions in laymen's terms and their primary language as to how to identify jaundice and when to notify the newborn healthcare provider. Parents must also receive clear instructions regarding the timing of follow-up. The AAP recommends that newborns discharged prior to 24 hours after birth return for a follow-up visit at 72 hours of age. If discharged between 24 and 47.9 hours of age, the newborn should return for follow-up at 96 hours; when the newborn is discharged between 48 and 72 hours, the follow-up should occur at 120 hours (AAP, 2004). Follow-up should occur earlier than the recommended hours if risk factors for hyperbilirubinemia are present. Assessment of the newborn should include current weight, which is compared with the percentage of change from the birth weight; review for adequacy of intake; evaluation of patterns of voiding and stooling; and assessment for presence or absence of jaundice. During the follow-up, if there is doubt about jaundice, the healthcare practitioner should measure TSB or TcB (AAP, 2004).

Pathologic Jaundice

Pathologic jaundice is defined by the timing of jaundice or by the rate of rise of total TSB. Jaundice is pathologic when it occurs within the first 24 hours of life, when it occurs after the first week of life, or when it lasts longer than 2 weeks. It can also be defined as a TSB rise of 5 mg/dL or more per day of life or a TSB greater than 18 mg/dL. Newborns with suspected pathologic jaundice should be cared for by a newborn specialist (i.e., neonatal nurse practitioner, pediatrician, or neonatologist).

Conjugated hyperbilirubinemia is always considered to be pathologic, and TSB levels over 14 mg/dL are probably not physiologic. When more than 15% of the total bilirubin is direct, the jaundice is categorized as conjugated hyperbilirubinemia. Pathologic causes can include isoimmunization, erythrocyte biochemical defects, structural abnormalities, infection, and sequestered blood. While the comprehensive list of causes for pathologic jaundice can seem daunting, limited examples of each are reviewed here.

Isoimmunization

Isoimmunization is most commonly a result of incompatible blood types between the mother and the fetus (i.e., a mother with O blood type and a fetus with A or B blood type), or incompatible Rh factor (the mother is Rh negative and her fetus is Rh positive). While more than 50 antibodies can cause hemolytic disease of the newborn, RhD alloimmunization is the most common etiology. In the past, Rh disease was the most common cause of hemolytic hyperbilirubinemia and kernicterus in newborns. Today, however, a combination of prophylactic methods—prenatal administration of anti-D immunoglobulin G (Rhogam), postpartum Rhogam administration for appropriate candidates, heightened neonatal surveillance, and early aggressive therapy—has decreased the incidence of severe hyperbilirubinemia and kernicterus in this population. Early laboratory evaluation is indicated when the maternal blood type is unknown or when the mother has O blood type or is Rh negative. Directed labs include ABO/Rh type along with antibody screening in the following circumstances:

- When the maternal blood type and Rh status are unknown
- When the newborn blood type and Rh status (obtained from cord blood) is associated with
  - An unknown maternal blood type and Rh status or
  - A maternal O blood type or Rh-negative status

The newborn should also have a Coombs test to determine presence of ongoing hemolysis. The newborn with ABO or Rh incompatibility who has a positive direct Coombs test and rapidly increasing bilirubin levels should be referred to a newborn specialist immediately for a higher level of care (Kaplan, Hammerman, Vreman, Wong, & Stevenson, 2010).

Erythrocyte Biochemical Defects

Erythrocyte destruction can also occur from nonimmune processes such as erythrocyte enzymatic defects. The most common erythrocyte enzyme defect, which affects hundreds of millions of people, is glucose-6-phosphate dehydrogenase (G6PD) deficiency. While G6PD deficiency has long been associated with populations in Africa, southern Europe, Mediterranean countries, the Middle East, and India, it is now a globally recognized problem due to immigration patterns and interracial childbearing.

The G6PD enzyme is a major contributor to the stability of the RBC membrane and protects against oxidative damage. Oxidative damage may be manifested as hemolysis. G6PD deficiency decreases reserves against the oxidation process, leaving the newborn more prone to increased hemolysis and extreme neonatal hyperbilirubinemia. Decreased protection from oxidation increases vulnerability to ABE.

Evaluation of the newborn for G6PD deficiency should be undertaken if G6Pd deficiency is suspected (review the family's geographic origins) or if the newborn's response to phototherapy is poor (AAP, 2004).

Structural Abnormalities

Structural abnormalities that involve obstruction of the upper intestinal tract are associated with elevated unconjugated hyperbilirubinemia; such abnormalities may include cholestasis, pyloric stenosis, and duodenal or jejunal obstruction. Physical findings may include right upper quadrant tenderness, hepatomegaly, anorexia, acholic (white) stools, and vomiting (Muchowski, 2014). Surgical correction results in a decline of TSB with rapid return to normal levels.

Infection

Erythrocytes are susceptible to injury, and bacterial infection is a known cause of hemolysis. Sepsis may also impair conjugation of bilirubin. Both processes—hemolysis and impaired conjugation—increase enterohepatic circulation. The increased hemolysis makes the newborn prone to disseminated intravascular coagulation (DIC). Newborns with elevations of direct-reacting or conjugated bilirubin should have a urinalysis and urine culture to rule out sepsis.

Sequestered Blood

Sequestered blood is blood that collects within a body cavity. Examples include cephalohematoma and excessive bruising with precipitous delivery. Birth trauma can result in the sequestration of RBCs within layers of the tissues covering the skull and brain. Bilirubin increases as the body metabolizes the erythrocytes and heme is released.

Management of Pathologic Jaundice

All newborns receiving phototherapy whose TSB level is rising rapidly and not following the expected trajectory (i.e., crossing percentiles), or is not explained by history or physical examination, should be evaluated for additional causes for hyperbilirubinemia (AAP, 2004; Noble, 2012). Results of the newborn thyroid and galactosemia screen should be reviewed, and other causes of jaundice should be sought and treated as indicated. Sick newborns and those who are jaundiced at or beyond 3 weeks of age should have a measurement of total and direct/conjugated bilirubin to screen for cholestasis.

Student Practice Activities

Case Study 1

You are assessing an apparently healthy male baby. A review of the chart reveals that the baby has a gestational age of 37 weeks and is of Greek descent. The mother's blood type is O negative. The baby was born vaginally with assistance of vacuum. His Apgar scores at delivery were 9 and 9 at 1 and 5 minutes, respectively. Birth weight was 8 lb, 2 oz. Currently, the baby is 22 hours old and weighs 7 lb, 10 oz. The physical assessment is normal with the exception of a notable cephalohematoma and visible jaundice. The baby is exclusively breastfeeding; he latches and coordinates suck and swallow well.

1. Which risk factors are identified?
2. Which laboratory tests are indicated?
3. Using the nomogram for initiating phototherapy, which TSB result would prompt you to consider phototherapy for this baby?
4. Access the online BiliTool (http://bilitool.org), and use the first option. Populate the birth date and time and current date and time to reflect a 22-hour newborn.
   A. Scroll down to the follow-up section. When should you follow up with TSB?
   B. Scroll to the phototherapy section.
      □ Because this baby is at higher risk, should you consider phototherapy?
      □ If the baby were medium risk, should phototherapy be considered?

Case Study 2

You are assessing a newborn girl who was born at 35 weeks' gestation. A review of her history reveals that the baby was born by normal spontaneous vaginal delivery and received Apgar scores of 8 and 9 at 1 and 5 minutes, respectively. Her mother's blood type is O negative and she received Rhogam after her first delivery. The mother did not receive Rhogam during this pregnancy. The blood type of the newborn's older sibling is O positive, and at birth she had a positive Coombs test. The sibling also received phototherapy at 48 hours that continued for 3 days. The newborn is currently 26 hours old and is exclusively breastfed. She is breastfeeding well, has had 4 wet diapers, and has passed

3 meconium stools. The newborn's physical assessment is normal except for significant jaundice over the face and chest.

1. What are the identified risk factors?
2. Which laboratory tests are indicated?
3. The newborn's TcB reading is 12 mg/dL. Based on the nomogram, what is your next step?
4. At 48 hours, after 24 hours of phototherapy, the newborn's TSB is 16. Based on the BiliTool app, what is your next step? Should the mother continue breastfeeding?
5. When should you refer this baby?

References

American Academy of Pediatrics (AAP), Subcommittee on Hyperbilirubinemia: Clinical Practice Guideline. (2004). Management of hyperbilirubinemia in the newborn infant 35 or more weeks of gestation. *Pediatrics, 114*(1), 297–316.

Bhutani, V. K., & the Committee on Fetus and Newborn of the American Academy of Pediatrics. (2011). Phototherapy to prevent severe neonatal hyperbilirubinemia in the newborn infant 35 or more weeks of gestation. *Pediatrics, 128*(4), 1046–1052.

Bhutani, V. K., Vilms, R. J., & Hamerman-Johnson, I. (2010). Universal bilirubin screening for severe neonatal hyperbilirubinemia. *Journal of Perinatology*, 30 (suppl), S6-15.

Bhutani, V. K., & Johnson, L. (2006). Kernicterus in late-preterm infants cared for as term healthy infants. *Seminars in Perinatology, 30*(2), 89–97.

Bhutani, V. K., Stark, A. R., Lazzeroni, L. C., Poland, R., Gourley, G. R., Kazmierczak, S., & The Initial Clinical Testing Evaluation and Risk Assessment for Universal Screening for Hyperbilirubinemia Screening Group. (2013). Predischarge screening for severe neonatal hyperbilirubinemia identifies infants who need phototherapy. *Journal of Pediatrics, 162*(3), 477–482.

Bromiker, R., Bin-Nun, A., Schimmel, M. S., Hammerman, C., & Kaplan, M. (2012). Neonatal hyperbilirubinemia in the low–intermediate-risk category on the bilirubin nomogram. *Pediatrics, 130*(3), 470–475.

Lee Wan Fei, S., & Abdullah, K. L. (2015). Effect of turning vs. supine position under phototherapy on neonates with hyperbilirubinemia: A systematic review. *Journal of Clinical Nursing, 24*(5–6), 672–682.

Kaplan, M., Hammerman, C., Vreman, J. J., Wong, R. J., & Stevenson, D. K. (2010). Hemolysis and hyperbilirubinemia in antiglobulin positive, direct ABO blood group heterospecific neonates. *Journal of Pediatrics, 157*(5), 772–777.

Kaplan, M., Wong, R., Sibley, E., & Stevenson, D. (2015). Neonatal jaundice and liver diseases. In R. J. Martin, A. A. Fanaroff, & M. C. Walsh (Eds.), *Fanaroff & Martin's neonatal–perinatal medicine* (pp. 1618–1673). Philadelphia, PA: Elsevier.

Maisels, M. J., & Kring, E. (2006). Transcutaneous bilirubin levels in the first 96 hours in a normal newborn population of >35 weeks gestation. *Pediatrics, 117*(4), 1169–1173.

Muchowski, K. (2014). Evaluation and treatment of neonatal hyperbilirubinemia. *American Family Physician, 89*(11), 873–878.

Noble, J. E. (2012). Breastfeeding. In C. D. Berkowitz, *Berkowitz's pediatrics: A primary care approach* (4th ed., pp. 133–136). Elk Grove Village, IL: American Academy of Pediatrics.

Taylor, J. A., Burgos, A. E., Flaherman, V., Chung, E. K., Simpson, E. A., Goyal, N. K., . . . Better Outcomes through Research for Newborns Network. (2015). Discrepancies between transcutaneous and serum bilirubin measurements. *Pediatrics, 135*(2), 224–231.

Wallenstein, M. B., & Bhutani, V. K. (2013). Jaundice and kernicterus in the moderate preterm infant. *Clinics in Perinatology, 40*(4), 679–688.

CHAPTER 10

I INFECTION IN THE NEONATE

Sandra L. Gardner and B. J. Snell

Worldwide, 4 million newborns die during the neonatal period (Lawn, Cousens, & Zupan, 2005). Approximately 25% to 45% of deaths occur on the first day of life, and 75% occur during the first week of life (World Health Organization [WHO], 2006; Young Infants Clinical Signs Study Group, 2008). The Centers for Disease Control and Prevention (CDC) estimates that 20,000 newborns die in their first month of life.

Severe neonatal infections account for 38% of deaths in the first month of life (Lawn et al., 2005). In the United States, 1 to 5 of every 1000 live births are affected by neonatal infection. Although preterm infants are more prone to infection, late-preterm and full-term newborns with certain risk factors also have a higher risk of neonatal infection (**Box 10-1**). Prior to the development of antibiotics, mortality rates from this cause were in the range of 95% to 100%. After the introduction of antibiotics and with improved care for newborns with infection, mortality rates for full-term infants have decreased 3% in the past 20 years (Leonard & Dobbs, 2015). Lowering the mortality rate in neonatal infection is the result of early case-finding, timely diagnostic evaluation, and initiation of empiric antibiotic therapies (Gardner, 2009; Polin & Committee on Fetus and Newborn, 2012).

Definition and Etiology

Newborns and neonates may be infected with bacteria, viruses, or fungi. Infected newborns easily become septic because of the immaturity of their immune systems and inability to

Box 10-1: Risk Factors for Infection in Late-Preterm and Term Newborns

- Immature immune system that is gestational age specific:
  - Less nonspecific (inflammatory) immunity
  - Less specific (humoral) immunity
  - Less passive immunity
- No local inflammatory reaction to portal of entry of infection
- Signs and symptoms are vague and nonspecific—mimic other common morbidities
- Sex difference: 2:1 male-to-female incidence of infection
- Method of feeding—breastfeeding is protective against infection
- Multiple pathways of acquiring infection: transplacental, perinatal, and postpartal
- Antibiotic use
- Low socioeconomic status
- Low birth weight (LBW) or intrauterine growth restriction (IUGR)—underweight or malnourished infants of any gestational age
- Intrapartum complications/instrumentation: maternal temperature/infection (chorioamnionitis), maternal colonization with group B *Streptococcus*, premature rupture of membranes, prolonged rupture of membranes (more than 18 hours), low Apgar scores, internal monitor electrode, resuscitation
- Congenital malformations such as neural tube defects or gastroschisis
- Procedures: invasive procedures such as intravenous lines, lumbar puncture, or surgery

Data from Gardner, S. L. (2008a). How will I know my newborn is sick? *Nurse Currents, 2*(2), 1–8; Gardner, S. L. (2009). Sepsis in the neonate. *Critical Care Clinics of North America, 21*(1), 121–141.

localize infection (Box 10-1). Left untreated, infection becomes septicemia—a life-threatening condition when it occurs in the first 28 days of life. Commonly called "blood poisoning" by lay people, septicemia is a generalized bacterial infection in the bloodstream.

Neonates may be infected transplacentally (before birth), intrapartally, or postpartally. Neonatal infections are categorized as early or late infections, and their timing gives the healthcare provider clues as to the causative agent (**Box 10-2**). Both transplacental and intra-partal infections manifest in the first 3 days (before 72 hours) of life; these so-called early in-fections are associated with higher morbidity and mortality (Pammi, Brand, & Weisman, 2016; Polin & Committee on Fetus and Newborn, 2012). Late-onset infections may occur as early as the third day of life, but more frequently occur after the first week of life. Newborns dis-charged within 24 to 48 hours of birth rely on the recognition of early-onset infection by their

Box 10-2: Causative Agents of Early- and Late-Onset Neonatal Infections

Early-Onset Sepsis

Common organisms:

- Group B *Streptococcus* (GBS)
- *Escherichia coli*
- Coagulase-negative *Staphylococcus*

Unusual organisms:

- *Staphylococcus aureus*
- *Neisseria meningitides*
- *Streptococcus pneumoniae*
- *Haemophilus influenzae* (type B and non-typeable)

Rare organisms:

- *Klebsiella pneumoniae*
- *Pseudomonas aeruginosa*
- *Enterobacter* species
- *Serratia marcescens*
- Group A *Streptococcus*
- *Anaerobic* species

Late Onset Sepsis

- Coagulase –negative *Staphylococcus*
- *Escherichia coli*
- *Klebsiella* species
- *Enterobacter* species
- *Candida* species
- *Malassezia furfur*
- Group B *Streptococcus*
- Methicillin-resistant *Staphylococcus aureus*

Reproduced from Pammi, M., Brand, M. C., &Weisman, L. E. (2016). Infection in the neonate. In S. L. Gardner, B. S. Carter, M. Enzman Hines, & J. A. Hernandez (Eds.), *Merenstein and Gardner's handbook of neonatal intensive care* (8th ed., pp. 537–563). St. Louis, MO: Mosby-Elsevier.

parents and by their primary caregivers during early follow-up or at home visits (Gardner, 2008a).

Prevention

Knowledgeable neonatal care providers are essential in preventing infections and recognizing infections quickly. Care providers also advocate for the newborn to receive a timely diagnostic assessment and the initiation of empiric antibiotics (Gardner, 2008a, 2009). Knowledge of at-risk groups and factors that increase a newborn's risk of infection enable neonatal caregivers to maintain a high level of suspicion when assessing and interacting with the neonate and the family. Prompt notification of the newborn's primary care provider coupled with prompt action by the primary provider will result in better outcomes for infected newborns.

Universal precautions and hand hygiene (hand washing/hand rubs) are essential when caregivers are in direct contact with the newborn and family. Using appropriate infection control principles and practices and control measures and techniques at birth can prevent and control the spread of infection (Pammi et al., 2016).

Data Collection

History

A history of maternal bacterial, viral, or fungal infections (**Table 10-1** and **Table 10-2**), in combination with the risk factors in Box 10-1, increases the risk of neonatal infection.

Signs and Symptoms

In the neonate, signs and symptoms of infection may be subtle, are typically nonspecific, and may mimic other neonatal morbidities such as hypoglycemia, hypothermia, respiratory distress, neurologic conditions, or cardiac disease (Polin & Committee on Fetus and Newborn, 2012). **Box 10-3** lists the most common signs and symptoms of neonatal infection.

Mothers are experts on their babies—they will notice a change in feeding behavior, alertness, and muscle tone. Wise primary-care providers listen intently to the mother's concerns: "Something is wrong" or "The baby just isn't doing well." Even if the baby's vital signs are normal, heeding subtle signs and vague complaints and feelings of parents will enable earlier identification of infection. Indeed, infection in the newborn can occur in the absence of any clinical signs or symptoms (Ottolini, Lundgren, Mirkinson, Carson, & Ottolini, 2003; Polin & Committee on Fetus and Newborn, 2012). In a neonate, by the time signs and symptoms are

Table 10-1: Congenital Viral Infections: TORCHS Infections

Organism	Incidence	Perinatal Presentation	Neonatal Symptoms	Treatment	Parent Education
Toxoplasmosis	30% of newborns have congenital birth defects; 70–90% are asymptomatic at birth	Asymptomatic in the mother	Prematurity; IUGR; hydrocephalus; chorioretinitis; seizures; cerebral calcifications; hepatosplenomegaly; thrombocytopenia; jaundice; rash; general lympadenopathy	Sulfadiazine (100–200 mg/kg/day PO divided every 12 h) and pyrimethamine (1 mg/kg/day PO divided every 12 h) and folic acid (1 mg/day) (Pammi et al., 2016) Prolonged treatment (as long as 1 year) results in better neurologic, ocular, cognitive and auditory outcomes (McLeod et al., 2006)	Prevention: Pregnant women to avoid contact with cat feces (changing litter box; gardening) and eating raw/undercooked meat.
Other: includes enteroviruses such as Coxsackie A and B, echovirus, poliomyelitis, and others	Frequent illness in infants and young children (hand–foot–mouth disease; conjunctivitis) spread by fecal–oral/respiratory routes and from infected fomites Newborns who acquire infection (without maternal antibody) are at risk for severe disease (sepsis, meningitis, myocarditis, pneumonia,	Symptom/disease processes include those related to: • Respiratory functions (common cold, sore throat, stomatitis, pneumonia, herpangina, pleurodynia) • Neurologic functions (aseptic meningitis, encephalitis, paralysis) • Skin (exanthema) • Gastrointestinal functions (vomiting, diarrhea, abdominal pain, hepatitis)	Signs and symptoms of neonatal sepsis Risk factors for severe infection include prematurity, early onset (< 7 days of age), perinatal history of disease, high WBC count (≥ 15,000/mm³), and low Hgb (< 10/7 gm/dl) (Lin et al., 2003)	Pleconaril, an antiviral, prevents viral attachment and entry into host cells (Abzug et al., 2003); it is being assessed in a phase 2, multicenter, RCT for newborns with sepsis characterized by myocarditis, hepatitis or coagulopathy (Abzug, 2014) IVIG may also be effective in severe enteroviral infection (Abzug, 2014; Rotbart, 2000)	Pregnant women are infected by young children, then infect their fetus Pregnant women and all childcare workers must be taught the importance of universal/contact precautions and hand hygiene (hand washing/hand rubs), especially when changing diapers and dealing with respiratory, eye,

(Continued)

Table 10-1: Congenital Viral Infections: TORCHS Infections (*continued*)

Organism	Incidence	Perinatal Presentation	Neonatal Symptoms	Treatment	Parent Education
	hepatitis, and coagulopathy) with high mortality (Abzug, 2004)	• Ocular functions (conjunctivitis) • Cardiac functions (myopericarditis)			and gastrointestinal secretions
Rubella	Incidence declined 99% from prevaccine (MMR) to vaccine era Fewer than 25 cases/year in United States	Maternal infection asymptomatic or only slight disease ("3-day measles"). First-trimester infection is teratogenic to the fetus in 85% of cases.	IUGR; deafness; cataracts; jaundice; purpura ("blueberry muffin" syndrome); microcephaly; hepatosplenomegaly; bone lesions; chorioretinitis; pneumonitis; cardiac defects (PDA; pulmonic stenosis)	Prevention with MMR immunizations Supportive care	Women without immunity during or after birth should receive rubella immunization postpartally, even if breastfeeding Discharge teaching: Infected infant/child sheds live virus for 2–5 years in body fluids
Cytomegalo-virus (CMV)	50–80% of childbearing women carry CMV. CMV is most common congenital infection of the newborn (0.2–2.2% in the United States)	Majority of infected mothers are asymptomatic Symptoms include malaise, fever, lymphadenopathy, hepatosplenomegaly Neonatal sequelae most common after maternal primary infection	Majority have no signs or symptoms at birth; 12–18% are symptomatic at birth 9% have transient thrombocytopenia ("blueberry muffin" syndrome). Congenital manifestations: IUGR; developmental delays; micro/	Antiviral therapy with ganciclovir, valganciclovir, cidofovir is approved for life- and sight-saving therapy Ganciclovir decreases progression of hearing loss, but 6-week therapy is associated with significant neutropenia (Kimberlin et al., 2003)	Discharge teaching: Infected infant/child sheds live virus for 2–5 years in body fluids, such as urine and saliva (CDC, 2015a) Proper hand hygiene with washing or rubs

Infection	Incidence/Transmission	Maternal Signs and Symptoms	Neonatal Signs and Symptoms	Treatment	Nursing Care/Discharge Teaching
(continued)			hydrocephaly; seizures; jaundice; deafness; hepatosplenomegaly; chorioretinitis; cerebral calcifications and progressive sensorineural hearing loss (Boppana, Fowler, Britt, Stagno, & Pass, 1999)	Infants with CNS involvement, including sensorineural hearing loss and end-organ disease (hepatitis, pneumonia, thrombocytopenia), should be treated with antivirals (Swanson & Schleiss, 2013)	Discharge teaching: Good hand hygiene with antiseptic gels/hand washing. Do *not* breastfeed if there are breast lesions. Call healthcare provider for treatment. Pump and dump breast milk until lesions are healed
Herpes (herpes simplex virus [HSV])	1 of 3000–20,000 live births; incidence increases with prematurity, infected birth canal: 33–50% risk of acquiring herpes with maternal primary genital infection: < 5% risk of acquiring herpes with maternal reactivated infection	Primary and recurrent infections may be asymptomatic or present with vaginal discharge, genital pain, or shallow ulcerations. 75% of neonates who contract herpes are born to mothers who have no history or clinical manifestations of herpes during pregnancy; 90% of pregnant women infected with herpes virus are unaware of their infection	Symptoms appear at any time from birth to 4 weeks of age. Disseminated infection appears earlier—in the first week of life. One-third of herpes cases are localized, one-third are systemic, and one-third are CNS infections. Localized skin lesions and/or systemic infections increase morbidity and mortality	Antiviral: Acyclovir (IV 20 mg/kg/dose every 8 h for 14 days) for skin and/or mucous membrane involvement and for 21 days for CNS involvement (Pammi et al., 2016)	
Syphilis	Transmission to fetus occurs at any stage of maternal disease	Primary stage: Painless indurated ulcer(s) (chancre) of the skin/mucous membrane at infection site. Secondary stage (occurs 1–2 months after	Asymptomatic at birth	Antibiotic therapy: • CNS involvement (neonate): Aqueous penicillin G (IV 100,000–150,000 units/kg/day divided	Skin lesions and nasal secretions are highly infective (until after 24 h of antibiotic treatment)

(Continued)

Table 10-1: Congenital Viral Infections: TORCHS Infections (*Continued*)

Organism	Incidence	Perinatal Presentation	Neonatal Symptoms	Treatment	Parent Education
	Early, untreated syphilis results in spontaneous abortion, stillbirth, or perinatal death in 40% of pregnancies Primary/secondary syphilis results in 65–100% transmission Early latent infection results in 40% transmission; late latent infection results in 8% transmission	primary stage): rash, fever, mucocutaneous lesions, malaise, splenomegaly, headache, sore throat, arthralgia, lymphadenopathy Latent stage (seroreactive, but without clinical manifestations): • Early: Latent infection acquired within preceding year • Late: All other latent infections, after the first year Tertiary stage (occurs decades after primary infection): Gumma formation and cardiovascular disease	Symptomatic at birth or within the first 4–8 weeks of life Involves organ sys:ems: hepatitis, pneumonitis, bone marrow failure, myocarditis, meningitis, nephritic syndrome, rash (palms, soles), bone les ons, rhinitis (snuffles)	into every 12 h doses for 7 days; then every 8 h/day for a total of 10 days); LP must be repeated every 6 months until normal results (Pammi et al., 2016) • Without CNS involvement (infants): Penicillin G procaine 50,000 units/kg/ day IM in a single dose for 10–14 days (Pammi et al., 2016) If more than 1 day of treatment is missed in either regimen, the entire course of therapy must be restarted	Importance of contact precautions and hand hygiene (wash and rubs) Importance of continued follow-up care at 1, 2, 4, 6, and 12 months of age to evaluate growth, development, serum titers, CBC and CSF exam, if CSF was initially positive

Abbreviations: CBC, complete blood culture; CFS, cerebrospinal fluid; CNS, central nervous system; Hgb, hemoglobin; IM, intramuscular; IV, intravenous; IUGR, intrauterine growth restriction; IVIG, intravenous immune globulir; LP, lumbar puncture; MMR, measles–mumps–rubella; PDA, patent ductus arteriosus; RCT, randomized controlled trial; WBC, white blood count.

Reproduced from Gardner, S. L. (2009). Sepsis in the neonate. *Critical Care Nursing Clinics of North America, 21,* 126–129. Copyright 2009, with permission from Saunders/Elsevier.

Table 10-2: Acquired Neonatal Infections: Viral, Bacterial, and Fungal

Agent	Incidence	Perinatal Presentation	Neonatal Symptoms	Treatment	Parent Education
Virus					
Human immunodeficiency virus (HIV) (causative agent of AIDS)	Mother-to-newborn transmission rates: Untreated HIV+ mother-to-fetal transmission: 13–39% Antepartal: Treatment with antiretrovirals reduces transmission rate from 30% to 8% Intrapartal: 70% decrease with administration of antiretrovirals to mother/baby Postpartal: 16% with breastfeeding Increased perinatal transmission: High maternal viral load, low CD4+ lymphocyte count, advanced maternal illness, increased exposure of fetus to maternal blood, placental inflammation, preterm birth, prolonged labor, and prolonged	Risk factors: IV drug use (MOC/FOC); promiscuity; gay/bisexual sex/multiple heterosexual partners; Haitian ethnicity; parental blood transfusion prior to 1985 MOC may be asymptomatic so antenatal testing/counseling/treatment recommended (AAP, 2008; AAP & ACOG, 2012; Thorne & Newell, 2007)	Usually asymptomatic in the neonatal period Majority of infected infants present with symptoms by 2 years of age, with median age of presentation being 11–12 months of age	Antiretroviral therapy: Zidovudine (AZT) alone or in combination with other retrovirals, started at 8–12 hours of life and continued for 6 weeks (2 mg/kg/dose PO every 6 h) (Pammi et al., 2016) Untreated HIV-infected mothers: ZDV for 6 weeks, and 3 doses of nevirapine (NVP) (12 mg/dose PO for infants > 2 kg) in the first week of life (at birth [as soon as possible] 48 h, and 96 h after second dose) (Pammi et al., 2016) Prophylaxis for *Pneumocystis jiroveci* pneumonia (begun at 4–6 weeks of life through the first year of age or until HIV infection is excluded): trimethoprim (5 mg/kg/day PO) and sulfamethoxazole	Live HIV virus is present in human milk. HIV+ mothers in developed countries are advised not to breastfeed: (1) Formula is a safe alternative to breast feeding, (2) safe water supply, (3) twice the risk of postpartal transmission of HIV virus to the infant with breastfeeding (AAP, 2013) Instruct parents about: • Ongoing follow-up care and immunizations • Prevention of infections with good hand hygiene, regular bathing and skin care, clean food preparation

(continued)

Table 10-2: Acquired Neonatal Infections: Viral, Bacterial, and Fungal (*continued*)

Agent	Incidence	Perinatal Presentation	Neonatal Symptoms	Treatment	Parent Education
	rupture of membranes and mode of delivery (cesarean section or vaginal delivery) (AAP, 2008; Pickering, Baker, Kimberlin, Long, & AAP, 2012; Thorne & Newell, 2007)			(25 mg/kg/day PO) in 2 divided doses for 3 consecutive days in a week (Pammi et al., 2016) Early treatment (within the first 3 months of life) of HIV+ infants with antiretroviral drugs reduces mortality rate by 75% (Volari, 2007)	
Varicella	Congenital varicella syndrome (1–25%) when mother has varicella at delivery and infection occurs before 20 weeks' gestation Nosocomially acquired infections in preterms born of susceptible mothers, infants who are severely preterm regardless of maternal status, and immunocompromised infants	Generalized, pruritic, vesicular skin rash with lesions in various stages of development and resolution (crusting), mild fever, malaise	Congenital varicella is rare: Teratogen with malformations of limbs (atrophy), skin scars, CNS and eye abnormalities Symptoms are indistinguishable from other causes of septicemia	Maternal infection within 5 days before or 7 days after birth may be fatal for newborn Administer zoster immune globulin (ZIG) (2 mL IM) within 72 h of birth (Pammi et al., 2016) Rapid diagnostic tests so that unnecessary antibiotics are not used and antivirals are administered (Strikas, CDC, ACIP Child/ Adolescent Immunization Work Group, 2015)	ZIG gives passive immunization so parents need to screen themselves and all visitors who have been exposed to varicella. Non-immune varicella-exposed individuals should not be around a newborn for the incubation period of 21 days.

| Influenza A and B | Twin pregnancy: Risk factor for neonatal influenza (Yusuf, Soraisham, & Fonseca, 2007)

Incubation period 1–4 days; maximum viral shedding in first 3 days, but duration may be as long as 7 days or much longer in young infants (AAP, Committee on Infectious Diseases, 2014) | Immunizing pregnant women is the single most important factor in decreasing influenza (71% effective) (Dabrara et al., 2014) and hospitalization of infants < 6 months (64% effective) (Dabrara et al., 2014) and ≤ 1 year of age

Maternal influenza immunization during pregnancy protects newborns from influenza by bestowing higher levels of specific immunoglobulin G antibodies

Late-preterm infants may not have received sufficient amounts of these antibodies because of their shortened gestation (AAP, Committee on Infectious Diseases, 2014; Strikas et al., 2015) | | Importance of infection control measures—do not expose newborns to *any* respiratory infection; hand hygiene; droplets and contaminated fomites are infectious

Influenza immunizations essential in anyone around young infants: parents, grandparents, childcare providers, healthcare providers |

(Continued)

Table 10-2: Acquired Neonatal Infections: Viral, Bacterial, and Fungal (*Continued*)

Agent	Incidence	Perinatal Presentation	Neonatal Symptoms	Treatment	Parent Education
Human papillomavirus (HPV)	75% of sexually active adults will develop HPV Most have no symptoms, and the immune system clears the virus before symptoms or detection 30 types of HPV; HPV is one of the most common sexually transmitted diseases Neonatal HPV occurs after birth through the infected mother's birth canal and has occurred after cesarean section birth	Asymptomatic or presence of infectious genital warts	HPV infection of epithelium results in laryngeal warts and recurrent respiratory papillomatosis	Surgical removal (may need to be repeated)	Gardasil is approved by the FDA as a vaccine to prevent 4 high-risk strains of HPV virus, thus preventing cervical, vulvar/vaginal, and anal cancers caused by these 4 strains of HPV. Gardasil does not treat HPV if it is already present Vaccination is recommended for young girls, boys, and women (Petrosky et al., 2015)
Respiratory syncytial virus (RSV)	Major risk factor for RSV is chronologic age: 2–3% of infants (≤ 12 months of age) are hospitalized with RSV infection yearly in the United States (AAP, Committee on Infectious Diseases & Bronchiolitis Guidelines Committees, 2014)	Parents, siblings, family, and visitors present with a "cold," an upper respiratory infection	Pneumonia, bronchiolitis, and otitis media Respiratory symptoms: Tachypnea, apnea, cyanosis, cough, choking and vomiting from strenuous coughing	Palivizumab (15 mg/kg IM once a month during RSV season for prevention of serious lower respiratory tract infections • AAP (2014) recommendations: Prophylaxis in first year of life to preterm infants born < 29 weeks'	Infection control principles to prevent RSV: • Good hand hygiene (washing/rubs) • Restrict contacts with the infant (no one with a "cold") • Avoid crowds— church nurseries, childcare

	...occur in the first 5 months of life; most hospitalizations occur in the first 3 months of life (AAP, Committee on Infectious Diseases & Bronchiolitis Guidelines Committees, 2014)		Poor oxygenation and ventilation	gestation; those with chronic illnesses (e.g., congenital heart disease, chronic lung disease) • Give qualifying infants no more than 5 monthly doses during RSV season • Broader use of prophylaxis may be indicated for Alaskan Natives and American Indian infants due to the heavy burden of RSV and costs for transport from remote areas	programs, shopping areas • Reduce/eliminate childcare or use programs with < 2–3 children • Eliminate second-hand smoke exposure • Stress importance of influenza immunizations for all infants (beginning at 6 months of age) and all infant contacts Breastfeeding offers passive immunity from maternal antibodies
Bacteria					
Chlamydia	50% transmission rate to infants born vaginally through an infected birth canal 25–50% conjunctivitis risk 5–20% pneumonia risk	Most common STI MOC may be asymptomatic or have vaginitis, urethritis, cervicitis	Conjunctivitis at 1–2 weeks after birth; pneumonia with staccato cough, tachypnea, hypoxemia, eosinophilia, otitis, bronchiolitis	Conjunctivitis: erythromycin 50 mg/kg/day PO in 4 divided doses for 14 days (Pammi et al., 2016) Pneumonia: Erythromycin 50 mg/kg/day in 4 divided doses for 14 days (Pammi et al., 2016)	Screen/treat pregnant women before birth through an infected birth canal Teach parents the signs and symptoms of infantile hypertrophic pyloric stenosis, which has been associated with the use of oral erythromycin

(Continued)

Table 10-2: Acquired Neonatal Infections: Viral, Bacterial, and Fungal (Continued)

Agent	Incidence	Perinatal Presentation	Neonatal Symptoms	Treatment	Parent Education
Group B Streptococcus (GBS)	Incidence has declined due to prevention and treatment guidelines (Baker, Byington, Polin, & AAP, 2011; CDC, 2010) 70% of early-onset GBS cases are term newborns (≥37 weeks GA); mortality rates are 2–3% (Baker et al., 2011; CDC, 2010) Mortality rates are higher among preterm infants: 20% to as high as 30% for preterm ≤ 33 weeks GA (CDC, 2010) Risk factors for early-onset GBS: • Preterm/late-preterm (<37 weeks) with obstetric complications such as PROM ≥ 18 hours; chorioamnionitis; maternal fever; preterm labor; UTI; fetal distress; neonatal aspiration • African American ethnicity	MOC often colonized in birth canal (10–30%), but asymptomatic Transmission: 1-in-100 chance of infecting newborn if colonized during labor/birth	Majority (98%) of colonized newborns are asymptomatic Early-onset (first 24 hours to first week of life); 2% of colonized neonates develop fulminate, multisystem illness (pneumonia, septicemia, meningitis); signs and symptoms of neonatal sepsis Late-onset (7 day –3 month of life): Present with sepsis or meningitis	CDC-recommended maternal intrapartum antibiotic prophylaxis: At least 1 dose of IV penicillin, given 4 h before birth; incomplete adherence to maternal antibiotic prophylaxis may not prevent early-onset GBS sepsis CDC-recommended neonatal management: (Baker et al., 2011; CDC, 2010) Signs of sepsis: Sepsis workup (blood cultures; CBC with differential and platelets; chest x-ray [if respiratory symptoms] and spinal tap) and antibiotic therapy • Maternal chorioamnionitis: Limited evaluation (blood culture, CBC with differential and platelets at birth and 6–12 h of age) and antibiotic therapy	80% of early-onset neonatal GBS sepsis can be prevented by use of CDC guidelines (AAP & ACOG, 2012; CDC, 2010) CDC guidelines for prevention of GBS infection (Baker et al., 2011; CDC, 2010): Perform universal prenatal screening with vaginal/rectal GBS cultures of all pregnant women at 35–37 weeks' gestation Indications for intrapartum antibiotic prophylaxis: • Previous infant with invasive GBS GBS bacteriuria during current pregnancy Positive GBS screening culture during current pregnancy

• Young maternal age • Low antibody level to GBS capsular polysaccharide (indicating immunologic vulnerability)		• Mother received antibiotic therapy for ≥ 4 h prior to delivery: Observe for ≥ 48 h* • > 37 weeks and duration of ruptured membranes < 18 h: Observe for ≥ 48 h* • Either < 37 weeks or duration of rupture ≥ 18 h: Limited evaluation and observe for ≥ 48 h* Empiric antibiotic therapy (for 48–72 h) (Baker et al., 2011; CDC, 2010): Ampicillin 50 mg/kg/dose IV every 12 h (for sepsis); 100 mg/kg/dose IV every 12 h (for meningitis) Gentamicin 2.5 mg/kg/dose IV every 12–24 h depending on gestational age If laboratory results/clinical presentation are negative for sepsis, discontinue antibiotics If symptomatic or laboratory results suggest sepsis, treat with antibiotics for 7–10 days; treat 14 days for meningitis	Unknown GBS status and any of the following: (1) delivery at < 37 weeks' gestation, (2) membranes ruptured ≥ 18 h, (3) intrapartum temperature > 38°C

(Continued)

Table 10-2: Acquired Neonatal Infections: Viral, Bacterial, and Fungal (*Continued*)

Agent	Incidence	Perinatal Presentation	Neonatal Symptoms	Treatment	Parent Education
Hepatitis B	High-risk mothers: Asian, African, Eskimo, Haitian, Pacific Islanders	History of maternal liver disease, IV drug use, exposure to blood in medical/dental settings HBsAG-positive mothers may pass the infection to their infants at birth	Asymptomatic Occasional acute fulminate hepatitis with elevated liver enzymes Neonatal infection results in chronic carrier status that is implicated in the development of primary hepatocellular carcinoma later in life	Immunizations (Pammi et al., 2016): • Active: For newborns with HBsAG-positive and HBsAG-negative mothers, give 3 separate doses—as soon as possible after birth, at 1 month, and at 6 month—Recombivax 0.25–0.5 mL IM, or Energix-B 0.5 mL IM • Passive: For newborns whose mothers have acute type B infection or mothers who are antigen positive, give within 12 h of birth hepatitis B immune globulin 0.5 mL/kg IM	Immunization (both active and passive) is indicated for newborns whose mothers are HBsAG positive because most newborns are at risk of becoming infected from their mothers Untreated newborns may become HBsAg positive at 4–12 weeks of age, become lifelong asymptomatic carriers, or develop hepatitis B (Pickering et al., 2012)
Gonorrhea	Highest incidence of infection in females 15–18 years of age Concurrent infection with chlamydia may exist	80% of mothers are asymptomatic	Purulent eye conjunctivitis at 2–5 days after birth Scalp abscess with use of internal fetal monitoring (Pickering et al., 2012)	Eye prophylaxis: • Antibiotics: 1% tetracycline or 0.5% erythromycin ophthalmic ointment • Silver nitrate: 1% solution	Eye prophylaxis to prevent ophthalmia neonatorum and blindness is required by state law; is administered after the first hour of life (to facilitate parent–infant bonding)

			Systemic infection may present as arthritis, bacteremia, pneumonia, endocarditis, or meningitis	Term newborns born to mothers with known gonococcal infection: Ceftriaxone 125 mg IV/IM × 1 (Pammi et al., 2016)	Eye prophylaxis minimizes but does not guarantee freedom from eye infection
Tuberculosis (TB)	Resurgence of active disease in at-risk mothers: Asian, Native American, HIV positive. 4.4 cases/100,000 people—lowest TB rate on record in United States	May be asymptomatic or have respiratory or systemic symptoms (fever, weight loss). Mother with active disease should be separated from the newborn until not contagious (sputum negative with treatment)	Maternal pulmonary TB does not infect fetus; newborns may be infected by droplet infection after birth by their mothers. Congenital TB is rare but can occur after maternal bacillemia. Signs and symptoms: Same as neonatal sepsis and failure-to-thrive in infancy	Mother: Isoniazid and rifampin with pyridoxine supplementation in pregnant and breastfeeding women. Newborn: Isoniazid at 10 mg/kg/day. Active immunization (Pammi et al., 2016) for selected infants at risk for contracting TB; give as soon as possible after birth—Bacille Calmette-Guérin (BCG) 0.1 mL intradermally and divided into 2 sites over the deltoid muscle	Teach parents infection control measures, including need for good hand hygiene (washing/rubs) and wearing face mask. Infants require pyridoxine supplementation if they are treated with isoniazid or are breastfeeding from a mother being treated with isoniazid (Pickering et al., 2012)
Methicillin-resistant *Staphylococcus aureus* (MRSA), including hospital-acquired (HA-MRSA) and MRSA	Hospital-acquired: Antepartal invasive procedures, postpartal mastitis, skin, wound infections	Mother may have mastitis; MRSA-positive breastmilk with no symptoms; skin/wound infection; infection after antepartal invasive procedure	Skin and soft-tissue infections; abscess; bacteremia/septicemia/meningitis; purulent conjunctivitis;	HA-MRSA is resistant to more antibiotics; treat infections with vancomycin IV; add gentamicin or rifampin for serious systemic infections (Pickering et al., 2012)	Transmission by direct contact with parents, staff, infected skin lesions, contaminated fomites, overcrowding

(Continued)

Table 10-2: Acquired Neonatal Infections: Viral, Bacterial, and Fungal (*Continued*)

Agent	Incidence	Perinatal Presentation	Neonatal Symptoms	Treatment	Parent Education
community-acquired (CA-MRSA)	Community-acquired: Parents, siblings, family, healthcare workers; most often causes skin and soft-tissue infections	Colonization increases risk of infection in both mothers and newborns	orbital cellulitis; necrotizing fasciitis; septic arthritis; subglottic stenosis (Gardner, 2008b)	CA-MRSA infections more susceptible to ciprofloxacin, clindamycin, gentamicin, and trimethoprim–sulfamethoxazole DS (double strength), tetracycline, linezolid, and vancomycin with or without rifampin (Pickering et al., 2012) Alternative drugs (e.g., trimethoprim–sulfamethoxazole, linezolid, quinapristin/dalfopristin, fluoroquinolones) should be used after susceptibility testing is complete and after consultation with a pediatric infectious diseases specialist (Pickering et al., 2012) Neither sulfa drugs nor tetracycline are used in the neonate or in the breastfeeding mother because of their adverse effects on the infant	50% transmission rate between healthy lactating mothers and their breastfeeding infants (Kawada, Okuzumi , Hitomi, & Sugishita, 2003); antibodies against MRSA also obtained by breastfeeding infants Education to prevent/control spread of MRSA (Gardner, 2008b): Infection control guidelines; contact isolation and universal precautions; strict adherence to hand hygiene (washing/rubs) (Romero, Treston, & O'Sullivan, 2006); covering all skin lesions with impermeable dressing; not sharing personal care items

Pertussis (whooping cough)	Highly contagious—spread by coughing or sneezing while in close contact (CDC, 2015b) Source of infection: Mothers and siblings (Skoff et al., 2015) A resurgence of pertussis in the United States resulted in 2269 cases of pertussis in infants < 3 months of age in 2012; 15 of these infected infants died (CDC, 2015b)	Whooping cough presents with severe coughing, difficulty breathing, vomiting, sleep disturbance, and weight loss Infants are most at risk for severe complications from pertussis (hospitalization for apnea, pneumonia)	Supportive, with monitoring, oxygen, fluids, and hospitalization	Pregnant women should receive a dose of tetanus–diphtheria–pertussis (Tdap) vaccine during the third trimester with every pregnancy to protect the newborn from pertussis (CDC, 2015c) Cocooning: Immunizing fathers, siblings, and all adults who will be in close contact to an infant < 12 months of age also recommended (CDC, 2015c) Transplacental passage of maternal pertussis antibodies to the fetus results in high concentrations of pertussis antibodies in infants during the first 2 months of life and does not alter infant responses to Tdap (Munoz et al., 2014)

(Continued)

Table 10-2: Acquired Neonatal Infections: Viral, Bacterial, and Fungal (*Continued*)

Agent	Incidence	Perinatal Presentation	Neonatal Symptoms	Treatment	Parent Education
					Vaccination with Tdap does not increase adverse events such as rates of preterm or SGA births or maternal hypertensive disorders in pregnancy (Kharbanda et al., 2014; Munoz et al., 2014)
Fungus					
Candida albicans (thrush; diaper dermatitis)	Thrush: yeast infection of the tongue, cheeks, and mouth	Maternal antibiotics may have caused yeast infection in birth canal Yeast infection causes a burning sensation in the nipple, a stabbing pain throughout the breast, shiny appearance Edematous skin or flaking skin on the nipple and/or areola (Gardner & Lawrence, 2016)	White patches scattered over tongue, gums, cheeks, and palate of newborn's mouth White patches do not wipe off and, when wiped, may bleed Mouth may be sore, resulting in feeding refusal	Term newborn: Nystatin 2 mL of 100,000 units/mL suspension divided and applied with swab to each side of the mouth and on the infant's tongue every 6 hours; continue treatment for 3 days after symptoms (white patches and sore mouth) subside Maternal nipples: Apply topical cream 100,000 units/g to both nipples every 6 h; continue treatment for 3 days after symptoms subside	Breastfeeding mothers *and* their breastfeeding babies must be simultaneously treated for yeast infection to effect a cure. Nipples are treated with a topical antifungal, nystatin, while the infant's mouth is swabbed with oral nystatin

| Diaper dermatitis caused by yeast infection | Intense inflammation of the skin that is bright red, sharply demarcated on the buttocks, thighs, inguinal folds, abdomen, and genitalia, with red pustular satellite lesions extending into the periphery | Nystatin ointment applied to affected areas every 6 h; continue treatment for 3 days after symptoms subside | Persistent yeast infections are treated with oral fluconazole, which is considered safe for nursing infants (Gardner & Lawrence, 2016) |

Abbreviations: AIDS, acquired immune deficiency syndrome; CBC, complete blood count; CDC, Centers for Disease Control and Prevention; CNS, central nervous system; FDA, Food and Drug Administration; FOC, father of the child; GA, gestational age; IM, intramuscular; IV, intravenous; MOC, mother of the child; PO, per os; PROM, premature rupture of membranes; SGA, small for gestational age; STI, sexually transmitted infection.

*If greater than 37 weeks' gestation, observation may occur at home after 24 hours if other discharge criteria have been met, access to medical care is readily available, and a person who is able to comply fully with instructions for home observation will be present. If any of these conditions is not met, the infant should be observed in the hospital for at least 48 hours and until discharge criteria are achieved.

Reproduced from Gardner, S. L. (2009). Sepsis in the neonate. *Critical Care Nursing Clinics of North America, 21,* 130–137. Copyright 2009, with permission from Saunders/Elsevier.

Box 10-3: Signs and Symptoms of Neonatal Infections

- Temperature instability: hypothermia or hyperthermia
- Respiratory distress: tachypnea, apnea, use of accessory muscles (grunting, flaring, retracting), cyanosis
- Cardiovascular changes: tachycardia, bradycardia, hypotension, pallor, poor peripheral perfusion (capillary refill time > 3 seconds), weak pulses, decreased urine output
- Neurologic changes: irritability, lethargy, seizures, apnea as a manifestation of seizure
- Feeding abnormalities: change in feeding behaviors, poor feeding, vomiting, abdominal distention, diarrhea
- Jaundice: progression of jaundice from head to toe; increase in direct or indirect bilirubin levels
- Skin changes: rash, purpura, erythema, petechiae
- Metabolic changes: acidosis (metabolic and/or respiratory), hypoglycemia, hypoxia

Data from Gardner, S. L. (2007). Late-preterm ("near-term") newborns: A neonatal nursing challenge, *Nurse Currents, 1*(1), 1–7; Gardner, S. L. (2008a). How will I know my newborn is sick? *Nurse Currents, 2*(2), 1–8; Pammi, M., Brand, M. C., &Weisman, L. E. (2016). Infection in the neonate. In S. L. Gardner, B. S. Carter, M. Enzman Hines, & J. A. Hernandez (Eds.), *Merenstein and Gardner's handbook of neonatal intensive care* (8th ed., pp. 537–563). St. Louis, MO: Mosby-Elsevier.

"obvious," a baby can be moribund and overwhelmingly septic (Gardner, 2008a, 2009; Polin & Committee on Fetus and Newborn, 2012).

According to WHO, improving identification of infants who are severely ill (and in danger of dying) in the first week of life is a major public health issue worldwide. To clarify signs and symptoms of neonatal sepsis, WHO conducted several multisite studies of the clinical features and causes of serious bacterial disease in infants (younger than 2 months of age) (WHO Young Infants Study Group, 1999; Young Infants Clinical Signs Study Group, 2008). In these studies, the mother or other caretaker had already decided that the infant was ill and needed to be seen by a healthcare provider. From an initial list of 20 signs and symptoms of neonatal illness, 7 were found to be independent clinical predictors of severe illness requiring hospitalization for neonates (0 to 7 days old) and for infants (7 days to 59 days old) (Young Infants Clinical Signs Study Group, 2008). The presence of *any one sign* listed in **Box 10-4** has high sensitivity and specificity for severe illness requiring hospitalization in the first 2 months of life (Gardner, 2009; Young Infants Clinical Signs Study Group, 2008). Based on these data, WHO (2009) developed an algorithm intended for all infants younger than 2 months of age who have been brought to a health facility for an illness.

Recognizing a neonate with infection is challenging, and making an incorrect diagnosis can be devastating. Although neonatal care is replete with scoring systems (i.e., Apgar, Neonatal Abstinence Scale [NAS], Crib score, and numerous pain scores), there was never an

Box 10-4: Signs and Symptoms Predictive of Serious Neonatal Illness and the Need for Hospitalization in Infants from 0 to 59 Days of Age

- History of feeding difficulty
- Movement only when stimulated
- Temperature < 35.5°C
- Temperature ≥ 37.5°C
- Respiratory rate > 60 breaths/min
- Severe chest indrawing (retractions)
- History of convulsions

Data from Young Infants Clinical Signs Study Group. (2008). Clinical signs that predict severe illness in children under age 2 months: A multi-center study. *Lancet, 371*(9607), 135–142.

objective, reliable, and validated scoring tool for neonatal infection until the Rubarth Newborn Scale of Sepsis (RNSOS) was introduced (**Figure 10-1**). The RNSOS was developed to assist nurses in looking for neonatal sepsis by using both clinical and laboratory data (Rubarth, 2005). This scale is an objective tool that can be used by nurses and advanced practice primary care providers to identify newborns who need to be evaluated for sepsis. It is an assessment rather than a diagnostic tool (Rubarth, 2008).

When using the RNSOS, the maximum possible score is 55: 20 points for the laboratory markers and 35 points for clinical indicators. A total clinical score less than 10 indicates that the newborn does not have sepsis—a judgment that has a predictive value of 97% (Rubarth, 2005, 2008). A total clinical score greater than 10 indicates a "sick" newborn, possibly with sepsis; it also indicates that the newborn needs further diagnostic evaluation.

Physical Examination

Evaluate vital signs, including blood pressure, while the infant is quiet. Neonates who are infected can be either hypothermic or hyperthermic. Of the two findings, hypothermia is the most common, with the baby feeling cold to touch, an axillary temperature less than 36°C, and an inability to warm the baby. The most common reason for hyperthermia in a neonate is environmental—the baby is dressed too warmly—but neonates can also have fever. If a newborn with a developmentally immature immune system has fever (axillary temperature ≥ 37.5°C), the baby is extremely sick!

Tachypnea (a respiratory rate greater than 60 breaths/min) is an early sign of many illnesses and is often accompanied by use of accessory muscles (grunting, flaring, and retracting) with respiration. Respiratory distress may also include apnea. In a term baby, apnea should be considered a seizure until proven otherwise—healthy late-preterm and term babies do *not* have apnea.

Newborn Scale Of Sepsis (SOS)

Rubarth © 2005

NAME		DATE OF EXAM	AGE AT EXAM (HOURS)

CLINICAL INDICATORS: | *Score*

Skin Color *Ashen/Grey =* **5** *Dusky =* **3** *Mottled =* **2** *Acrocyanosis =* **1** *Pink =* **0**	
Perfusion (Cap. Refill) *Poor > 7 sec =* **5** *Moderate 6–7 sec =* **3** *Fair 4–5 sec =* **1** *Good < 4 sec =* **0**	
Muscle Tone *Flaccid =* **5** *Low tone =* **3** *Good tone =* **0**	
Responsiveness to Pain *No response =* **5** *Some response (withdrawal) =* **2** *Active crying =* **0**	
Respiratory Distress *Present with grunting =* **5** *Present no grunting =* **3** *None =* **0**	
Respiratory Rate *Respiratory rate ≥ 100 =* **5** *RR 60–99 =* **3** *RR < 60 =* **0**	
Temperature *Low temp < 97°F =* **3** *High temp < 99°F =* **2** *Normal 97–99°F =* **0**	
Apnea *Present =* **2** *Absent =* **0**	

+

LABORATORY FINDINGS:

White Blood Cell Count *< 5,000 =* **5** *> 30,000 =* **2** *5,000–30,000 =* **0**	
Immature: Total Neutrophil Ratio *< 0.3 =* **5** *0.2–0.3 =* **3** *< 0.2 =* **0**	
Platelet Count *< 100,000 =* **3** *≥ 100,000 =* **0**	
Blood Acidity *pH < 7.25 =* **2** *pH 7.25–7.34 =* **1** *pH normal 7.35–7.45 =* **0**	
Absolute Neutrophil Count *< 1000 =* **5** *1000–2000 =* **3** *> 2000 =* **0**	

=

Total score | |

Figure 10-1: Rubarth Newborn Scale of Sepsis. A total clinical score less than 10 indicates that the newborn does not have sepsis—a negative predictive value of 97%. Any newborn with a total clinical score greater than 10 is considered "sick," possibly with sepsis. A clinical score greater than 10 is also an indicator of the need for further diagnostic evaluation.

Reproduced from Rubarth, L. B. (2005). Nursing patterns of knowing in assessment of newborn sepsis, Doctoral Dissertation, University of Arizona, with permission.

Cyanosis, a late sign of respiratory distress, is present when fetal hemoglobin is desaturated and oxygen saturation falls to 60% to 65% and the PaO_2 is 30 mm Hg. Central cyanosis, affecting the perioral and periorbital areas, and general body cyanosis are pathologic and must be distinguished from acrocyanosis of the hands and feet, which is normal.

Infected infants may be tachycardic as a result of temperature instability. Septic shock presents with tachycardia, hypotension, and poor color (mottling, pallor); the last finding represents poor peripheral perfusion—poor capillary refill time (CRT) of more than 3 seconds.

Neurologic changes are often noticed first by the mother/parents. Feeding behavior often changes in such a case: a vigorously crying baby who once demanded feeding now does not awaken to feed, falls asleep while feeding, or refuses to eat. Diminished activity, lethargy, less "quiet alert" behavior, and failure to respond to noxious stimuli or pain are all abnormal central nervous system (CNS) signs. Conversely, inconsolable crying and fussiness may be a behavioral manifestation of infection.

Skin changes can accompany neonatal infection. Every jaundiced baby needs to be evaluated for infection. Neonatal care providers need to ask themselves, "Is this jaundiced baby septic?", as part of the assessment for both jaundice and sepsis. Petechiae on the presenting part during birth (i.e., head for vertex presentation, face for face presentation, buttocks for breech presentation) is normal, but the presence of petechiae on the hard palate or the baby's skin (other than the presenting part) may be a symptom of infection. Omphalitis presents with erythema and induration of the skin around the umbilicus. Community-acquired methicillin-resistant *Staphylococcus aureus* (MRSA; Table 10-2) most often presents as a skin or soft-tissue infection—there will be an erythematous rash or an erythematous area on the skin.

Infected neonates who are very sick will present with metabolic alterations such as acidosis, hypoglycemia, and hypoxia. Infection and sepsis cause metabolic acidosis. If the neonate has respiratory distress caused by a pulmonary infection, such as pneumonia, there may be a combined metabolic acidosis (from infection) and respiratory acidosis (from hypoventilation and retained carbon dioxide). Hypoxia (pulse oximetry less than 90%) may also be present.

Diagnostic Evaluation

When it goes undiagnosed and untreated, neonatal infection has a high mortality rate; clearly, then, identifying who is and is not infected is imperative. A diagnostic workup, which is outlined in **Box 10-5**, is required in all neonates exhibiting signs and symptoms of infection or sepsis. Unfortunately, there is no laboratory test that is 100% sensitive and 100% specific for neonatal sepsis (Borna & Borna, 2004). *Laboratory tests with normal results do not rule out infection and sepsis in the neonate.* Results of a complete blood count (CBC) with differential may be difficult to interpret due to variations in normal values based on (1) birth weight, (2) gestational age, (3) postconceptual age, (4) physiologic stress, and (5) intrapartum

Box 10-5: Diagnostic Evaluation

Physical examination: by the healthcare provider

Noninvasive monitoring: pulse oximetry to assess oxygenation

Sepsis workup

Laboratory tests:

- Complete blood count with (WBC) differential and platelet count
- Cultures of nonpermissive sites (blood, urine, cerebrospinal fluid [CSF], closed body cavity)
- Chemistries: electrolytes, glucose, CSF (glucose/protein)
- Arterial blood gases: acid–base status; oxygenation
- Gram stain
- C-reactive protein (CRP); serum procalcitonin level
- Tests for presence of bacterial antigens/endotoxins: counter-immunoelectrophoresis (CIE); latex agglutination (LA); limulus lysate

Radiologic tests: chest, abdomen, joint

Data from Pammi, M., Brand, M. C., &Weisman, L. E. (2016). Infection in the neonate. In S. L. Gardner, B. S. Carter, M. Enzman Hines, & J. A. Hernandez (Eds.), *Merenstein and Gardner's handbook of neonatal intensive care* (8th ed., pp. 537–563). St. Louis, MO: Mosby-Elsevier.

complications such as low Apgar scores or pregnancy-induced hypertension (Pammi et al., 2016). Use of surface cultures yields colonization, but does not necessarily identify the cause of active infection.

Blood culture is the gold standard for diagnosing and detecting bacteremia. Isolating, growing, and identifying bacteria from a nonpermissive site (e.g., urine, cerebral spinal fluid, blood) is the most valid method of diagnosing bacterial sepsis (Pammi et al., 2016). In the neonate, blood culture time to positivity is 71% at 24 hours, 95% at 36 hours, and 97% at 48 hours (Janjindamai & Phetpisal, 2006). Even in the presence of neonatal sepsis, however, blood cultures are not always positive. Therefore, in this nonverbal, vulnerable population, a combination of clinical and laboratory evidence is required to diagnose and treat the neonate with suspected sepsis.

Some elements of the CBC are associated with bacterial sepsis. Leukopenia (less than 5000 cells/mm^3) and neutropenia (less than 1750 cells/mm^3) are predictive of bacteremia in the neonate (Johnson, Whitwell, Pethe, Saxena, & Super, 1997). The presence of neutropenia and an abnormal immature neutrophil-to-total neutrophil (I:T) ratio is most predictive of infection (Manroe, Weinberg, Rosenfeld, & Browne, 1979; Polin & Committee on Fetus and Newborn, 2012). In the presence of infection, the I:T ratio is elevated. If it is normal, there is a high likelihood that infection is absent (Edwards, 2011). A low platelet count (fewer than 100,000 cells/mm^3), which is known as thrombocytopenia, is also associated with neonatal sepsis.

When evaluating test results, a single laboratory test must not be relied upon, especially if it is "reassuring" and not reflective of the clinical picture of a symptomatic infant. In the neonate, laboratory tests are most useful when serial testing is performed and initial results are compared to follow-up tests performed 12 to 24 hours later (Pammi et al., 2016)

Several newer laboratory tests may not be available or be sensitive or specific enough on their own to influence clinical decision making (Christensen, Rothstein, Hill, & Hall, 1985; Engle & Rosenfeld, 1984; Pammi et al., 2016; Pickering et al., 2012). Findings of leukocytosis and leukopenia are insensitive and nonspecific for diagnosing neonatal infection and sepsis (Edwards, 2011).

Acute-phase reactant tests are diagnostic markers for infection. In particular, C-reactive protein (CRP) levels will be elevated in any acute inflammatory condition, including infection. An acute-phase reactant, CRP is synthesized in the liver in the first 6 to 8 hours of infection, although its level has a low sensitivity (60%) early in infection (Pammi et al., 2016). Serial CRP determinations at 24 and 48 hours improve sensitivity to 82% to 84%, while sensitivity and positive predictive values range from 83% to 100% with this approach (Ng, 2004; Pammi et al., 2016). A CRP level less than 1.0 mg/dL has a negative predictive value of 92% to 99% (Mathers & Pohlhandt, 1987). On the first and second days of life, normal CRP values are less than 1.6 mg/dL, but decrease to less than 1 mg/dL on subsequent days (Kapur, Yoder, & Polin, 2011). Serial CRP values are used to follow infection resolution and guide antibiotic therapy (Dollner, Vatten, & Austgulen, 2001; Franz, Steinback, Kron, Pohlandt, 1999; Hofer, Muller, & Resch, 2013; Kawamura & Nishida, 1995; Pammi et al., 2016; Polin & Committee on Fetus and Newborn, 2012; Weitkamp & Aschner, 2005). CRP levels are not affected by gestational age, have better sensitivity than leukocyte indices, and are higher in gram-negative infections (Pammi et al., 2016). Two normal CRP values (at 8 to 24 hours after birth and 24 hours later) have a negative predictive accuracy of 99.7% (Polin & Committee on Fetus and Newborn, 2012).

The level of another acute-phase reactant, serum procalcitonin, rises within 4 hours of exposure to bacterial endotoxin. Procalcitonin measurements have a sensitivity and specificity ranging from 83% to 100%, are better able to differentiate infection from inflammation, and may be superior to CRP levels for identifying neonatal infection (Pammi et al., 2016).

Differential Diagnoses

Because of the developmental immaturity of their immune system, neonates are unable to localize infection. In turn, meningitis is a frequent manifestation of sepsis, especially in symptomatic infants, those with group B *Streptococcus* (GBS) sepsis, and late-onset disease (Pammi et al., 2016). Meningitis may also be present without overt signs of CNS infection.

Lumbar puncture (LP) and examination of cerebrospinal fluid (CSF) is more common in neonatal care because meningitis is difficult to diagnose or exclude without an LP. In neonates with bacteremia, the incidence of meningitis may be as high as 23%, while blood cultures may be negative in as many as 38% of neonates with meningitis (Polin & Committee on Fetus and Newborn, 2012). The presence of meningitis affects the type of antibiotic used to treat the infection, its dose, and the length of therapy, as well as morbidity, mortality, and follow-up care (Gardner, 2009; Pammi et al., 2016; Ray, Mangalore, Harikumar, & Tuladhar, 2006; Smith et al., 2006).

Critical congenital heart disease (CCHD), in which systemic circulation is dependent on an intact or patent ductus arteriosus, often mimics septic shock. Current screening using pulse oximetry has been instituted to detect CCHD prior to discharge. When the ductus arteriosus closes, systemic circulation becomes severely compromised and the neonate goes into cardiogenic shock, which has the same symptoms (i.e., hypotension, poor peripheral perfusion, CRT greater than 3 seconds, pallor, mottling, tachypnea, apnea, poor/no urine output, hypoglycemia, acidosis, hypoxemia, hypothermia) and is indistinguishable from septic shock based on clinical presentation.

Many other neonatal conditions also mimic infection. The respiratory symptoms listed in Box 10-3, for example, could be caused by respiratory distress syndrome, meconium aspiration, transient tachypnea of the newborn, hypoglycemia, pneumonia, or air leak syndromes. Central nervous system symptoms (Box 10-3) may not be due to infection but rather to neonatal abstinence syndrome, intracranial hemorrhage, hypoglycemia, or inborn errors of metabolism (Edwards, 2011). The gastrointestinal symptoms listed in Box 10-2 could be caused by necrotizing enterocolitis, gastric perforation, or gastrointestinal abnormalities such as midgut volvulus, intestinal atresia, stenosis, and obstruction (Edwards, 2011). Neonatal infections may be caused by viruses and fungi as well as bacteria, and all of these conditions present with indistinguishable symptoms.

Standard of Care for Treatment

Localized infections such as oral thrush, diaper dermatitis, and conjunctivitis may be treated locally with topical or oral antibiotics or antifungals (Table 10-2). In contrast, empiric antibiotics are the cornerstone of therapy for both presumed and confirmed neonatal infection and sepsis (Pammi et al., 2016; Pickering et al., 2012; Polin & Committee on Fetus and Newborn, 2012). Upon completion of a sepsis workup, broad-spectrum antibiotics against both gram-positive and gram-negative bacteria should be started *immediately* and given *intravenously*. Usually ampicillin (for gram-positive bacteria) and an aminoglycoside (for gram-negative bacteria) are the drugs of choice pending culture and sensitivity results (Pammi et al., 2016; Pickering et al., 2012; Polin & Committee on Fetus and Newborn, 2012). Use of a third-generation cephalosporin, such as cefotaxime, is associated with rapid development of resistance (Bryan, John, Pai, & Austin, 1985; Polin & Committee on Fetus and Newborn, 2012) and twice the risk of neonatal mortality (Clark, Bloom, Spitzer, & Gerstmann, 2006). For this reason, the AAP recommends limiting cefotaxime use to those neonates with gram-negative meningitis (Pickering et al., 2012; Polin & Committee on Fetus and Newborn, 2012). Identification of the causative agent(s) of an infection is followed by administration of the most effective, least toxic antibiotic or antibiotic combination for the appropriate period of time (bacteremia: up to 10 days; meningitis: 14–21 days) (Pammi et al., 2016; Polin & Committee on Fetus and Newborn, 2012).

Empiric antibiotics are necessary because if therapy for infection or sepsis is delayed pending culture results (which become available only after 24 to 72 hours), infected/septic neonates will die (Polin & Committee on Fetus and Newborn, 2012). Intravenous antibiotic or antiviral therapies are the standard of care for both inpatient and outpatient neonatal sepsis/infection. Neonatal infection/sepsis is *not* treated with oral antibiotics and discharge to home. If a neonate is thought to be infected at the physical examination, the infant should *immediately* be sent to the hospital for admission, diagnostic workup, intravenous empiric antibiotics, and supportive care. If after diagnostic workup and 48 hours of antibiotic treatment, the late-preterm or term infant does not have infection, the antibiotics are discontinued (Polin & Committee on Fetus and Newborn, 2012).

Typically, febrile infants suspected of infection are hospitalized for 36 to 48 hours pending culture results (Biondi, Murzycki, Ralston, & Gigliotti, 2013; Remington, 2011), and some guidelines recommend hospitalization for 96 hours (Kara, Kanra, Cengiz, Apis, & Gur, 2004; Randhawa, Sherwal, & Mehta, 2006). A recent study of febrile infants younger than 90 days of age found that 91% of blood cultures became positive within 24 hours of hospitalization on a generalized pediatric unit (these infants were not "sick enough" to be in an intensive care unit) (Biondi et al., 2014). By 36 and 48 hours, 96% and 99%, respectively, had become positive. The researchers concluded that inpatient observation of febrile infants for more than 24 hours may be unnecessary in most infants. "Well" infants with negative cultures may, indeed, be discharged earlier than infants who are still symptomatic and "ill appearing."

With severe neonatal infection and sepsis, numerous physiologic derangements occur, including apnea, seizures, hypoglycemia, temperature instability (hypothermia or hyperthermia), hypoxemia and hypoventilation, acidosis, hypovolemia, and hypotension. These severely ill infants require intensive monitoring; supportive care; attention to fluid, calories, and electrolyte management; ventilation; temperature support; and medication administration (Gardner, 2008a, 2009; Pammi et al., 2016). Until they have recovered (i.e., are feeding well and gaining weight, with normal vital signs) and have completed the prescribed course of antibiotics, these infants should remain hospitalized.

Cultural Considerations

Every culture has beliefs and traditions about health, illness, and causes of illness. Some common beliefs about illness in newborn infants are described here (Gardner, Voos, & Hills, 2016; Moore, 1981).

The "evil eye" (*mal ojo*) is a magical look that heats up the newborn's blood, causing fever, crying, diarrhea, vomiting, and aches and pains. Effects of the "evil eye" are ascribed to admiration of or coveting of a newborn baby. As a consequence, many Spanish-speaking groups do not praise or admire another's baby so as not to bring sickness to the infant. Spanish-speaking parents may also delay seeking care from an Anglo provider because they believe that someone of this ethnic group will not know or believe in *mal ojo* and, therefore, cannot cure it. Help from a folk healer may be tried before bringing the baby for "Western" care. A traditional folk healer (*curandero*) treats evil eye by performing a healing ceremony or by placing a healing amulet (*azabache*) or leather strap on the infant for protection.

A fallen fontanel (*mallera caida*) is believed to occur when the breast or bottle are removed too quickly and the baby becomes dehydrated. The soft palate is believed to sink in, causing feeding and swallowing problems. Treatments for *mallera caida* include sucking the fontanel, pushing up on the soft palate, or pulling the hair.

"Bad air" (*mal aire*), especially night air, is thought to enter the baby's body through the umbilical cord and cause illness. Covering the baby's umbilical stump serves to protect the baby from *mal aire*. Belief in *mal aire* increases concerns about air entering the body through the incision.

In Spanish-speaking cultures that revere *la familia*, the entire family—not just the baby's parents—is involved in making crucial decisions, including hospitalization for sick newborns. Parents and families believe that the "healer" gives advice and that the final decision is made by the family. Honoring this tradition enables parents to follow advice, administer medications, and comply with follow-up care.

Native Americans have ideas and beliefs as varied as the numerous tribes. However, most native peoples believe that illness and health are connected to their religious life. The tribal medicine man may treat an infant with traditional rites before sending parents and baby to a clinic, then complete the traditional healing when the baby returns home. Some traditional care practices for Native American mothers may include delaying breastfeeding until the milk comes in and use of a cradle-board for carrying and securing babies.

Middle and Far Eastern cultures share some common cultural beliefs that influence maternal–newborn care. Traditionally in these varied cultures, female relatives (mother, sisters, cousins, aunts), rather than the father of the baby, provide support during pregnancy. Traditional male partners view pregnancy and babies as "women's work," although male partners who were born or have been in the United States for years may wish to participate more fully. The desires of each individual family must be explored, acknowledged, and accommodated.

Having a sick infant is very stressful. Parents are rightfully worried and need constant communication, support, and reassurance from their healthcare providers (Gardner, 2008a, 2009). In many cultures, parents stay with their sick baby 24 hours a day, yet many hospitals are not prepared to have rooming-in parents. Involving the family in care planning and decision making is as important as having them participate in the care of their sick, hospitalized child. Using "infection control" as an excuse for excluding parents from care of their sick child should never occur (Gardner, 2008a, 2009). There is no evidence to support exclusion of parents as a safe or effective method of infection control.

Parent Education

As the primary teacher for parents, the healthcare provider is in a key position to utilize every encounter with parents as a "teaching opportunity" to familiarize parents with their infant, infant behaviors, and reading newborn cues. Table 10-1 and Table 10-2 contain parental education specifics related to bacterial, viral, and fungal diseases.

Teaching hand hygiene to parents and encouraging the continuation of hand hygiene after discharge helps to prevent community-acquired infections. Encouraging breastfeeding, cautioning parents about restricting visitors who are "sick" with infectious diseases, and avoiding taking newborns into crowds (i.e., shopping areas, church nurseries, childcare programs, children's parties) will arm parents with the knowledge they need to protect their infant and prevent infections after discharge.

Every parent taking a newborn home must be taught how to recognize a sick newborn, be given written instructions about how a sick newborn behaves and appears, and be provided with clear instructions about who to notify if they have concerns (Gardner, 2008a, 2009). Parents should be encouraged to call their baby's healthcare provider if they are the least bit concerned about the baby's behavior or condition. "Waiting until morning" or fear of "disturbing" the baby's healthcare provider should never be a concern for parents. Together, parents and professionals who recognize a sick neonate, and who advocate for prompt diagnosis and treatment, will ensure timely interventions and a positive outcome.

Student Practice Activities

Case Study 1

The mother of a 10-day-old male term infant appears at your clinic complaining that "My baby just will not eat." The baby was born by vaginal birth, with Apgar scores of 8 and 9 at 1 and 5 minutes, respectively. The baby is breastfeeding, and the mother says that he was eating well until yesterday, when he did not awaken to feed. The mother attempted to awaken him, but he was "so sleepy at the breast that he really did not get much."

On physical examination, the baby's axillary temperature is 35.5°C, and he is cool to the touch with pale, mottled skin. His respiratory rate is 80 breaths/min with grunting, flaring, and retractions. His pulse oximetry reading in your clinic is 85%. His blood sugar is 40, and he did not respond to the heel lance for blood draw. He is tachycardic, hypotensive, and lethargic and has poor muscle tone.

1. Is this baby infected?
2. Does the baby need a sepsis workup?
3. Will you do the sepsis workup?
4. Does this baby need to be referred? If so, where and when?

Case Study 2

Baby Andrea is a 3-week-old, formula-fed term neonate who is visibly jaundiced and has an indirect bilirubin level of 15mg/dL; her direct bilirubin level is 0.2 mg/dL. She is alert, is feeding well, and has been gaining 1 oz/day since the fifth day of life. None of her three older siblings had difficulty with jaundice; her mother's blood type is O negative and Andrea's blood type is O negative. The baby's blood sugar is 35. Her vital signs are normal and her pulse oximetry is 95% in room air.

1. Is this baby infected?
2. Does the baby need a sepsis workup?
3. Will you do the sepsis workup?
4. Does this baby need to be referred? If so, where and when?

Create a tool or handout for parents so that they can recognize that their baby is sick.

Multiple Choice

1. Place the following steps in the appropriate order for caring for an infected neonate:
    A) Discharge home
    B) Sepsis workup
    C) Perinatal history
    D) Physical examination
    E) Empiric antibiotics

2. All of the following are symptoms of neonatal sepsis except:
    A) Jaundice
    B) Poor feeding
    C) Temperature of 36.5°C
    D) Hypotonia
    E) Tachypnea
    F) Hypotension

3. Mothers of babies born with congenital TORCH viral infection may have no perinatal history of infection.
    A) True
    B) False

4. A parent's statement that "Something is wrong" or "My baby is not doing well" warrants the baby being seen by you:
    A) In 2 hours when you have an opening
    B) Tomorrow at the 1500 open slot
    C) As soon as possible
    D) At the next regularly scheduled visit

5. Neonates with infection are more often:
    A) Hypothermic
    B) Hyperthermic

6. The change in the behavior of an infected baby most often first noticed by the mother/parents is:
    A) Temperature change
    B) Irritability
    C) Jaundice

D) Change in feeding behavior

E) Crying

7. One CRP value is diagnostic of neonatal sepsis.
   A) True
   B) False

8. Skin changes that accompany infection may include all of the following except:
   A) Acrocyanosis
   B) Jaundice
   C) Rash
   D) Erythema
   E) Purpura

9. Early-onset sepsis occurs in the first:
   A) 24 hours of life
   B) Month of life
   C) 3 days of life
   D) 2 weeks of life

References

Abzug, M. J. (2004). Presentation, diagnosis, and management of enterovirus infections in neonates. *Paediatric Drugs, 6*(1), 1–10.

Abzug, M. J. (2014). The enteroviruses: problems in need of treatments. *Journal of Infection, 68*(suppl 1), S108–S114.

Abzug, M. J., Cloud, G., Bradley J., Sanchez, P. J., Romero, J., Powell, D., & The National Institute of Allergy and Infectious Diseases Collaborative Antiviral Study Group. (2003). Double blind placebo-controlled trial of plecoonaril in infants with enterovirus meningitis. *Pediatric Infectious Disease Journal, 22*(4), 335 –341.

American Academy of Pediatrics (AAP), Committee on Infectious Diseases. (2014). Recommendations for prevention and control of influenza in children, 2014–2015. *Pediatrics, 134*(5), e1503–31519.

American Academy of Pediatrics (AAP), Committee on Infectious Diseases & Bronchiolitis Guidelines Committees. (2014). RSV policy statement: Updated guidance for palivizumab prophylaxis among infants and young children at increased risk of hospitalization for respiratory syncytial virus infection. *Pediatrics, 134*(2), 415–420.

American Academy of Pediatrics (AAP), Committee on Pediatric AIDS. (2008). HIV testing and prophylaxis to prevent mother-to-child transmission in the United States. *Pediatrics, 122*(5), 1127–1134.

American Academy of Pediatrics (AAP), Committee on Pediatric AIDS. (2013). Infant feeding and the transmission of human immunodeficiency virus in the United States. *Pediatrics, 131*(2), 391–396.

American Academy of Pediatrics (AAP) & American College of Obstetricians and Gynecologists (ACOG). (2012). *Guidelines for perinatal care* (7th ed.). Elk Grove Village, IL: Authors.

Baker, C. J., Byington, C. L., Polin, R.A., & Committee on Infectious Diseases & Committee on the Fetus and Newborn of the American Academy of Pediatrics (AAP). (2011). Policy statement: Recommendations for the prevention of perinatal group B streptococcal (GBS) disease. *Pediatrics, 128*(3), 611–616.

Biondi, E., Murzycki, J., Ralston, S., & Gigliotti, F. (2013). Fever and bacteremia. *Pediatric Reviews, 34*(3), 134–136.

Biondi, E. A., Mischler, M., Jerardi, K. E., Statile, A. M., French, J., Aligne C. A., & The Pediatric Research in Inpatient Settings (PRIS) Network. (2014). Blood culture time to positivity in febrile infants with bacteremia. *JAMA Pediatrics, 168*(9), 844–849.

Boppana, S. B., Fowler, K. B., Britt, W. J., Stagno, S., & Pass, R. F. (1999). Symptomatic congenital cytomegalovirus infection in infants born to mothers with preexisting immunity to cytomegalovirus. *Pediatrics, 104*(1 pt 1), 55–60.

Borna, H., & Borna, S. (2004). Value of laboratory tests and C-reactive proteinin the detection of neonatal sepsis. *International Journal of Pediatrics and Neonatology, 5*(2), 1–6.

Bryan, C. S., John, J. F., Pai, M. S., & Austin, T. L. (1985). Gentamicin vs cefotaxime for therapy of neonatal sepsis: Relationship to drug resistance. *American Journal of Disease in Childhood, 139*(11), 1086–1089.

Centers for Disease Control and Prevention (CDC). (2010). Prevention of perinatal group B streptococcal disease: Revised guidelines of CDC, 2010. *Morbidity and Mortality Weekly Report, 59*(RR-10), 1–36.

Centers for Disease Control and Prevention (CDC). (2015a). Cytomegalovirus (CMV) and pregnancy: Facts and prevention. Retrieved from http://www.cdc.gov/cmv/index.html

Centers for Disease Control and Prevention (CDC). (2015b). *Pregnancy and whooping cough.* Retrieved from http://www.cdc.gov/pertussis/pregnant/hcp/rationale-vacc-pregnant-women.html

Centers for Disease Control and Prevention (CDC). (2015c). *Tdap vaccine: What you need to know?* Washington, DC: U.S. Department of Health and Human Services.

Christensen, R. D., Rothstein, G., Hill, H. R., & Hall, R. T. (1985). Fatal early onset group B streptococcal sepsis with normal leukocyte counts. *Pediatric Infectious Disease Journal, 4*(3), 242–245.

Clark, R. H., Bloom, B. T., Spitzer, A. R., & Gerstmann, D. R. (2006). Empiric use of ampicillin and cefotaxime, compared to ampicillin and gentamicin, for neonates at risk for sepsis is associated with an increased risk of neonatal death. *Pediatrics, 117*(1), 67–74.

Dabrara, G., Zhao, H., Andrews, N., Begum, F., Greene, H., Ellis, J., & Pebody, R. (2014). Effectiveness of seasonal influenza vaccination during pregnancy in preventing influenza infection in infants, England 2013/2014. *European Surveillance, 19*(45), 20959.

Dollner, H., Vatten, L., & Austgulen, R. (2001). Early diagnostic markers for neonatal sepsis: Comparing C-reactive protein, interleukin-6, soluble tumour necrosis factor receptors and soluble adhesion molecules. *Journal of Clinical Epidemiology, 54*(12), 1251–1257.

Edwards, M. S. (2011). Postnatal bacterial infections. In R. J. Martin, A. A. Fanoroff, & M. C. Walsh (Eds.), *Fanaroff and Martin's neonatal–perinatal medicine* (9th ed., pp. 793–830). Philadelphia, PA: Elsevier-Mosby.

Engle, W. D., & Rosenfeld, C. R. (1984). Neutropenia in high risk neonates. *Journal of Pediatrics, 105*(6), 982–986.

Franz, A. R., Steinbach, G., Kron, M., & Pohlandt, F. (1999). Reduction of unnecessary antibiotic therapy in newborn infants using interleukin-8 and C-reactive protein as markers of bacterial infections. *Pediatrics, 104*(3 pt 1), 447–453.

Gardner, S. L. (2008a). How will I know my newborn is sick? *Nurse Currents, 2*(2), 1–8.

Gardner, S. L. (2008b). Methicillin-resistant *Staphylococcus aureus* (MRSA) infections in maternal–newborn nursing practice. *Nurse Currents, 1*(2), 1–7.

Gardner, S. L. (2009). Sepsis in the neonate. *Critical Care Clinics of North America, 21*(1), 121–141.

Gardner, S. L., & Lawrence, R. A. (2016). Breastfeeding the neonate with special needs. In S. L. Gardner, B. S. Carter, M. Enzman Hines, & J. A. Hernandez (Eds.), *Merenstein and Gardner's handbook of neonatal intensive care* (8th ed., pp. 419–463). St. Louis, MO: Mosby-Elsevier.

Gardner, S. L., Voos, K., & Hills, P. (2016). Families in crisis: Theoretical and practical considerations. In S. L. Gardner, B. S. Carter, M. Enzman Hines, & J. A. Hernandez (Eds.), *Merenstein and Gardner's handbook of neonatal intensive care* (8th ed., pp. 821–864). St. Louis, MO: Mosby-Elsevier.

Hofer, N., Muller, W., & Resch, B. (2013, April 30). The role of C-reactive protein in the diagnosis of neonatal sepsis. *INTECH, Open Science*. Retrieved from http://dx.doi.org/10.5772/54255

Janjindamai, W., & Phetpisal, S. (2006). Time to positivity of blood culture in newborn infants. *Southeast Asian Journal of Tropical Medicine and Public Health, 37*(1), 171–176.

Johnson, C. E., Whitwell, J. K., Pethe, K., Saxena, K., & Super, D. M. (1997). Term newborns who are at risk for sepsis: are lumbar punctures necessary? *Pediatrics, 99*(4), E10.

Kapur, R., Yoder, M. C., & Polin, R. A. (2011). The immune system. In R. J. Martin, A. A. Fanaroff, & M. C. Walsh (Eds.), *Fanaroff and Martin's neonatal–perinatal medicine* (9th ed., pp. 761–792). Philadelphia, PA: Elsevier-Mosby.

Kara, A., Kanra, G., Cengiz, A. B., Apis, M., & Gur, D. (2004). Pediatric blood culture: Time to positivity. *Turkish Journal of Pediatrics, 46*(3), 251–255.

Kawada, M., Okuzumi, K., Hitomi, S., & Sugishita, C. (2003). Transmission of *Staphylococcus aureus* between healthy lactating mothers and their infants by breastfeeding. *Journal of Human Lactation, 19*(4), 411–417.

Kawamura, M., & Nishida, H. (1995). The usefulness of serial C-reactive protein measurement in managing neonatal infection. *Acta Paediatrica, 84*(1), 10–13.

Kharbanda, E. O., Vazquez-Benitez, G., Lipkind, H. S., Klein, N. P., Cheetham, T. C., Naleway, A., & Nordin, J. D. (2014, November 11). Evaluation of the association of maternal pertussis vaccination with obstetric events and birth outcome. *Journal of the American Medical Association*. doi: 10.1001/jama.2014.14825. http://dx.doi.org/doi:10.1001/jama.2014.14825

Kimberlin, D. W., Lin, C. Y., Sánchez. P. J., Demmler, G. J., Danker, W Shelton, M., & The National institute of Allergy and Infectious Diseases Collaborative Antiviral Study Group. (2003). Effect of ganciclovir therapy on hearing in symptomatic congenital cytomegalovirus disease involving the central nervous system: A randomized, controlled trial. *Journal of Pediatrics, 143*(1), 16–25.

Lawn, J. E., Cousens, S., & Zupan, J. (2005). 4 million neonatal deaths: When? Where? Why? *Lancet, 365*(9462), 891–900.

Leonard, E. G., & Dobbs, K. (2015). Postnatal bacterial infections. In R. J. Martin, A. A. Fanaroff, & M. C. Walsh (Eds.), *Fanaroff and Martin's neonatal–perinatal medicine* (10th ed., pp. 734–750). Philadelphia, PA: Elsevier-Mosby.

Lin, T. Y., Kao, H. T., Hsieh, S. H., Huang, Y. C., Chiu, C. H., Chou, Y. H., & Chang, L. Y. (2003). Neonatal enterovirus infections: Emphasis on risk factors of severe and fatal infections. *Pediatric Infectious Disease Journal, 22*(10), 889–894.

Manroe, B. L., Weinberg, A. G., Rosenfeld, C. R., & Browne, R. (1979). The neonatal blood count in health and disease. I. Reference values for neutrophilic cells. *Journal of Pediatrics, 95*(1), 89–98.

Mathers, N. J., & Pohlhandt, F. (1987). Diagnostic audit of C-reactive protein in neonatal infection. *European Journal of Pediatrics, 146*(2), 147–151.

McLeod, R., Boyer, K., Karrison, T., Kasza, K., Swisher, C., Roizen, N., & The Toxoplasmosis Study Group. (2006). Outcome of treatment for congenital toxoplasmosis, 1984–2004: The National Collaborative Chicago-Based Congenital Toxoplasmosis Study. *Clinical Infectious Disease, 42*(10), 1383–1394.

Moore, M. L. (1981). *Newborn family and nurse* (2nd ed.). Philadelphia, PA: W. B. Saunders.

Munoz, F. M., Bond, N. H., Maccato, M., Pinell, P., Mammill, H. A., Swamy, G. K., & Baker, C. J. (2014). Safety and immunogenicity of tetanus, diphtheria, and acellular pertussis (Tdap) immunization during pregnancy in mothers and infants: A randomized clinical trial. *Journal of the American Medical Association, 311*(17), 1760–1769.

Ng, P. C. (2004). Diagnostic markers of infection in neonates. *Archives of Disease of Childhood—Fetal and Neonatal Edition, 89*(3), F229–F235.

Ottolini, M. C., Lundgren, K., Mirkinson, L. J., Cason, S., & Ottolini, M. G. (2003). Utility of complete blood count and blood culture screening to diagnose neonatal sepsis in the asymptomatic at risk newborn. *Pediatric Infectious Disease Journal, 22*(5), 430–434.

Pammi, M., Brand, M. C., &Weisman, L. E. (2016). In S. L. Gardner, B. S. Carter, M. Enzman Hines, & J. A. Hernandez (Eds.), *Merenstein and Gardner's handbook of neonatal intensive care* (8th ed., pp. 537–563). St. Louis, MO: Mosby-Elsevier.

Petrosky, E., Bocchini, J. A., Jr., HarirI, S., Chesson, H., Curtis, C. R., Saraiya, M., & Centers for Disease Control and Prevention (CDC). (2015). Use of 9-valent human papillomavirus (HPV) vaccine: Updated HPV vaccination recommendations of the advisory committee on vaccination practices. *Morbidity and Mortality Weekly Report, 64*(11), 300–304.

Pickering, L. K., Baker, C. J., Kimberlin, D. W., & Long, S. S. (Eds.); American Academy of Pediatrics. (2012). *Red book 2012: 2012 report of the Committee on Infectious Disease* (29th ed.). Elk Grove Village, IL: American Academy of Pediatrics.

Polin, R. A., & Committee on Fetus and Newborn. (2012). Management of neonates with suspected or proven early-onset bacterial sepsis. *Pediatrics, 129*, 1006–1015.

Randhawa, V. S., Sherwal, B. L., & Mehta, G. (2006). Incubation period for culture positivity to detect septicaemia in neonates. *Indian Journal of Medical Microbiology, 24*(3), 237–238.

Ray, B., Mangalore, J., Harikumar, C., & Tuladhar, A. (2006). Is lumbar puncture necessary for evaluation of early neonatal sepsis? *Archives of Disease of Childhood, 91*, 1033–1038.

Remington, J. S. (2011). *Infectious diseases of the fetus and newborn infant* (7th ed.). Philadelphia, PA: Saunders/Elsevier.

Romero, D., Treston, J., & O'Sullivan, A. (2006). Hand-to-hand combat: Preventing MRSA infection. *Nurse Practitioner, 31*(3), 16–18, 21–23.

Rotbart, H. A. (2000). Antiviral therapy for enteroviral infections. *Pediatric Infectious Disease Journal, 18*(7), 632–633.

Rubarth, L. B. (2005). *Nursing patterns of knowing in assessment of newborn sepsis.* Doctoral dissertation, University of Arizona.

Rubarth, L. B. (2008). Infants in peril: Assessing sepsis in newborns. *American Nurse Today, 3*(4), 14–18.

Skoff, T. H., Kenyon, C., Cocoros, N., Liko, J., Miller, L., Kudish, K., . . . Martin, S. (2015). Sources of infant pertussis infection in the United States. *Pediatrics, 136*(4), 634–641.

Smith, P. B., Cotton, C. M., Garges, H. P., Tiffany, K. F., Lenfestey, R. W., Moody, M. A., & Benjamin, D. K., Jr. (2006). A comparison of neonatal gram-negative rod and gram positive cocci meningitis. *Journal of Perinatology, 26*(2), 111–114.

Strikas, R. A., Centers for Disease Control and Prevention (CDC), Advisory Committee on Immunization Practices (ACIP), & ACIP Child/Adolescent Immunization Work Group. (2015). Advisory Committee on Immunization Practices recommended immunization schedules for persons aged 0 through18 years—United States, 2015. *Morbidity and Mortality Weekly Report, 64*(4), 93–94.

Swanson, E. C., & Schleiss, M. R. (2013). Congenital cytomegalovirus infection: New prospects for prevention and therapy. *Pediatric Clinics of North America, 60*(2), 335–349.

Thorne, C., & Newell, M. L. (2007). HIV. *Seminars in Fetal and Neonatal Medicine, 12*(3), 174–181.

Volari, A. (2007, August). *Early treatment of HIV-infected infants reduces mortality risk: Results of CHER study.* Presentation at International AIDS Society Conference.

Weitkamp, J. H., & Aschner, J. L. (2005). Diagnostic use of C-reactive protein (CRP) in assessment of neonatal sepsis. *NeoReviews, 6,* e508.

WHO Young Infants Study Group. (1999). Clinical prediction of serious bacterial infections in young infants in developing countries. *Pediatric Infectious Disease Journal, 18*(10 suppl), S23–S31.

World Health Organization (WHO). (2006). *World health report 2005: Make every mother and child count.* Geneva, Switzerland: Author.

World Health Organization (WHO). (2009). IMCI chart booklet. Retrieved from http://who.int?child-adolescent-health/publications/IMCI/chartbooklet.htm

Young Infants Clinical Signs Study Group. (2008). Clinical signs that predict severe illness in children under age 2 months: A multi-center study. *Lancet, 371*(9607), 135–142.

Yusuf, K., Soraisham, A. S., & Fonseca, K. (2007). Fatal influenza B virus pneumonia in a preterm neonate: Case report and review of the literature. *Journal of Perinatology, 27*(10), 623–625.

11

GENERAL CONSIDERATIONS OF THE NEWBORN WITH COMPLICATIONS

Sheron Bautista and Curry J. Bordelon

Some complications of the neonate are able to be anticipated; other neonatal problems occur at birth or are unable to be anticipated. This chapter briefly discusses factors affecting the developing fetus, fetal growth, delivery complications, genetic and structural factors, and their consequences for neonatal health, referral, and a specialized level of caretaking.

Factors Affecting the Developing Fetus

Placental Complications

The placenta provides the fetus with its blood supply containing nutrients for growth and oxygen; it also provides for the removal of waste products (Harmon, 2013). Placental abnormalities result in inadequate blood flow to the fetus and inadequate or interrupted oxygen and carbon dioxide exchange. Such abnormalities may contribute to adverse neonatal outcomes including preterm birth, birth asphyxia, and diminished fetal brain and body growth. Placental complications that result in a disruption of the normal function of the placenta are listed in **Table 11-1** and **Figure 11-1**.

Inadequate placental flow contributes to hypoxic–ischemic encephalopathy (HIE) both before and during birth. HIE ranges in seriousness from mild to severe, with possible

Table 11-1: Placental Complications

Type	Definition
Accreta	Placenta attaches to the myometrium of the uterine wall, which can lead to severe hemorrhage, perforated uterus, or uterine infection
Previa	Abnormal implantation of the placenta near or over the cervical opening; common finding in the second trimester but decreases with increasing gestational age
Insufficiency	Abnormal development of the placenta, causing a decrease in the maternal blood supply
Abruption	Premature separation of the placenta from the uterus, resulting in hemorrhage, increased risk for preterm delivery, stillbirth, and neurologic deficits in the infant

Reproduced from Harmon, J. S. (2013). High-risk pregnancy. In C. Kenner & J. W. Lott (Eds.), *Comprehensive neonatal nursing: A physiologic perspective* (5th ed.). New York, NY: Springer. Reproduced with permission of Springer Publishing Company.

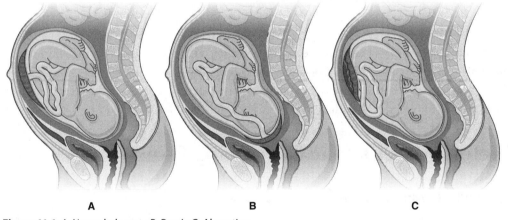

A   **B**   **C**

Figure 11-1: A. Normal placenta B. Previa C. Abruption.

long-term adverse consequences including cerebral palsy, feeding difficulties, and poor neurodevelopmental outcomes. Premature infants (those born prior to 35 weeks' gestation) are at increased risk for respiratory distress syndrome, hypoglycemia, sepsis, hypothermia, feeding difficulties, and intraventricular hemorrhage.

Both birth-asphyxiated and preterm infants require specialized care in the neonatal intensive care unit (NICU) immediately after birth, early childhood intervention, and follow-up to optimize their outcomes and help them meet developmental milestones. Early parent education and anticipatory guidance are essential in preparing parents to take home a potentially medically fragile infant.

Multifetal Pregnancy

Most human conceptions (more than 99.2%) emerge from a single zygote (i.e., fertilization of a single egg by a single spermatozoon). In other cases, however, more than one egg is released during ovulation and fertilization of multiple eggs occurs, resulting in a multifetal pregnancy. The exact mechanism of this phenomenon is unknown. One known factor of multifetal pregnancies is infertility treatment—a therapy in which the ovaries are stimulated and polyovulation occurs. **Table 11-2** provides a brief overview of the classifications of twins. **Figure 11-2** shows twinning pregnancies.

Multiple-gestation pregnancies may result in maternal and fetal complications due to the overwhelmed maternal homeostasis. Notably, maternal hypertensive diseases related to pregnancy are more likely to occur with multifetal pregnancies. For example, both preeclampsia and pregnancy-induced hypertension are more frequently seen in multiple-gestation pregnancies. HELLP syndrome (i.e., **h**emolysis, **e**levated **l**iver enzymes, **l**ow **p**latelet count) occurs earlier and more frequently in multifetal pregnancies when compared to singleton pregnancies (Blickstein & Shinwell, 2015). In addition, hypertensive mothers are more likely to develop preterm labor and deliver preterm. After 28 weeks of a multifetal gestation, the overwhelmed maternal system must support two to three times the fetal mass that develops in a singleton pregnancy.

Table 11-2: Twin Gestation Classification

Type	Definition
Monozygotic	Fertilization and subsequent division of a single egg.
Dizygotic	Fertilization and subsequent division of two eggs. Twins of a different sex are dizygotic. Twins of the same sex can be monozygotic or dizygotic.
Dichorionic/diamniotic	The fertilized egg splits 0–3 days after fertilization. Accounts for approximately 30% of twins.
Monochorionic/diamniotic	The fertilized egg splits 4–8 days after fertilization. Accounts for approximately 70% of twins.
Monochorionic/monoamniotic	The fertilized egg splits 8–12 days after fertilization. Rare occurrence that carries higher mortality, increased risk for neurologic problems, discordant growth, and co-twin death in utero.

Reproduced from Blickstein, I., & Shinwell, E. S. (2015). Obstetric management of multiple gestation and birth. In R. J. Martin, A. A. Fanaroff, & M. C. Walsh (Eds.), *Neonatal–perinatal medicine* (10th ed., pp. 312–320). St. Louis, MO: Mosby-Year Book.

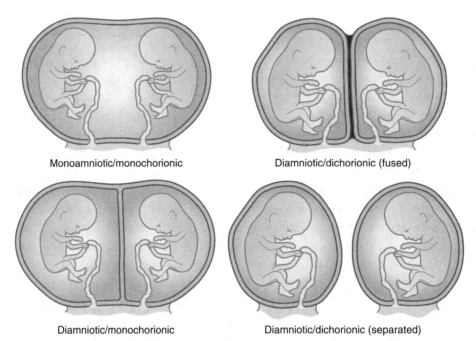

Monoamniotic/monochorionic

Diamniotic/dichorionic (fused)

Diamniotic/monochorionic

Diamniotic/dichorionic (separated)

Figure 11-2: Twin Gestation Classification.

The higher risk and incidence of structural abnormalities in twins corresponds to the type of twinning that has occurred (**Table 11-3**). Multiple-gestation pregnancies often result in deceleration of fetal growth leading to low-birth-weight neonates, intrauterine growth-restricted newborns, and/or discordance in birth weights. More serious complications of multifetal pregnancies include increased mortality related to twin-to-twin transfusion syndrome (TTTS), twin embolization syndrome, umbilical cord entanglement or prolapse, and preterm birth (Blickstein & Shinwell, 2015).

Because of the increased risk of maternal and fetal complications during pregnancy and labor, delivery of multifetal pregnancies occurs by 37 to 38 weeks' gestation. Preterm infants born at less than 34 weeks' gestation require admission to the NICU; delivery between 34 0/7 and 36 6/7 weeks' gestation results in the birth of late-preterm infants.

Fetal Growth

Intrauterine Growth Restriction

Fetal growth is dependent on a variety of genetic, placental, and maternal factors. Intrauterine growth restriction (IUGR), defined as a fetus less than the 10th percentile for estimated fetal

Table 11-3: Structural Defects in Twins

Category	Defect
Malformation common in twins	Neural tube defects
	Hydrocephaly
	Congenital heart disease
	Esophageal atresia
Malformations in monozygotic twins	Amniotic band syndrome
	TRAP sequence
	Conjoined twins
	Twin embolization syndrome
Placental malformations	Twin-to-twin transfusion syndrome
	Single umbilical cord
	Velamentous cord insertion
Intrauterine crowding	Clubfoot
	Positional abnormalities

Abbreviation: TRAP, twin reversed arterial perfusion sequence.
Reproduced from Blickstein, I., & Shinwell, E. S. (2015). Obstetric management of multiple gestation and birth. In R. J. Martin, A. A. Fanaroff, & M. C. Walsh (Eds.), *Neonatal–perinatal medicine* (10th ed., pp. 312–320). St. Louis, MO: Mosby-Year Book.

weight, may be either symmetric or asymmetric and results in higher morbidity and mortality (Peleg, Kennedy, & Hunter, 1998). Symmetric growth restriction results in the entire body of the fetus/newborn being proportionally small. Asymmetric growth restriction is preferential brain-sparing, most often as a consequence of placental insufficiency, resulting in a larger head circumference relative to the fetus's weight and length. If asymmetric growth is sustained, the fetus/newborn may develop symmetric growth restriction and compromised brain growth. In addition to placental insufficiency, other causes of IUGR include chronic maternal diseases (i.e., hypertension, diabetes) and abnormal placentae (i.e., previa, abruption, and accreta).

Small for Gestational Age

Small for gestational age (SGA), defined as a neonate with a birth weight less than the 10th percentile, is often seen in infants with a maternal history of hypertension, smoking, or cardiac and renal disease (Cochran & Lee, 2011). The birth of an SGA infant is also associated with maternal and congenital infections, chromosomal abnormalities, congenital anomalies, and maternal drug use (e.g., heroin, cocaine, alcohol). Multifetal pregnancies, placenta abruption, placenta previa, placental insufficiency, and maternal malnutrition are other maternal factors resulting in SGA infants. Early delivery of SGA infants may occur if there is an arrest in fetal growth, fetal distress, or maternal conditions that increase either maternal or neonatal risk for morbidity and mortality (Cochran & Lee, 2011).

The etiology for growth restriction is often unknown. SGA infants are admitted to the NICU for management of complications (i.e., hypoglycemia, hypothermia, nutrition), as well as evaluation for chromosomal abnormalities and congenital infections. Management of subsequent pregnancies includes high-risk maternal care, because SGA pregnancies often recur.

Appropriate for Gestational Age

Appropriate for gestational age (AGA) infants have achieved appropriate intrauterine growth (i.e., weight, length and head circumference) for gestational age. AGA infants are at the lowest risk for morbidity and mortality after birth.

Large for Gestational Age

Large for gestational age (LGA) infants have birth weights above the 90th percentile. Maternal conditions such as diabetes often result in LGA infants. Other causes include large parents, post maturity, and conditions such as Beckwith-Weidemann syndrome (Devaskar & Garg, 2015). Common morbidities for LGA newborns include hypoglycemia, management of respiratory distress, and examination for birth trauma (i.e., fractured clavicles, brachial plexus injury). After birth, prevention of hypoglycemia includes early feeding and ongoing monitoring of blood glucose levels.

Infants of Diabetic Mothers

Infants of diabetic mothers (IDMs) are at significant risk for increased morbidity and mortality (Hay, 2012). Because maternal diabetes is associated with delayed fetal lung maturity, good glucose control is important for improved fetal outcomes. In contrast, poor glucose management increases neonatal risks for complications such as respiratory distress syndrome (RDS), hypoglycemia, hypocalcemia, polycythemia, perinatal asphyxia, birth injuries due to macrosomia, and congenital malformations including cardiac defects.

Care of the IDM neonate focuses on ensuring adequate cardiorespiratory adaptation at birth, possible birth injuries, maintenance of normal glucose metabolism, and close observation for polycythemia, hyperbilirubinemia, and feeding intolerance. Rigorous management of IDM infants can improve outcomes and may decrease length of stay in the NICU. Parents should be provided information on the disease processes affecting these infants and should employ strategies to improve mother–infant bonding after birth.

IDMs may be LGA, SGA, or AGA infants, as well as infants born prematurely. When diabetic mothers have renal, retinal, or cardiac disease, SGA infants and preterm births commonly occur. Hyperglycemia in the mother tends to result in hyperglycemia in the fetus, with increased fetal insulin secretion resulting in macrosomia and an increase in adipose tissue. Macrosomic, LGA infants are at risk for birth trauma such as shoulder dystocia and may require cesarean-section delivery.

After birth, infants experience significantly reduced plasma glucose levels between 30 minutes to 90 minutes of life. Some newborns recover from this decrease in plasma glucose, whereas others require management of hypoglycemia either in or out of the NICU.

Cardiac septal hypertrophy and cardiomegaly are direct consequences of poor maternal glucose control (Devaskar & Garg, 2015). Both of these conditions may present as cardiac failure in the newborn, which increases morbidity and mortality in the neonatal period. Despite monitoring of fetal cardiac growth and good maternal glucose control, some IDMs may develop heart enlargement. Cardiomyopathy in the infant may be asymptomatic and/or transient, spontaneously resolving within 6 months.

Fetal hyperinsulinemia results in increased oxygen demand and consumption, hypoxemia, and suppression of surfactant production in the fetal lungs. Relative hypoxemia increases erythrocyte production, resulting in polycythemia at birth. Infants of mothers with Class A, B, and C diabetes are at greater risk for decreased surfactant production, which in turn predisposes them to development of respiratory distress syndrome (Devaskar & Garg, 2015). Some of these infants will require mechanical ventilation and exogenous surfactant administration to improve their respiratory function.

Delivery Complications

During the birth process, birth injuries occur in approximately 2 to 7 of every 100 live births. Predisposing factors for birth injuries include macrosomia, prolonged labor, shoulder dystocia, breech presentation, and cephalopelvic disproportion. Most birth injuries are not life threatening and do not require intervention. If birth injuries are expected, however, clinicians must perform a thorough assessment immediately after birth to properly identify injuries and provide necessary interventions. Birth injuries that require immediate intervention include subgaleal hemorrhage, skull fractures, spinal cord injuries, shoulder dystocia, subdural bleed, and damage to internal organs. Management of infants with birth injuries requires care in the NICU and treatment of associated symptoms. Perinatal history to ascertain whether assistive devices (i.e., forceps or vacuum) were used for delivery of the infant and whether the delivery was traumatic is essential.

Shoulder Dystocia

The incidence of shoulder dystocia is related to fetal weight, with such injuries being more common in LGA infants and IDMs. Because these newborns are large, shoulder dystocia is associated with the use of assistive devices (vacuum and forceps) during delivery. Other risk factors include macrosomia, post-term birth, and previous shoulder dystocia. Maternal complications of shoulder dystocia include third- or fourth-degree lacerations, hemorrhage, and uterine rupture. Neonatal complications may include brachial plexus palsy, hypoxia (with or without associated neurologic damage), or death (Baxley & Gobbo, 2004). Newborns in respiratory failure require mechanical ventilation, cardiac support, and management of neurologic symptoms.

Intracranial Hemorrhage

Types of intracranial hemorrhage include subarachnoid, epidural, and subdural bleeds. Subarachnoid bleeds are typically asymptomatic, with complications occurring only rarely. Likewise, epidural bleeds are rare; they are often very difficult to diagnose because symptoms are delayed.

Subdural bleeds are the most serious types of intracranial hemorrhage and present shortly after birth with serious neurologic effects. Affected newborns are stuporous, have seizure activity, are unresponsive, have unresponsive pupils, and are comatose. Newborns with subdural bleeds require immediate interventions to support respiratory and cardiac function until surgical evacuation of the blood can be accomplished.

Subgaleal Hemorrhage

Subgaleal hemorrhage—that is, a rupture of the vein that connects the dural sinuses and scalp veins—is a rare occurrence that causes a life-threatening emergency. With this type of hemorrhage, blood accumulates between the scalp and periosteum and extends from the orbits of the eyes to the back of the neck and temporally over the entire scalp (Abdulhayoglu, 2011). In term babies, the subgaleal space holds a large volume of blood (as much as 25% of the newborn's blood volume), so the sequestration of blood there results in severe hypovolemic shock. Early recognition is essential to begin immediate management of respiratory and cardiac function as well as aggressive replacement of blood volume. Surgical intervention is indicated if bleeding does not subside. Thorough documentation and communication by delivery room and neonatal care personnel is crucial to ensure prompt examination, monitoring, and treatment that improve outcomes.

Genetic Complications

Approximately 1% to 3% of newborns have more than one major congenital anomaly present at birth. Such anomalies are classified based on the developmental process affected; **Table 11-4** provides an overview of the types of congenital anomalies. An understanding of the pathophysiology involved is necessary for appropriate diagnosis and treatment for infants with genetic disorders. Upon recognition of a possible congenital anomaly, genetic testing can provide valuable diagnostic information for clinicians and families.

Genetic alterations may involve chromosome material deletion (loss of chromosomal material), translocation (exchange of material between two different chromosomes), microdeletion (deletions too small for microscopic examination), duplication (extra copy of material), or mutation (change in DNA sequence) (Bajaj & Gross, 2015). The majority of congenital anomalies and syndromes are recognized in the neonatal period.

Chromosomal disorders may stem from an error in the number of chromosome material (aneuploidy), decrease in amount of material (monosomy), or extra material (polyploidy). Disorders resulting from single-gene errors are called Mendelian inheritance disorders; the most common single-gene disorder is cystic fibrosis. Inherited disorders can be autosomal dominant (affected children from one affected parent or spontaneous mutation), autosomal recessive (both parents must be carriers or be affected to have affected children), or X-linked (disorder located on X chromosome). Multifactorial disorders derive from a combination of genetic abnormalities and environmental factors. **Table 11-5** provides a general overview of the types of chromosomal disorders.

Table 11-4: Morphologies

Type	Genetic Alteration
Malformation	Abnormal tissue formation
Deformation	Alteration in mechanical forces (intrinsic or extrinsic)
Dysplasia	Abnormal, deregulated cellular organization
Disruption	Destructive breakdown of tissue
Syndrome	Many primary malformations related to one etiology
Sequence	Primary defect with secondary effects
Association	Collection of malformations without specific genetic or chromosome complication

Reproduced from Parikh, A. S., & Mitchell, A. L. (2015). Congenital anomalies. In R. J. Martin, A. A. Fanaroff, & M. C. Walsh (Eds.), *Neonatal–perinatal medicine* (10th ed., pp. 436–459). St. Louis, MO: Mosby-Year Book.

Table 11-5: Congenital Anomalies

Category	Disorder Examples
Trisomy	Trisomy 13 (Patau), trisomy 18 (Edwards), trisomy 21 (Down)
Deletion	Cri-du-chat, 13q deletion
Microdeletion	Angelman (majority are 15q11-13 deletions), DiGeorge (22q11.2 deletion), Prader-Willi, Williams
Autosomal dominant	Beckwith-Wiedemann, Noonan, Marfan, Holt-Oram, osteogenesis imperfecta, Treacher Collins, Aperts, retinoblastoma, Crouzon, myotonic dystrophy, neuro-fibromatosis, protein C and S deficiencies, aplasia cutis, adult polycystic kidney disease
Autosomal recessive	Thrombocytopenia–radial aplasia (TAR) syndrome, cystic fibrosis, inborn errors of metabolism (majority are autosomal recessive), alpha and beta thalassemias, congenital muscular dystrophy, 21-hydroxylase deficiencies, sickle cell disease, Smith-Lemli-Opitz, Meckel-Gruber syndrome
X linked	Hunter disease, Menkes disease, glucose-6-phosphate dehydrogenase (G6PD) deficiency, Duchenne muscular dystrophy, fragile X, nephrogenic diabetes insipidus, red-green color blindness, hemophilia A and B
Sequence	Mobius, Pierre Robin
Associations	CHARGE, Cornelia de Lange, Goldenhar, Klippel-Feil, Klippel-Trenaunay Weber, Poland, VACTERL (VATER)
Other syndromes	Klinefelter, Turner, cat-eye

Abbreviations: CHARGE, a genetic syndrome characterized by coloboma of the eyes, heart defects, atresia of the choanae, retardation of growth and/or development, genital and/or urinary abnormalities, and ear abnormalities and deafness; VACTERL or VATER, syndrome characterized by vertebral, anal, cardiac, tracheal, esophageal, and renal anomalies.

Reproduced from Parikh, A. S., & Mitchell, A. L. (2015). Congenital anomalies. In R. J. Martin, A. A. Fanaroff, & M. C. Walsh (Eds.), *Neonatal–perinatal medicine* (10th ed., pp. 436–459). St. Louis, MO: Mosby-Year Book.

Genetic testing identifies genetic alterations and their specific location on the involved chromosomes. Prenatal tests such as amniocentesis, non-invasive prenatal testing (NIPT), alpha-fetoprotein levels, and sonographic findings can aid in early identification of possible genetic disorders. Clinicians can request specific testing for suspected anomalies based on the use of fluorescent in situ hybridization (FISH), disorder panel groupings (i.e., metabolic disorder panel, hypotonia panel), infectious disease panels (i.e., CHARGE, TORCH), or microarray studies (Bajaj & Gross, 2015).

Structural Complications

Cardiac

Congenital heart disease (CHD) is divided into two main categories: cyanotic and acyanotic heart lesions. Cyanotic heart lesions involve cardiac defects that result in deoxygenated blood being shunted away from the pulmonary circulation and into the systemic circulation. Shunting may be complete when no mixing of oxygenated and deoxygenated blood occurs without open fetal shunts (parallel circulation). Incomplete shunting occurs when there is partial mixing of deoxygenated and oxygenated blood through open fetal shunts. Acyanotic heart lesions are typically less critical at birth and may not be evident on prenatal fetal echocardiogram. Infants with acyanotic lesions may become symptomatic only after their pulmonary vascular and systematic vascular resistance changes hours after birth (Ashwath & Snyder, 2015). **Table 11-6** lists cyanotic and acyanotic structural cardiac diseases.

For newborns with cyanotic heart lesions, maintaining patency of the ductus arteriosus is paramount for survival; consequently, these lesions are called "ductal-dependent." Early

Table 11-6: Congenital Heart Disease

Cyanotic	Acyanotic
Tetralogy of Fallot (ToF)	Ventricular septal defect (VSD)
Transposition of the great arteries (TGA)	Atrial septal defect (ASD)
Total anomalous pulmonary venous return	Patent ductus arteriosus (PDA)
Tricuspid atresia	Atriovenous (AV) canal
Truncus arteriosus	Partial anomalous pulmonary venous return
Double outlet right ventricle	Coarctation of aorta (mild–moderate)
Ebstein's anomaly	Anomalous left coronary artery
Single ventricle	
Pulmonary atresia	
Coarctation of aorta (severe)	

Reproduced from Ashwath, R., & Snyder, C. S. (2015). Congenital defects of the cardiovascular system. In R. J. Martin, A. A. Fanaroff, & M. C. Walsh (Eds.), *Neonatal–perinatal medicine* (10th ed., pp. 1230–1249). St. Louis, MO: Mosby-Year Book.

recognition of cardiac disease by well-trained staff, restrictive oxygen use, and prostaglandin (PGE$_1$) therapy are the gold-standard care for stabilizing infants with cyanotic heart lesions in preparation for surgical intervention (Ashwath & Snyder, 2015). For infants whose CHD was not diagnosed prenatally, rapid recognition of cardiac disease by trained clinicians is important for infant survival. Auscultation of heart sounds and murmurs, electrocardiogram findings, radiography, vital signs (including blood pressures), and blood gas measurements are useful tools in identification of possible CHD. Other cardiac dysfunctions may occur from clinical conditions such as pulmonary disease, arrhythmias, shock, surgery, infection, or displaced indwelling catheters.

Pulmonary

During fetal development, a variety of bronchopulmonary malformations may result from disordered interactions between embryonic mesodermal and endodermal lung components. Congenital pulmonary abnormalities may be clinically unapparent at birth or manifest with life-threatening pulmonary failure (Crowley, 2015). Upper airway malformations influence the neonate's transition to extrauterine life and may affect pulmonary function. Choanal atresia (nasal occlusion), vascular ring (vascular tissue completely or incompletely encircling the tracheal and esophageal tissue), obstructions (supraglottic, laryngeal, intrathoracic), and weak structural support (tracheomalacia, laryngomalacia) are examples of upper airway structural complications. Congenital malformations of lung tissue include congenital cystic adenomatoid malformations (CCAM; usually only one lobe involved), congenital lobar emphysema (CLE; one or more lobes involved), bronchogenic cysts, bronchopulmonary sequestration (nonfunctional portions of lung tissue with aberrant blood supply), and pulmonary hypoplasia (abnormal and underdeveloped lung tissue). The specific disease pathology and diagnostic findings dictate the appropriate treatment and likely outcomes.

The transition from an intrauterine fluid environment to an oxygen-containing environment may be complicated by a variety of pulmonary diseases. In air leak syndromes, air leaks into extrapulmonary spaces. These conditions include pneumothorax (leakage of air into the space between the plural and visceral lining), pneumomediastinum (leakage of air into the mediastinal space), pneumopericardium (leakage of air into the pericardial sac), and pulmonary interstitial emphysema (PIE; leakage of air into the interstitial space). The significance of these syndromes depends on the status of the infant, the level of respiratory support, infectious disease status, and the volume of air accumulation. Radiographic findings with clinical assessment are used to determine the level of significance and treatment needs.

Neonates who require respiratory support may develop chronic lung disease. Lung tissue may become fibrotic in such infants, with cystic changes resulting in areas of atelectasis and hyperinflation. These infants are able to ventilate before they can adequately oxygenate themselves and may be dependent on supplemental oxygen after discharge.

Cranial and Facial

Infants with oral facial deformities may develop both feeding and respiratory complications. Cleft lip is an opening in the upper lip that may extend into nasal cavity; cleft palate may involve an opening of the soft and/or hard palate. Newborns with these anomalies may successfully feed orally with specialized bottles and nipples. Breastfeeding is also successful for some of these infants. Oral palate prosthetics may be required in the early newborn period to support feeding success. As the infant grows, surgical intervention to repair the anomaly is performed.

Craniosynostosis, the premature closing of suture lines, results in malformation of the cranium and possibly impaired brain growth (with an associated microcephaly) (Gressens & Huppi, 2015). This condition is usually an isolated occurrence but may be part of a genetic malformation; thus chromosomal testing is required in infants with such an abnormality.

Because ear and renal structures develop during the same embryonic stage, ear pits and ear tags require close examination for other congenital anomalies. Any significant abnormality of the external ear may indicate additional anomalies of the middle/inner ear and may be associated with hearing loss. Early hearing screening can identify newborns with hearing deficits (Parikh & Mitchell, 2015).

Musculoskeletal

Clavicle fractures are the most common musculoskeletal abnormalities (affecting as many as 3%) in the neonate (Abdulhayoglu, 2011). Decreased movement of the affected arm, crepitus, and visualization on x-ray are diagnostic for fracture. Comfort measures and immobilization are treatments for clavicle fracture. Other common musculoskeletal deformities in newborns include polydactyly (extra digit), infantile scoliosis (abnormal curvature of spine), and torticollis (limited motion of the neck from a shortened sternocleidomastoid muscle). Treatment for these conditions is based on severity of the disorder and level of skeletal involvement.

Congenital hip dysplasia involves dislocation of one or both hips. The initial diagnosis is made by physical examination of hip mobility by using Barlow's and Ortolani's tests. Barlow's test attempts to dislocate the hip, whereas Ortolani's test attempts to reduce a dislocated hip (**Figure 11-3**). Referral to a pediatric orthopedist is required for infants with dislocated hips. Universal screening with ultrasound is not recommended but may be necessary for infants

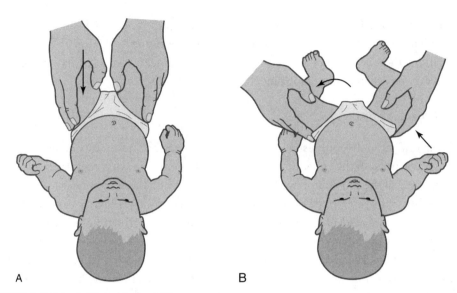

FIGURE 11-3: Ortolani's (A) and Barlow's (B) maneuver.

at increased risk for hip dysplasia (Kasser, 2011). Siblings or immediate family members with congenital hip dysplasia, breech positioning at birth, and abnormal findings on hip examination are risk factors warranting consultation and ultrasonography.

Genu recurvatum (hyperextension of the knee), metatarsus adductus (adducted metatarsals), and calcanevalgus deformities (malposition of foot) are positional deformities of the lower extremities (Kasser, 2011). These deformities will likely improve with positioning and range-of-motion exercises. In severe cases, consultation with an orthopedic specialist is recommended. Congenital club foot (talipes equinovarus), an inability to return the newborn's foot to a neutral position, requires early consultation with pediatric orthopedics.

Conclusion

Early recognition of complications after birth enables the neonatal healthcare provider to consult with and refer the newborn and family to appropriate specialists.

Student Practice Activities

Case Study 1

Clinical Presentation

B.T. is a 39-week-gestation male infant born to a 38-year-old G2, A1 mother. The mother presented to a birthing center with regular contractions following rupture of membranes at home. Her labor lasted 2 hours. Following delivery of the infant's head, the anterior shoulder of the right arm became lodged into the maternal symphysis pubis. The nurse–midwife was able to dislodge the infant's shoulder with moderate, direct pressure and a successful McRobert's maneuver. After delivery, there was no spontaneous movement of the newborn's right arm and inward rotation of the right hand. Grasp was intact but there was no movement of the upper and lower right arm. The physical exam of the infant was normal except for the right arm.

Prenatal History

Prenatal history included a healthy, nonsmoking, advanced-maternal-age mother with negative infectious disease history. She attended all prenatal visits as scheduled and denied any use of alcohol or illegal substances during pregnancy. Her pregnancy was unremarkable.

Clinical Interpretation

1. Based on B.T.'s history and clinical presentation, which diagnosis is most likely?
    A. Klumpke paralysis resulting from prolonged labor
    B. Cayler syndrome from renal anomalies
    C. Erb's paralysis resulting from brachial plexus nerve injury

Pathophysiology

Based on clinical presentation and examination findings, B.T. suffered a brachial plexus nerve injury from shoulder dystocia of the right arm during delivery. The incidence of shoulder dystocia is 0.6% to 3% in normal infants, with a higher incidence (up to 9%) if additional risk factors are present (Baxley & Gobbo, 2004). Additional risk factors include macrosomia, previous shoulder dystocia, maternal diabetes, abnormal pelvis, post-due dates, advanced maternal age, instrument-assisted delivery, epidural anesthesia, and secondary labor arrest. Brachial plexus nerve injury may also involve the cervical and thoracic nerves, affecting upper and lower arm mobility.

Klumpke paralysis is characterized by lower brachial nerve branch injury and loss of lower arm and hand control (Grossman et al., 2004). Erb's paralysis involves upper and middle nerve injury with sparing of the grasp reflex (Grossman et al., 2004). Overall outcomes are positive, with nearly 90% of infants experiencing a full recovery by 3 to 6 months of age (Grossman et al., 2004). In severe cases, neurosurgical intervention may be required.

Case Study 2

A.C. is a 36-week-gestation infant born to a G3, P2 mother who presented with spontaneous rupture of membranes. The birth, which was attended by a nurse–midwife, was uncomplicated. After birth, A.C. was placed on the mother's chest for skin-to-skin contact. A.C. breastfed within the first hour of life. At 2 hours of age, the father called the labor and delivery nurse because the baby was making "noise" with breathing. The nurse examined the infant and found mild intercostal retractions, grunting respirations, nasal flaring, and intermittent tachypnea. Pulse oximetry on the right hand showed a saturation greater than 90%, with brief decreases to 87% to 89% on room air. Heart rate and blood gases were normal. Chest x-ray showed no pneumothorax or pulmonary congenital malformation. Perihilar streakiness was visible bilaterally on the chest x-ray with hyperinflation. A.C. is an AGA infant with normal initial blood glucose.

Prenatal History
Prenatal history included a healthy mother with well-controlled gestational diabetes and no history of infection. The mother attended all prenatal visits and denied use of substances (i.e., alcohol and illegal drugs) during pregnancy.

Clinical Interpretation
1. Based on the clinical presentation and diagnostic findings, what is the most likely diagnosis for A.C.?
   A. Congenital heart disease
   B. Cleft palate
   C. Transient tachypnea of the newborn
2. Which treatment is likely needed for A.C.?
   A. Intubation with mechanical ventilation
   B. Keep prone with skin-to-skin care, maintain warmth, assess vital signs, and monitor with pulse oximetry
   C. Immediate transfer to the NICU

Pathophysiology

A.C. is a late-preterm infant with mild respiratory distress most likely caused by transient tachypnea of the newborn (TTN). The most common cause of respiratory distress in the newborn, TTN is characterized by periods of tachypnea, most often due to retained fetal lung fluid (Gardner, Enzman Hines, & Nyp, 2016). TTN is most common in late-preterm and term infants and infants born by cesarean section. This self-limiting condition resolves in 24 to 72 hours. Treatment is supportive care (i.e., warmth, fluids/calories, positioning, monitoring vital signs and oxygenation with noninvasive pulse oximetry, and supplemental oxygen) until the lung fluid clears and the tachypnea resolves (Gardner et al., 2016).

References

Abdulhayoglu, E. (2011). Birth trauma. In J. P. Cloherty, E. C. Eichenwald, & A. R. Stark (Eds.), *Manual of neonatal care* (7th ed.). Philadelphia, PA: Lippincott, Williams & Wilkins.

Ashwath, R., & Snyder, C. S. (2015). Congenital defects of the cardiovascular system. In R. J. Martin, A. A. Fanaroff, & M. C. Walsh (Eds.), *Neonatal–perinatal medicine* (10th ed., pp. 1230–1249). St. Louis, MO: Mosby-Year Book.

Bajaj, K., & Gross, S., J. (2015). Genetic aspects of perinatal disease and prenatal diagnosis. In R. J. Martin, A. A. Fanaroff, & M. C. Walsh (Eds.), *Neonatal–perinatal medicine* (10th ed., pp. 130–146). St. Louis, MO: Mosby-Year Book.

Baxley, E. G., & Gobbo, R. W. (2004). Shoulder dystocia. *American Family Physician, 69,* 7.

Blickstein, I., & Shinwell, E. S. (2015). Obstetric management of multiple gestation and birth. In R. J. Martin, A. A. Fanaroff, & M. C. Walsh (Eds.), *Neonatal–perinatal medicine* (10th ed., pp. 321–326). St. Louis, MO: Mosby-Year Book.

Cochran, W. D., & Lee, K. G. (2011). Assessment of the newborn. In J. P. Cloherty, E. C. Eichenwald, & A. R. Stark (Eds.), *Manual of neonatal care* (7th ed.). Philadelphia, PA: Lippincott, Williams, & Wilkins.

Crowley, M. A. (2015). Neonatal respiratory disorders. In R. J. Martin, A. A. Fanaroff, & M. C. Walsh (Eds.), *Neonatal–perinatal medicine* (10th ed., pp. 1113–1136). St. Louis, MO: Mosby-Year Book.

Devaskar, S. U., & Garg, M. (2015). Disorders of carbohydrate metabolism in the neonate. In R. J. Martin, A. A. Fanaroff, & M. C. Walsh (Eds.), *Neonatal–perinatal medicine* (10th ed., pp. 1434–1459). St. Louis, MO: Mosby-Year Book.

Gardner, S. L., Enzman Hines, M., & Nyp, M. (2016), Respiratory diseases. In S. L. Gardner, B. S. Carter, M. Enzman-Hines, & J. A. Hernandez (Eds.), *Merenstein and Gardner's handbook of neonatal intensive care* (8th ed., pp. 565–643). St. Louis, MO: Elsevier-Mosby.

Gressens, P., & Huppi, P. S. (2015). Normal and abnormal brain development. In R. J. Martin, A. A. Fanaroff, & M. C. Walsh (Eds.), *Neonatal–perinatal medicine* (10th ed., pp. 836–865). St. Louis, MO: Mosby-Year Book.

Grossman, J. A., DiTaranto, P., Yaylali, I., Alfonso, I., Ramos, L. E., & Price, A. E. (2004). Shoulder function following late neurolysis and bypass grafting for upper brachial plexus birth injuries. *Journal of Hand Surgery (British)*, *29*(4), 356–358.

Harmon, J. S. (2013). High-risk pregnancy. In C. Kenner & J. W. Lott (Eds.), *Comprehensive neonatal nursing: A physiologic perspective* (5th ed.). New York, NY: Springer.

Hay, W. H. (2012). Care of the infant of diabetic mother. *Current Diabetes Reports, 12*, 1.

Kasser, J. R. (2011). Orthopaedic problems. In J. P. Cloherty, E. C. Eichenwald, & A. R. Stark (Eds.), *Manual of neonatal care* (7th ed.). Philadelphia, PA: Lippincott, Williams & Wilkins.

Parikh, A. S., & Mitchell, A. L. (2015). Congenital anomalies. In, R. J. Martin, A. A. Fanaroff, & M. C. Walsh (Eds.), *Neonatal–perinatal medicine* (10th ed., pp. 436–459). St. Louis, MO: Mosby-Year Book.

Peleg, D., Kennedy, C. M., & Hunter, S. K. (1998). Intrauterine growth restriction: Identification and management. *American Family Physician, 58*(2), 453–460.

CHAPTER 12

HEALTH MAINTENANCE VISITS IN THE FIRST MONTH OF LIFE

Karla Reinhart and Sandra L. Gardner

Introduction

Ideally, outpatient follow-up of the newborn begins at 3 days of age and continues through a routine set of visits throughout childhood. Health maintenance—that is, well-child visits—consists of comprehensive assessment of the newborn's health, as well as the parent's or guardian's role in providing an environment for optimal growth, development, and health. During the first month of life, visits in the outpatient setting are routinely performed at 3 days, 2 weeks, and 1 month of age. The goal of well-child care is to periodically monitor and screen for normal progression in growth and development and to ensure early detection of deviations.

Somatic history and physical examination of the neonate are important parts of each visit. In addition, anticipatory guidance and discussions about nutrition, development, safety, and behavior are crucial. All visits should be seen as teaching opportunities, because the processes of growth and development are interrelated. At every health supervision visit, accurate measurements of length, weight, and head circumference are obtained and plotted on specific growth charts for males and females, and the results are shared with parents. As clinicians become familiar with normal patterns of growth and development, the ability to recognize and manage abnormal variations will become easier.

Outpatient Visits

Each visit consists of an evaluation and management of parental concerns. The interval history includes inquiry about any illness since the last health maintenance visit. A thorough physical examination follows the anthropometric measurements, evaluation of growth, and the administration of age-appropriate screening tests. Anticipatory guidance and teaching about expected development, nutrition, and safety concerns is completed before the administration of recommended immunizations.

Bright Futures, a national health promotion and prevention initiative, provides theory-based and evidence-based guidance for pediatric health maintenance visits. Led by the American Academy of Pediatrics (AAP) and supported by the Maternal and Child Health Bureau, Health Resources and Services Administration, Bright Futures provide resources for working with children and families (AAP, 2015). Each health maintenance visit is optimized by utilizing the innovative health promotion curriculum developed to incorporate Bright Futures principles into clinical practice (http://brightfutures.aap.org/Pages/default.aspx). The six core concepts of each health maintenance visit are listed in **Box 12-1**.

Pediatric health promotion visits are key times for communication between parents/guardians and healthcare providers. Discussion topics include normal development, nutrition, sleep, safety, local diseases, anticipatory guidance, and parental questions and concerns. Whether the infant is meeting normal developmental milestones is of special concern. Well-child visits are also an opportune time to screen mothers and families for factors that can affect the infant's growth and development, such as depression and intimate partner violence.

A balance between the internal and external environmental forces affecting the infant is essential to promote and maintain health during infancy. A safe and secure source of attachment and interaction between parents and infant is paramount to healthy infant development. Observing and commenting on aspects of the infant's development during the office visit

Box 12-1: Core Concepts for Each Pediatric Health Maintenance Visit

- Communication
- Partnership
- Health promotion and illness prevention
- Time management
- Education
- Advocacy

Modified from Hagan, J. F., Shaw, J. S., Duncan, P. (Eds.), & American Academy of Pediatrics. (2015). *Bright Futures: Guidelines for health supervision of infants, children, and adolescents (3rd ed.). Pocket Guide.* Elk Grove Village, IL: American Academy of Pediatrics.

becomes a teachable moment, enabling the provider to initiate discussions with parents about concerns or anticipatory guidance topics (Burns, Dunn, Brady, Starr, & Blosser, 2013). Providing parents with health education and anticipatory guidance promotes knowledge about their infant's needs, capabilities, and future development.

Newborn Development

Newborn development is usually divided into four areas: cognitive, language, physical (i.e., fine and gross motor skills), and social.

Physical Development

Development progresses in an orderly fashion from (1) cephalocaudal—beginning at the head and progressing downward (from head to foot), to (2) centripetal—from the outside toward the center, to (3) gross to specific (e.g., peripheral to central to lateralization). Developmental competencies of the newborn and neonate are listed in **Box 12-2**.

Box 12-2: Developmental Competencies of Newborns and Neonates

> ### Behavior (based on six states of consciousness)
> - Active crying
> - Active sleep
> - Drowsy waking
> - Fussing
> - Quiet alert
> - Quiet sleep
>
> ### Sensory/Cognitive
> - Piaget's sensorimotor phase (Ball, Bindler, & Cowen, 2013).
> - Hearing: Begins before birth, and is mature at birth. Recognizes familiar sounds heard during pregnancy, such as parental and sibling voices, music, and stories. Turns toward familiar voices; prefers higher-pitched sounds.
> - Touch, taste, smell: Mature at birth. Prefers sweet taste; keen sense of smell; able to recognize familiar smell of mother's breastmilk.
> - Vision: Notes bright objects and faces within a range of 8 to 10 inches. Vision 20/100. Eyes may appear to cross, which is normal because of immature eye muscles that mature by 3 to 4 months of age. Eyes fix and follow horizontally and vertically.

(Continued)

Box 12-2: Developmental Competencies of Newborns and Neonates (*Continued*)

- Inner ear: Calmed and soothed by rocking and changes in position.
- Obligate nasal breathers.
- Able to self-console by hand-to-mouth behaviors.
- Able to habituate to noxious stimuli.

Language

- Awakens and demands feedings
- Makes small, throaty sounds
- Crying is important way to communicate needs to caregivers; uses a range of noises to signal needs, such as when hungry or uncomfortable
- Alerts to voices

Motor Skills

- Lifts and turn the head when lying (supervised) in a prone position
- Hands are fisted, arms are flexed
- Neck supports the head for only a short period of time when the newborn is pulled into a sitting position

Primitive Reflexes

Dominant behaviors that include:

- Babinski reflex: Toes fan outward when sole of foot is stroked
- Moro reflex (startle): Extends arms, then bends and pulls them in toward body with a brief cry; often initiated by loud sounds or sudden movements
- Palmar grasp: Closes hand and "grips" the examiner's finger
- Placing: Leg extends when sole of foot is touched
- Plantar grasp: Flexes toes and forefoot
- Rooting: Turns head toward anything that strokes cheek or mouth
- Sucking: Begins to suck when anything touches the roof of the mouth
- Stepping/walking: Takes steps when both feet are placed on a surface, with body supported
- Tonic neck (fencing): Left arm extends when looking to the left, while right arm and leg flex inward; and vice versa
- Truncal (Galant): When skin alongside of back is stroked, will swing back toward side that was stroked

Initially, normal term newborns may lose as much as 10% of their birth weight before stabilizing and beginning to gain weight at the beginning of the second week of life. At the end of the second week of life, weight should be back to birth weight. Neonates are gaining weight appropriately if they gain ½ to 1 ounce per day. The neonatal period of rapid growth is characterized by a weight gain of 1½ pounds per month, a gain in length of 1 inch per month, and an increase in head circumference of 0.8 cm per month. This growth pattern continues for the first 6 months of life.

A normal growth trajectory includes a doubling of birth weight by 6 months of age and a tripling of birth weight by 1 year of age (Marcdante, Kliegman, Jensen, & Behrman, 2011).

Social/Cognitive Development

Neonatal behavior is based on the six states of consciousness listed in Box 12-2. Healthy babies with a normal nervous system move smoothly from one state to another. Each state is associated with varying heart rate, breathing, muscle tone, and body movements. Neonates with intact central nervous systems are also able to habituate—that is, turn off and cease responding—to noxious stimuli.

Bodily functions are unstable during the first months after birth—a normal finding that varies from infant to infant. Stress and stimulation affect bowel movements, gagging, hiccupping, skin color, temperature control, vomiting, and yawning.

Developmental Task

The primary developmental task of the newborn is to establish biorhythmic balance after birth (Gardner, Goldson, & Hernandez, 2016). As a result of the change from a dependent fetus to an independent newborn, all basic physiologic needs (i.e., breathing, eating, elimination, heat balance, and communication) must now be met in new and different ways. After birth, bodily contact with the infant's mother facilitates the establishment of the infant's biorhythmic balance.

The developmental task of infancy (birth to 1 year of age) is the development of a sense of self and a sense of trust versus mistrust (Ball et al., 2013; Gardner et al., 2016). Daily tactile caretaking and interaction with the parent/caregiver provides the infant with reciprocal stimuli for developing his or her identity and trust. The sense of trust versus mistrust in self and the environment is solidified during infancy (Gardner et al., 2016). The two major factors influencing this development of trust are (1) the ability of the infant to communicate needs and (2) the reliability and contingency of the responding caretakers in the environment (Gardner et al., 2016). Caretakers who contingently respond to the cries of their infant reinforce the development of a sense of self and trust. Noncontingent care occurs when caretakers ignore or delay need gratification of their infant's cues for care (Gardner et al., 2016).

Box 12-3: Safety Topics to Discuss with Parents of Newborns and Neonates

- Do not drink or carry anything hot while holding the infant to prevent burns.
- Do not leave the infant alone with siblings or pets. Pets may appear gentle and loving, but may react unexpectedly to an infant's cries or grabs, or may smother an infant by lying too closely. Siblings may attempt to feed, pick up, or quiet a crying infant.
- Do not leave an infant alone on a surface from which the infant may fall. To prevent falls, always have one hand on the baby!
- Back to Sleep: Place the infant only on the back to sleep. Supine, rather than prone, sleeping reduces the incidence of sudden infant death syndrome (SIDS) (Gardner et al., 2016).
- Know how to perform infant cardiopulmonary resuscitation (CPR) and handle a choking emergency.
- Never leave small objects within an infant's reach.
- Place the infant in a proper car seat for every car ride, no matter how short the distance. Make sure the car seat is rear facing and in the middle of the back seat. Do not use a car seat or infant swing for sleep.
- Do not heat formula or breastmilk in a microwave—hot spots in the liquid can burn the neonate's mouth and tongue.
- Be aware of poisons in the home and keep them out of the infant's reach. Post the national poison control number (1-800-222-1212) near the phone.

Safety

Newborns/neonates totally rely on their parents and caregivers to provide a safe environment. Basic safety topics to discuss with parents/caregivers during health maintenance visits are listed in **Box 12-3**.

Health Maintenance Visits

Social and emotional development are closely linked to the mother's emotional state. After birth, mood alterations are common:

- "Baby blues" affect 60% to 80% of mothers in the first 2 weeks of life.
- Postpartum depression affects 10% to 15% of new mothers.
- Postpartum psychosis affects 0.1% to 0.2% of new mothers (Burns et al., 2013).

Postpartum depression may occur at any time during the first year, whereas postpartum psychosis generally presents in the first weeks after delivery. Postpartum psychosis rates are higher in women with a history of schizophrenia, bipolar disease, or postpartum psychosis (Burns et al., 2013).

Postpartum mood disorders are characterized by the signs and symptoms listed in **Box 12-4**. Mothers at higher risk for postpartum mood disorders are those with the predictors listed in **Box 12-5**. Healthcare providers should screen new mothers for postpartum depression using the Postpartum Depression Predictors Inventory—Revised (**Table 12-1**) or the Edinburgh Postnatal Depression Scale (**Table 12-2**). Intervention and referral for depressed mothers are important because of the deleterious effects that the mother's illness may have on the behavioral, cognitive, emotional, and social development of the infant (Alhusen, Gross, Hayes, Rose, & Sharp, 2012; Alhusen, Hayat, & Gross, 2013; Huhtala et al., 2012; Letourneau, Tramonte, & Willms, 2013).

Three-Day-Old Visit

After discharge from the hospital or birthing center, or following a home birth, the initial health maintenance visit for the newborn usually occurs at 3 days of age. Late-preterm infants or those with specific health issues (e.g., at risk for the development of significant hyperbilirubinemia) needing close supervision may be seen for their initial visit at 24 to 48 hours after discharge (AAP, 2004; Association of Women's Health, Obstetric, and Neonatal Nurses [AWHONN], 2014; Engle, Tomashek, & Committee on Fetus and Newborn of the AAP, 2007). The initial visit establishes a relationship between the healthcare provider and family that guides future visits. The specific areas for this visit focus on weight change, evaluation for jaundice, CCHS screening, feeding success, cord and circumcision care, and adaptation to family life. Observation of parent–child interaction focuses on noting parental recognition and response to newborn needs and the parent's comfort level during feeding, holding, and caring. Assessment of parental and family support systems is also important.

History A complete health history includes a review of the newborn's chart and interviewing parents or guardians. Assessment of the neonatal chart includes a review of prenatal care,

---

Box 12-4: Features of Postpartum Mood Disorders

- Overly concerned for the baby or excessive anxiety over the infant's health
- Guilt, inadequacy, worthlessness, especially feeling like a failure at motherhood
- Fear of losing control or "going crazy"
- Lack of interest in the baby
- Fear of harming the baby
- Obsession

Reproduced from Gardner, S. L., Voos, K., & Hills, P. (2016). Families in crisis: Theoretical and practical considerations. In S. L. Gardner, B. S. Carter, M. Enzman-Hines, & J. A. Hernandez (Eds.), *Merenstein and Gardner's handbook of neonatal intensive care* (8th ed., pp. 821–864). St. Louis, MO: Mosby-Elsevier.

Box 12-5: Significant Predictors of Postpartum Mood Disorders

- History of previous depression (before and during pregnancy; bipolar disorder) (Alhusen et al., 2012; Janssen, Heaman, Urquia, O'Campo, & Thiessen, 2012; Liu & Tronick, 2013)
- Present depression and anxiety disorders (panic, post-traumatic stress and obsessive–compulsive disorders; phobias) (Hynan, Mounts, & Vanderbilt, 2013)
- Depression and anxiety associated with previous prenatal loss that continues after the birth of a subsequently healthy infant (Blackmore et al., 2011)
- Low quality of prenatal attachment (Goecke et al., 2012; Rowe , Wynter, Steele, Fischer, & Quinlivan, 2013)
- Nonworking women with a history of emesis during pregnancy and depression (Goker et al., 2012)
- Low self-esteem
- Negative, stressful life events such as childhood physical abuse (Plaza et al., 2012); intimate partner violence (Janssen et al., 2012); mode of delivery that entails maternal lack of control, such as primary (Rauh et al., 2012) or emergency cesarean section (Goecke et al., 2012); preterm birth (Gulamani, Premji, Kanji, & Azam, 2013)
- Marital discord
- Poor social support (Alhusen et al., 2013; Gulamani et al., 2013)
- Difficult infant temperament
- Childcare stresses
- History of endocrine dysfunction
- Maternity blues
- Single marital status
- Adolescent pregnancy (Clare & Yeh, 2012; Rowe et al., 2013)
- Unplanned/unwanted pregnancy
- Low socioeconomic status
- Minority race and ethnic groups (Native Americans, African Americans, Hispanic) (Clare & Yeh, 2012; Liu & Tronick, 2013)
- Immigrant women (Clare & Yeh, 2012; Gulamani et al., 2013; Lucero, Beckstrand, Callister, & Sanchez Burkhead, 2012)

Reproduced from Gardner, S. L., Voos, K., & Hills, P. (2016). Families in crisis: Theoretical and practical considerations. In S. L. Gardner, B. S. Carter, M. Enzman-Hines, & J. A. Hernandez (Eds.), *Merenstein and Gardner's handbook of neonatal intensive care* (8th ed., pp. 821–864). St. Louis, MO: Mosby-Elsevier.

Table 12-1: Postpartum Depression Predictors Inventory (PDPI)—Revised and Guide Questions for Its Use

During Pregnancy	Check One	
Marital Status		
1. Single	○	
2. Married/cohabiting	○	
3. Separated	○	
4. Divorced	○	
5. Widowed	○	
6. Partnered	○	
Socioeconomic Status		
Low	○	
Middle	○	
High	○	
Self-Esteem	Yes	No
Do you feel good about yourself as a person?	○	○
Do you feel worthwhile?	○	○
Do you feel you have a number of good qualities as a person?	○	○
Prenatal Depression		
1. Have you felt depressed during your pregnancy?	○	○
If yes, when and how long have you been feeling this way?		
If yes, how mild or severe do you consider your depression?		
Prenatal Anxiety		
Have you been feeling anxious during your pregnancy?	○	○
If yes, how long have you been feeling this way?		
Unplanned/Unwanted Pregnancy		
Was the pregnancy planned?	○	○
Is the pregnancy unwanted?	○	○

(Continued)

Table 12-1: Postpartum Depression Predictors Inventory (PDPI)—Revised and Guide Questions for Its Use (*Continued*)

During Pregnancy	Check One	
History of Previous Depression		
1. Before this pregnancy, have you ever been depressed?	○	○
If yes, when did you experience this depression?		
If yes, have you been under a physician's care for this past depression?	○	○
If yes, did the physician prescribe any medication for your depression?	○	○
Social Support		
1. Do you feel you receive adequate emotional support from your partner?	○	○
2. Do you feel you receive adequate instrumental support from your partner (e.g., help with household chores or baby sitting)?	○	○
3. Do you feel you can rely on your partner when you need help?	○	○
4. Do you feel you can confide in your partner?	○	○
(Repeat same questions for family and again for friends)		
Marital Satisfaction		
1. Are you satisfied with your marriage (or living arrangement)?	○	○
2. Are you currently experiencing any marital problems?	○	○
3. Are things going well between you and your partner?	○	○
Life Stress		
1. Are you currently experiencing any stressful events in your life such as:		
Financial problems	○	○
Marital problems	○	○
Death in the family	○	○
Serious illness in the family	○	○
Moving	○	○
Unemployment	○	○
Job change	○	○

Table 12-1: Postpartum Depression Predictors Inventory (PDPI)—Revised and Guide Questions for Its Use (*Continued*)

During Pregnancy	Check One	
After delivery, add the following items: Child Care Stress		
1. Is your infant experiencing any health problems?	○	○
2. Are you having problems with your baby feeding?	○	○
3. Are you having problems with your baby sleeping?	○	○
Infant Temperament		
1. Do you consider your baby irritable or fussy?	○	○
2. Does your baby cry a lot?	○	○
3. Is your baby difficult to console or soothe?	○	○
Maternity Blues		
1. Did you experience a brief period of tearfulness and mood swings during the first week after delivery?	○	○
Comments		

Reproduced from Beck, C. (2002). Revision of the Postpartum Depression Predictors Inventory. *Journal of Obstetric, Gynecologic, & Neonatal Nursing, 31*(4), 394–402. Copyright 2002, with permission from Elsevier.

pregnancy history including any maternal illnesses, family health conditions, delivery history including gestational age, Apgar scores, and hospital course. The hospital course comprises a review of any completed laboratory tests—specifically, blood type and Coombs results. Environmental history is also important, including the number and ages of those in the household, type of household, sleeping arrangements for the newborn, type of heating, safety, and presence of substance (i.e., tobacco, alcohol, drugs) use in the home.

Physical Examination Assessment of a newborn may not progress in as orderly a fashion as assessment of an older child or adult. Observation and assessment of the newborn may be completed while the infant is asleep or breastfeeding. Primitive reflexes are elicited while

Table 12-2: Edinburgh Postnatal Depression Scale

Health Visitor	Number
Today's date _____	Baby's age _____
Baby's date of birth _____	Birth weight _____
Triplets/twins/single _____	Male/female _____

How are you feeling?	
As you have recently had a baby, we would like to know how you are feeling now. Please <u>underline</u> the answer that comes closest to how you have felt in the past 7 days, not just how you feel today.	

Here is an example already completed:	
I have felt happy:	
Yes, most of the time	
<u>Yes, some of the time</u>	
Not very often	
No, never	
This means: "I have felt happy some of the time" during the past week.	
Please complete the other questions in the same way.	

In the past 7 days:	Number
1. I have been able to laugh and see the funny side of things:	
As much as I always could	0
Not quite so much now	1
Definitely not so much now	2
Not of all	3
2. I have looked forward with enjoyment to things:	
As much as I ever did	0
Rather less than I used to	1
Definitely less than I used to	2
Hardly at all	3
3. I have blamed myself unnecessarily when things went wrong:	
Yes, most of the time	0
Yes, some of the time	1
Not very often	2
No, never	3

Table 12-2: Edinburgh Postnatal Depression Scale (*Continued*)

4. I have felt worried and anxious for no good reason:	
No, not at all	0
Hardly ever	1
Yes, sometimes	2
Yes, very often	3
5. I have felt scared or panicky for no very good reason:	
Yes, quite a lot	3
Yes, sometimes	2
No, not much	1
No, not at all	0
6. Things have been getting on top of me:	
Yes, most of the time I haven't been able to cope at all	3
Yes, sometimes I haven't been coping as well as usual	2
No, most of the time I have coped quite well	1
No, I have been coping as well as ever	0
7. I have been so unhappy that I have had difficulty sleeping:	
Yes, most of the time	3
Yes, some of the time	2
Not very often	1
No, not at all	0
8. I have felt sad or miserable:	
Yes, most of the time	3
Yes, some of the time	2
Not very often	1
No, not at all	0
9. I have been so unhappy that I have been crying:	
Yes, most of the time	3
Yes, some of the time	2
Not very often	1
No, not at all	0
10. The thought of harming myself has occurred to me:	
Yes, quite often	3
Sometimes	2
Hardly ever	1
Never	0

Reproduced from Beck, C. (2002). Revision of the Postpartum Depression Predictors Inventory. *Journal of Obstetric, Gynecologic, & Neonatal Nursing, 31*(4), 394–402. Copyright 2002, with permission from Elsevier.

handling the neonate and performing the physical examination. The most invasive and uncomfortable parts of the examination are performed at the end.

Four basic techniques are used during a physical exam: inspection, auscultation, percussion, and palpation. Examination of the newborn or neonate should be a complete head-to-toe assessment, including measurement of length, weight, and head circumference. Postnatal growth charts can be used to compare the infant's growth at specific intervals with standardized norms. Recording of temperature, respirations, and heart rate should be completed at each visit. The exam should begin with assessment and observation of alertness, distress, and congenital anomalies, which is then followed by a detailed systematic head-to-toe exam as outlined in **Box 12-6**.

Box12-6: Important Elements of the Physical Examination of the Newborn

- **Skin.** Approximately 50% of newborns develop a rash about 24 hours after birth called erythema toxicum, which disappears in 7 to 14 days. Note skin color—jaundice, cyanosis, or slate gray areas depending on ethnicity. Inspect skin appearance, folds, and turgor.
- **Head.** Inspect the hair. Palpate the head and face, checking for symmetry. Lightly palpate the fontanels, noting soft and flat areas; palpate suture lines.
- **Ears.** Inspect and palpate the external and internal ears. Review the results of the initial newborn hearing screen.
- **Eyes.** Inspect and palpate the external eyes, eyelids, lacrimal ducts, conjunctiva, and sclera, and elicit the red reflex.
- **Nose.** Inspect the nose and check its patency. Teach parents use of a suction bulb to maintain nasal patency, because infants are nasal breathers.
- **Mouth.** Inspect the oral cavity, including the palate, tongue, gums, and tonsils. Suck should be strong; the palate should be intact to inspection and palpation.
- **Neck.** Palpate clavicles especially in a neonate weighing more than 4 kg. Abnormalities of the newborn/neonatal neck are listed in Table 4-6.
- **Chest.** Inspect the size, shape, and symmetry of the neck. Palpate the chest and back, checking for thrills and fremitus. Auscultate breath sounds anterior and posteriorly.
- **Cardiovascular.** Auscultate the apical pulse, and palpate peripheral pulses.
- **Abdominal.** Inspect the shape, size, and symmetry of the abdomen. Inspect the umbilicus for any signs of infection or hernias. Palpate the liver, spleen, kidneys, and bladder. Auscultate bowel sounds.
- **Genitalia.** In *boys*, inspect and palpate the penis and urethra, observing the location of the urethra; palpate the testes. In *girls*, inspect external genitalia.
- **Anus/rectum.** Check for patency; observe for sacral dimple, sinus, or hair tufts.
- **Extremities.** Inspect the hands, arms, feet, legs, and hips. Test range of motion; perform Ortolani's and Barlow's maneuvers.
- **Neurologic.** Inspect and test muscle strength, sensory function, and primitive reflexes.

Box 12-7: Three-Day-Old Visit

Developmental Surveillance

- Shows responsiveness to parental voice and touch
- Has periods of wakefulness
- Calms when picked up
- Moves in response to visual or auditory stimuli
- Looks at caregiver when awake

Anticipatory Guidance

- *Family readiness:* Family support, maternal wellness, transition, sibling relationships, family resources.
- *Infant behaviors:* Infant capabilities, parent–child relationship, sleep (location, position, crib safety), sleep–wake states (calming).
- *Feeding:* Patterns of weight gain, changes in milk for breastfeeding mothers. Assess for pain with nursing. Evaluate the frenulum. Address difficulties with breastfeeding and problem-solve or refer to a lactation specialist/consultant. Counsel formula-feeding mothers about the proper mixing of formula, frequency of feeding (i.e., 8 to 12 feedings in 24 hours), and amount to be taken by the infant. Discuss burping and spitting up—normal versus abnormal.
- *Safety:* Car safety seats, tobacco smoke, falls, home safety.
- *Routine baby care:* Infant supplies, skin care, illness prevention, introduction to practice/early intervention referrals.

Screening

- *Genetic:* Perform first blood draw if the baby was born in a birth center or at home.
- *Hearing:* Perform/refer for hearing screen if the baby was born in a birth center or at home.
- *Critical congenital heart disease (CCHD):* Perform/refer for CCHD screen if the baby was born in a birth center or at home.

Data from Hagan, J. F., Shaw, J. S., Duncan, P. (Eds.), & American Academy of Pediatrics. (2015). *Bright Futures: Guidelines for health supervision of infants, children, and adolescents* (3rd ed.). *Pocket Guide.* Elk Grove Village, IL: American Academy of Pediatrics.

Box 12-7 outlines developmental surveillance, anticipatory guidance, and screening activities for the 3-day-old visit.

First to Second Week of Life Visit

Observation Observe parent–child interactions:

- Do parents and newborn respond to each other?
- Do parents appear content, depressed, angry, fatigued, or overwhelmed?
- Are parents responsive to the newborn's distress?

- Do parents appear confident in caring for the newborn?
- Do parents support each other?

Physical Examination   Perform the same examination as done during the initial health maintenance visit at 3 days of age, so that a full head-to-toe examination is completed during the visit. **Box 12-8** outlines developmental surveillance, anticipatory guidance, and screening activities for the first to second week of life visit.

Box 12-8: First to Second Week of Life Visit

Developmental Surveillance

- Sustains periods of wakefulness for feeding
- Gradually will become able to establish longer sleep periods at night
- Turns toward parent voice, calms when hearing parent voice
- Communicates needs through behaviors
- Briefly fixes and follows on objects or faces
- Sucks, swallows, and breathes effectively to breastfeed or formula feed
- Shows strong primitive reflexes
- Lifts head briefly in the prone position

Anticipatory Guidance

- *Parental (maternal) well-being:* Assess for health and depression, family stress, uninvited advice, and parent roles.
- *Newborn transition:* Assess daily routines, sleep (location, position, crib safety, co-sleeping), state modulation (calming), parent–child relationship, and early developmental referrals.
- *Nutritional adequacy:* Assess feeding success (weight gain), feeding strategies (holding, burping), hydration/jaundice, hunger/satiation cues, and feeding guidance (breastfeeding, formula).
- *Safety:* Assess for car seats, infant swings, and infant seats; tobacco smoke; hot liquids (water temperature; not using microwave to heat expressed breastmilk or formula); and siblings.
- *Newborn care:* Educate parents about when to call (fever), emergency readiness (CPR), illness prevention (hand washing, outings), and skin care (sun exposure).

Screening

- *Genetic:* Perform second blood draw, if indicated.
- *Hearing:* Perform/refer for hearing screen if not done after a birth center or home birth. Refer for a repeat test if the infant failed to "pass" the first screening.

Data from Hagan, J. F., Shaw, J. S., Duncan, P. (Eds.), & American Academy of Pediatrics. (2015). *Bright Futures: Guidelines for health supervision of infants, children, and adolescents* (3rd ed.). *Pocket Guide.* Elk Grove Village, IL: American Academy of Pediatrics.

One Month Visit

Observation Observe parent–child interactions:

- Do parents seem uncertain or nervous?
- How do the parent and infant interact?
- How do parents respond to infant cues?
- Do parents appear comfortable with each other and with the baby?

Physical Examination Perform the same examination as done during the initial health maintenance visit at 3 days of age, so that a full head-to-toe examination is completed during the visit. **Box 12-9** outlines developmental surveillance and anticipatory guidance activities for the first month visit.

Box 12-9: One Month Visit

Developmental Surveillance

- Responsive to calming actions when upset
- Fixes and follows parents with eyes
- Recognizes parent's voices
- Has started to smile
- Lifts head when on stomach

Anticipatory Guidance

- *Parental (maternal) well-being:* Assess maternal health (maternal postpartum checkup, depression, substance abuse) and return to work/school (breastfeeding plans, child care).
- *Family adjustment:* Assess family resources, family support, parent roles, domestic violence, and community resources.
- *Infant adjustment:* Assess sleep–wake cycles, sleep position (back to sleep, location, crib safety), state modulation (crying, consoling, shaken baby), developmental changes (bored baby, tummy time), and early developmental referrals.
- *Feeding routines:* Assess feeding frequency (growth spurts), feeding choices (types of foods/fluids), hunger cures, feeding strategies (holding, burping), pacifier use (cleanliness), and feeding guidance (breastfeeding, formula).
- *Safety:* Assess for car seats, infant swings, and infant seats; tobacco smoke; falls; hot liquids (water temperature; not using microwave to heat expressed breastmilk or formula); toys and window blinds with loops or strings; and siblings.

Data from Hagan, J. F., Shaw, J. S., Duncan, P. (Eds.), & American Academy of Pediatrics. (2015). *Bright Futures: Guidelines for health supervision of infants, children, and adolescents* (3rd ed.). *Pocket Guide.* Elk Grove Village, IL: American Academy of Pediatrics.

Standard of Care/National Guidelines for Care

The AAP's Bright Futures guidelines set the national standard for the content of health maintenance visits/well-child care for infants, children, and adolescents. *Healthy People 2020*, the health policy statement for the United States, created the objectives for newborn, infant, and child health promotion and care; these objectives are listed in **Box 12-10**.

Cultural Considerations

From the moment of conception, the fetus/newborn is subject to influences of culture. The familial environment is the setting within which the infant experiences overall cultural attitudes. Cultures form around language, gender, disability, sexual orientation, religion, or socioeconomic status.

Provision of culturally competent care for parents and their newborns includes three key aspects: (1) understanding the dimensions of their culture, (2) moving beyond the biophysical to a more holistic approach, and (3) increasing knowledge and perfecting clinical skills, while addressing the needs of diverse populations (Callister, 2001). Cultural or

Box 12-10: *Healthy People 2020* **Objectives**

- Increase proportion of infants who are put to sleep on their back
- Increase percentage of infants who are breastfed, especially those exclusively breastfed
- Increase percentage of infants and children who are screened appropriately and referred for autism spectrum disorder and other developmental delays
- Increase percentage of infants and children who have an ongoing source of medical care
- Decrease blood lead levels in infants and children
- Achieve and maintain effective vaccination coverage levels for universally recommended vaccines among young children
- Decrease deaths caused by unintentional injuries
- Increase use of age-appropriate vehicle restraint systems
- Increase proportion of newborns who are screened for hearing loss by no later than 1 month, have audiology evaluation by 3 months, and are enrolled in appropriate intervention services no later than 6 months

Data from Office of Disease Prevention and Health Promotion. (1999). Healthy People, 2020.
2020 Topics & objectives. Maternal, infant, and child health. Retrieved from https://www.healthypeople.gov/2020/topics-objectives/topic/maternal-infant-and-child-health/objectives.

ethnic influences may affect assessment findings as well as the acceptability of recommended interventions.

Knowledge of normal variations among races and cultures can help the healthcare provider avoid mistaking these variations for abnormal findings. Health assessment skills, therefore, should include knowledge of biologic and physiologic variations among ethnic and racial groups. For example, the blue–gray discolorations found on various parts of the skin of neonates from races with more pigmentation have been mistaken for bruising from nonaccidental trauma. Documentation of the site and size of these normal variations is essential.

Cultural influences are significant and unique, and may affect relationships between the infant and parent, thereby defining the roles of the parent and the infant within the family structure. Cultural influences also affect the infant's health and wellness. Common cultural and ethnic variations in infants are presented in **Box 12-11**. Factors influencing multicultural care are listed in **Box 12-12**.

Box 12-11: Common Cultural and Ethical Variations in Infants

- *African American:* Slate gray spots and/or other birthmarks more prevalent than in other ethnic groups.
- *Amish:* Babies seen as gifts from God. Have high birth rates, large families. Higher risk for maple syrup urine disease.
- *Appalachian:* Newborns wear bands around abdomen to prevent umbilical hernias and asafetida bags around neck to prevent contagious diseases.
- *Arab American:* Children "dearly loved." Male circumcision is a religious requirement.
- *Chinese American:* Children highly valued due to one-child rule in China. Slate gray spots occur in approximately 80% of infants. Bilirubin levels higher in Chinese newborns than in others, with higher rates noted on day 5 or 6.
- *Cuban American:* Childbirth is a celebration. Family cares for mother and infant for first 4 weeks. Preference for bottle-feeding over breastfeeding; if breastfeeding, infants are weaned early, around 3 months of age.
- *Egyptian American:* Children very important. Mother and infant are cared for by family for the first 50 days.
- *Filipino American:* Eyes are almond shaped; flat nose bridge with mildly flared nostrils is often present. Slate gray spots are common.
- *French Canadian:* Five mutations account for 90% of phenylketonuria (PKU) in French Canadians. Also have a high incidence of cystic fibrosis and muscular dystrophy.
- *Greek American:* High incidence of two genetic conditions: thalassemia and glucose-6-phosphate dehydrogenase (G6PD) deficiency.

(Continued)

Box 12-11: Common Cultural and Ethical Variations in Infants (*Continued*)

- *Iranian American:* Believe in hot and cold influences, with baby boys being considered hotter than baby girls. Infants are confined to home during their first 40 days. A ritual bath takes place sometime between days 10 and 40.
- *Jewish American:* Children are viewed as a valued treasure. High incidence of Tay-Sachs disease. Male circumcision is a religious ritual.
- *Mexican American:* Use of stomach belt to prevent umbilicus from protruding when the infant cries. Belief that trimming or cutting of nails first 3 months of age can cause blindness and deafness.
- *Navajo Native American:* Infants kept on cradle boards until able to walk. Slate gray spots are common.
- *Vietnamese American:* Slate gray spots are common.

Reproduced from Dillon, P. M. (2007). *Nursing health assessment: Clinical pocket guide* (2nd ed.). Philadelphia, PA: F. A. Davis, with permission.

Box 12-12: Factors Influencing Multicultural Health Care

- Self-exploration of values and beliefs concerning other cultures and their beliefs
- Knowledge of historical experience, both recent and long term, of ethnic groups that live in the community
- Knowledge of demographic data of various ethnic groups: family size, socioeconomic status, and future expectations
- Understanding and sensitivity to cultural healthcare practices different from one's own practices
- Recognition of beliefs and cultural attitudes toward health and illness
- Awareness of problems and barriers encountered by ethnic group members when they enter the healthcare system, which may include fear and distrust of healthcare professionals, language barriers, literacy levels, and discrimination by caregivers

Conclusion

The first month of life completes the transition from fetal life through the neonatal period. Frequent follow-up in the first month of life can confirm that the newborn is completing the transition without difficulties in physiologic adaptation, feeding efficiency, and integration into the family. The initial visit establishes care with a provider for ongoing assessment and developmental evaluation. Visits at 2 and 4 weeks ensure appropriate growth and provide an opportunity for intervention if growth is inadequate. A critical part of care during the first month of life is evaluation of the integration of the newborn into the family and provision of interventions if needed.

Student Practice Activities

Case Study: Down Syndrome

While maternal serum screening and prenatal ultrasound identify the majority of pregnancies at increased risk for Down syndrome, some cases are missed. Newborns with Down syndrome must be evaluated at birth for specific medical complications. Forthright presentation of the news that a child has Down syndrome is imperative to greater parental satisfaction.

The following physical features lead to the suspicion of Down syndrome at birth:

* Hypotonia
* A small brachycephalic head
* Epicanthic folds
* Flat nasal bridge
* Upward-slanting palpebral fissures
* Brushfield spots of the iris (gray–white specks of depigmentation seen in a ring around the pupil)
* Small mouth
* Small ears
* Excessive skin at the nape of the neck
* Single transverse palmar crease: simian crease
* Wide space between the first and second toes
* Short fifth finger with clinodactyly

Newborns with Down syndrome should be evaluated for some specific complications:

* Congenital heart defects (50% risk)
* Bowel obstruction (duodenal atresia, about 12% risk), usually evident by persistent vomiting
* Hearing loss (60% risk)
* Ocular abnormalities (congenital cataracts, strabismus)
* Constipation with an increased risk of Hirschsprung's disease (less than 1% risk)
* Leukemia (1% risk) and polycythemia (18% risk)
* Congenital hypothyroidism (1% risk)

All individuals with Down syndrome have some degree of cognitive impairment. Most often, mild to moderate developmental delays occur. Enrollment in an early intervention program should occur shortly after birth so that the child can receive physical, speech, and occupational therapies. Early intervention focuses on four main areas of development: fine and gross motor skills, language, social development, and self-help skills. Programs are individualized for each child.

1. How is Down syndrome diagnosed in the newborn period?
2. What is the treatment for Down syndrome?
3. What is the prognosis for a child with Down syndrome?

Multiple Choice

1. You are testing the reflexes of a neonate. One of the reflexes you test is the Babinski reflex. What is the physical response for the Babinski reflex?
   A) When the outer sole of foot is stimulated from the heel upward and across the ball of the foot toward the large toe, the large toe dorsiflexes and the toes flare.
   B) When startled (noise, jarring), the infant's arms extend and abduct, with the fingers forming a C, while the knees and hips flex slightly, and the arms return to chest in an embracing motion.
   C) When the infant's cheek or lips are touched, the head turns toward the touch and the mouth opens in attempt to suck.
   D) When the infant is supine with the head turned to one side, the extremities on the same side straighten and the extremities on the opposite side flex.

2. You are testing the reflexes of a neonate. One of the reflexes you test is the tonic neck reflex. What is the physical response for the tonic neck reflex?
   A) When the outer sole of foot is stimulated from the heel upward and across the ball of the foot toward the large toe, the large toe dorsiflexes and the toes flare.
   B) When startled (noise, jarring), the infant's arms extend and abduct, with the fingers forming a C, while the knees and hips flex slightly, and the arms return to chest in an embracing motion.
   C) When the infant's cheek or lips are touched, the head turns toward the touch and the mouth opens in attempt to suck.
   D) When the infant is supine with the head turned to one side, the extremities on the same side straighten and the extremities on the opposite side flex.

3. A baby still has her umbilical cord attached. Which special care would the cord need?

   A) No special care is needed; the cord will fall off in 10 to 14 days.

   B) Assess the cord for bleeding or infection. Clean the cord with soap and water after each diaper change, and apply a topical antibiotic if ordered. Place the diaper below the umbilical cord stump.

   C) Assess the cord for bleeding or infection. Clean the cord with soap and water daily, and apply a topical antibiotic if ordered. Place the diaper below the umbilical cord stump.

   D) Assess the cord for bleeding or infection. Clean the cord with soap and water daily, and apply a topical antibiotic if ordered. Place the diaper on the top of the umbilical cord stump.

4. You are measuring the vital signs of a newborn. He had an irregular heart rate when he was first born, and his parents are worried. What is the expected heart rate of a newborn?

   A) 50–90 beats/min

   B) 60–100 beats/min

   C) 60–110 beats/min

   D) 80–180 beats/min

References

Alhusen, J. L., Gross, D., Hayes, M. J., Rose, L., & Sharp P. (2012). The role of mental health on maternal–fetal attachment in low-income women. *Journal of Obstetric, Gynecologic, and Neonatal Nursing, 41,* e71.

Alhusen, J. L., Hayat, M. J., & Gross, D. (2013). A longitudinal study of maternal attachment and infant developmental outcomes. *Archives of Women's Mental Health, 16,* 521.

American Academy of Pediatrics (AAP). (2015). Bright futures. Retrieved from http://brightfutures.aap.org/materials

American Academy of Pediatrics (AAP), Subcommittee on Hyperbilirubinemia: Clinical Practice Guideline. (2004). Management of hyperbilirubinemia in the newborn infant 35 or more weeks of gestation. *Pediatrics, 114*(1), 297–316.

Association of Women's Health, Obstetric, and Neonatal Nurses (AWHONN). (2014). *Assessment and care of the late preterm infant.* Washington, DC: Author.

Ball, J. W., Bindler, R. C., & Cowen, K. J. (2013). *Child health nursing: Partnering with children and families* (3rd ed.). Upper Saddle River, NJ: Prentice Hall.

Blackmore, E. R., Cote-Arsenault, D., Tang, W., Glover, V., Evans, J., Golding, J., & O'Connor, T. G. (2011). Previous prenatal loss as a predictor of perinatal depression and anxiety. *British Journal of Psychiatry, 198,* 373.

Burns, C. E., Dunn, A. M., Brady, M. A., Starr, N. B., & Blosser, C. G. (2013). *Pediatric primary care* (5th ed.). Philadelphia, PA: Elsevier.

Callister, L. C. (2001, March/April). Culturally competent care of women and newborns: Knowledge, attitude, and skills. *Journal of Obstetric, Gynecologic, and Neonatal Nursing, 30*(2), 209–215.

Clare, C. A., & Yeh, J. (2012). Postpartum depression in special populations: A review. *Obstetrics & Gynecology Survey, 67,* 313.

Engle, W., Tomashek, K. M., Wallman, C., & Committee on Fetus and Newborn of the American Academy of Pediatrics (AAP). (2007). "Late-preterm": A population at risk. *Pediatrics, 120*(6), 1390–1401.

Gardner, S. L., Goldson, E., & Hernandez, J. A. (2016). The neonate and the environment: Impact on development. In S. L. Gardner, B. S. Carter, M. Enzman-Hines, & J. A. Hernandez (Eds.), *Merenstein and Gardner's handbook of neonatal intensive care* (8th ed., pp. 262–314). St. Louis, MO: Elsevier-Mosby.

Goecke, T. W., Voight, F., Faschingbauer, F., Spangler, G., Beckmann, M. W., & Beetz, A. (2012). The association of prenatal attachment and perinatal factors with pre- and postpartum depression in first-time mothers. *Archives of Gynecology and Obstetrics, 286,* 309.

Goker, A., Yanikkerem, E., Dermet, M. M., Dikayak, S., Yildirim, Y., & Koyuncu, F. M. (2012, December 13). Postpartum depression: Is mode of delivery a risk factor? *ISRN Obstetrics & Gynecology.* [Epub ahead of print]. doi: 10.5402/2012/616759

Gulamani, S. S., Premji, S. S., Kanji, Z., & Azam, S. I. (2013). A review of postpartum depression, preterm birth, and culture. *Journal of Perinatal and Neonatal Nursing, 27,* 52.

Huhtala, M., Korja, R., Lehtonen, L., Haataja, L., Lapinleimu, H., Rautava, P., & The PIPARI Study Group. (2012). Parental psychological well-being and behavioral outcome of very low birth weight infants at 3 years. *Pediatrics, 129,* e937.

Hynan, M. T., Mounts, K. O., & Vanderbilt, D. L. (2013). Screening parents of high-risk infants for emotional distress: rationale and recommendations. *Journal of Perinatology, 33,* 748.

Janssen, P. A., Heaman, M. I., Urquia, M. L., O'Campo, P. J., & Thiessen, K. R. (2012). Risk factors for postpartum depression among abused and nonabused women. *American Journal of Obstetrics & Gynecology, 207,* 489.

Letourneau, N. L., Tramonte, L., & Willms, J. D. (2013). Maternal depression, family functioning and children's longitudinal development. *Journal of Pediatric Nursing, 28,* 223.

Liu, C. H., & Tronick, E. (2013). Rates and predictors of postpartum depression by race and ethnicity: Results from the 2004 to 2007 New York City PRAMS survey (Pregnancy Risk Assessment Monitoring System). *Maternal and Child Health, 17,* 1599.

Lucero, N. B., Beckstrand, R. L., Callister, L. C., & Sanchez Birkhead, A. C. (2012). Prevalence of postpartum depression among Hispanic immigrant women. *Journal of the American Academy of Nurse Practitioners, 24,* 726.

Marcdante, K. J., Kliegman, R. M., Jensen, H. B., & Behrman, R. E. (2011). *Nelson essentials of pediatrics* (6th ed.). Philadelphia, PA: Saunders.

Plaza, A., Garcia-Esteve, L., Torres, A., Ascaso, C., Gelabert, E., Luisa Imaz, M., & Martin-Santos, R. (2012). Childhood physical abuse as a common risk factor for depression and thyroid dysfunction in the earlier postpartum. *Psychiatry Research, 200,* 329.

Rauh, C., Beetz, A., Burger, P., Engel, A., Haberle, L., Fasching, P. A., & Faschingbauer, F. (2012). Delivery mode and the course of pre- and postpartum depression. *Archives of Gynecology and Obstetrics, 286,* 1407.

Rowe, H. J., Wynter, K. H., Steele, A., Fischer, J. R., & Quinlivan, J. A. (2013). The growth of maternal–fetal emotional attachment in pregnant adolescents: A prospective cohort study. *Journal of Pediatric and Adolescent Gynecology, 26,* 327.

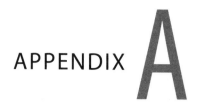

ANSWERS TO STUDENT PRACTICE ACTIVITIES

Chapter 2

Short Answer

1. The mother is most likely dependent on opioids. She had only one prenatal visit, at which time she had a positive urine toxicology screen for opiates. She may not have returned to the clinic for prenatal care because she feared prosecution or referral to child protective services. Although she has consistently denied drug use, you have evidence of two urine drug screens that were positive for opiates, and she has had several documented visits to different emergency departments for treatment of chronic pain, perhaps because she was seeking opiates. She may be obtaining opiates illegally since her last emergency department visit was 3 months ago.

2. Neonatal abstinence syndrome (NAS) is a combination of physiologic and neurobehavioral symptoms displayed by infants following the abrupt withdrawal of drug exposure at the time of birth. While cocaine and other stimulants, benzodiazepines, and selective serotonin reuptake inhibitors (SSRIs) have been implicated in this syndrome, NAS most commonly occurs in the context of prenatal opioid use. This may include the illicit use of prescribed substances or the licit use of prescribed opioids such as methadone and buprenorphine.

3. The gastrointestinal, respiratory, and autonomic and central nervous systems are affected, as are critical regulatory centers of postnatal adaptation. Infants with NAS have

increased morbidity, including poor weight gain, respiratory problems, feeding difficulties, and seizures. The intelligence of children with prenatal exposure to drugs appears to be affected, and some studies suggest the presence of long-term neurodevelopmental difficulties related to behavior, cognition, language, and achievement in infants with NAS (Hayes & Brown, 2012). Infants with NAS require prolonged hospitalizations (5 or more days) and may require treatment with opioids. Infants treated for methadone and buprenorphine typically require more than 28 days of observation, which may include a combination of inpatient and outpatient care, before the problem of NAS is resolved.

4. Scoring the severity of NAS is most often completed using the modified Finnegan Scoring Tool (FST), the instrument recommended by the American Academy of Pediatrics. The AAP identifies the FST as the gold standard for assessing the severity of neonatal withdrawal, and it is the most widely used tool for this purpose in the United States. The FST aids clinicians in determining whether nonpharmacologic interventions are sufficient to mitigate the effects of opioid withdrawal or whether pharmacologic adjuncts are necessary to ensure the safest wean from opioid addiction. Nonpharmacologic interventions include swaddling, rocking, soft music therapy, suckling by pacifier, skin-to-skin bonding with parent(s), and enteral feedings. Pharmacologic regimens may include the provision of methadone or morphine, with phenobarbital occasionally used as adjunct therapy. An infant's requirement for pharmacologic therapy and hospital length of stay are primarily dependent upon timely identification and accurate evaluation by way of the FST.

5. Obstetric providers should know which factors increase the likelihood of maternal ingestion of licit or illicit opioids alone or in combination with other substances such as heroin and cocaine. Prompt identification of at-risk maternal/infant dyads is key to the prompt initiation of screening and assessment of the severity of neonatal withdrawal. Even after discharge, newborns may require ongoing weaning of pharmacologic drugs before resolution of NAS is achieved. Timely and comprehensive assessments of parental understanding of NAS, compliance with medication regimens, and compliance with pediatric follow-up appointments are necessary aspects of follow-up care. Outpatient NAS clinics are a cost-effective alternative to lengthy inpatient hospitalizations (Backes, Backes, Gardner, Nankervis, & Giannone, 2012; Kelly, Knoppert, Roukema, Rieder, & Koren, 2015; Ramsey, 2015). Neonatal clinical nurse specialists, neonatal and pediatric nurse practitioners, and pediatricians may staff these clinics to provide ongoing continuity of care while encouraging family-centered care and bonding in the home environment.

Multiple Choice

1.	B	6.	D
2.	C	7.	B
3.	A	8.	C
4.	B	9.	A
5.	D	10.	D

Chapter 3

Short Answer

1. Thermoregulation; nasal and oral suction as necessary

2. Grunting, "singing"; retractions; circumoral cyanosis; lung fields

3. • Complete physical exam, including vital signs

   • Pulse oximeter reading with supplemental oxygen as needed

   • Thermoregulation ensured with radiant warmer

   • Glucose monitoring

   • Consult with physician for management

   • If at a birth center, prepare for transport

   • If in labor and delivery, prepare to have the baby closely observed or transferred to the nursery, where the baby can be monitored and watched continuously

4. Keep them informed and explain what is happening and the importance of changing the direction.

Multiple Choice

1.	A	4.	C
2.	B	5.	C
3.	B	6.	A

Chapter 4

1. A
2. B
3. B
4. C
5. C
6. A

Chapter 5

Case Study 1

1. Diagnosis: inadequate latch and expression of milk; cracked nipples

Recommendations:

- Examine the baby, paying special attention to the mouth, tongue, frenulum, and suck.
- Observe a full breastfeeding session.
- Observe the infant positioning; latch-on technique, including bringing the baby to breast; ability of the baby to "fish lip"; and sucking coordination.
- Adjust the positioning and assist with latch-on. Have the mother rate the "pain."
- Refer the mother to a lactation consultant prior to discharge. Recommend application of lanolin or vitamin E to her nipples (not the entire areola), air-drying her nipples, expressing milk with pump as needed to reduce engorgement, and connecting with a breastfeeding support group. Follow up with her in 24 hours.

2. Diagnosis: inadequate latch and expression of milk; tight frenulum

Recommendations:

- Refer the mother to a pediatric provider skilled with frenulum evaluation and clipping as soon as possible.
- Observe a breastfeeding session to assess correct positioning, latch-on technique, and so on.
- Use a breast pump as needed to support adequate milk supply.

- Apply lanolin or vitamin E to the nipples (not the entire areola); air-dry the nipples; make a referral to a lactation consultant who can evaluate and assist the mother.
- Follow up with the nursing couple in 24 hours for evaluation.

Case Study 2

1. Take a feeding history: Which formula is the baby receiving? How much is the baby taking? Take an elimination history: Why does mother think baby is constipated? What do the baby's stools look like? How often is baby stooling?

2. No evidence supports the contention that iron constipates babies. Use constipation algorithm in Figure 5-13.

Chapter 6

1. A
2. B
3. C
4. C
5. B

Chapter 7

1. C
2. D
3. B
4. A
5. C
6. D

Chapter 8

1. C. It has not yet been at least 2 hours since the circumcision procedure and the infant has not voided.

2. D. The only approved sleep position for an infant in the first year of life is supine ("Back to Sleep").

3. A. The infant should be placed into approximately 2 inches of warm (not hot or cool) water and should be bathed approximately 3 times per week; a bath ring should *not* be used with bathing of a newborn infant.

Chapter 9

Case Study 1

1. Male, less than 38 weeks' gestation, Greek ethnicity, maternal blood type O, maternal Rh negative, operative/vacuum delivery, blood sequestration, jaundiced at less than 24 hours of age, exclusive breastfeeding

2. Cord blood for newborn blood and Rh type with Coombs testing; bilirubin measurement by TcB or TSB

3. Approximately 7

4. A. 4–24 hours

   B. Yes; no

Case Study 2

1. Less than 38 weeks' gestation, maternal blood type of O negative, limited Rhogam prophylaxis, a sibling with hyperbilirubinemia, jaundiced at less than 24 hours.

2. Cord blood type and Rh, Coombs test, TSB or TcB bilirubin measurement.

3. Consider phototherapy. Ensure safety measures (e.g., eye mask), ensure adequate intake, monitor output, and monitor temperature to reduce risk of iatrogenic hyperthermia.

4. Continue with phototherapy. The baby should continue with breastmilk, but the phototherapy should not be interrupted because the bilirubin level is approaching

exchange transfusion levels. The mother should pump her breasts to promote milk production and feed the breastmilk to the newborn.

5.   Refer the baby now, as the bilirubin level is not responsive to phototherapy and is approaching exchange transfusion levels.

Chapter 10

1.   C, D, B, E, A
2.   C
3.   A, TRUE
4.   C
5.   A
6.   D
7.   B, FALSE
8.   A
9.   C

Chapter 11

Case Study 1

1.   C

Case Study 2

1.   C
2.   B

Chapter 12

Case Study

1.   Trisomy 21, Down syndrome, is diagnosed by chromosomal analysis in a newborn who presents with any of the physical characteristics of Trisomy 21 on physical examination.

2. Trisomy 21 is often associated with chronic medical conditions such as upper respiratory infections, pneumonia, congenital heart defects, gastrointestinal disorders, feeding difficulties, and developmental delays, which are treated. Trisomy 21 has no treatment or "cure."

3. The prognosis for a child with Trisomy 21 is individual and depends on numerous factors such as the "severity" of the syndrome; the presence and severity of medical conditions; early-childhood therapies such as physical, occupational, and speech-language; and the age and socioeconomic level of the mother.

Multiple Choice

1. A
2. D
3. B
4. D

References

Backes, C. H., Backes, C. R., Gardner, G., Nankervis, C. A., & Giannone, P. J. (2012). Neonatal abstinence syndrome: Transitioning methadone-treated infants from an inpatient to outpatient setting. *Journal of Perinatology, 32*(6), 425–430.

Hayes, M. J., & Brown, M. S. (2012). Epidemic of prescription opiate abuse and neonatal abstinence. *Journal of the American Medical Association, 307,* 1974–1975.

Kelly, L. E., Knoppert, D., Roukema, H., Rieder, M. J., & Koren, G. (2015). Oral morphine weaning for neonatal abstinence syndrome at home compared with in-hospital: An observational cohort study. *Pediatric Drugs, 17*(2), 151–157. doi: 10.1007/s40272-014-0096-y

Ram ey, K. (2015, October). *Examination of an outpatient approach to the treatment of neonatal abstinence syndrome.* Poster session presented at the meeting of the Vermont Oxford Network, Chicago, IL.

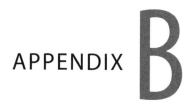

RESOURCES FOR PARENTS

Books and Pamphlets

American Academy of Pediatrics: Parent Education Materials
    Care of the Uncircumcised Penis: Fact Sheet
    Circumcision: Information for Parents
    Diaper Rash
    Early Arrival: Information for Parents of Premature Infants
    Infant Sleep Positioning and SIDS: Fact Sheet
American Academy of Pediatrics, Meek, J. Y., & Yu, W. (2011). *New mother's guide to breast feeding* (2nd ed.). New York, NY: Bantam Books.
American Academy of Pediatrics, Shelov, S. (Ed.). (2010). *Your baby's first year* (3rd ed.). Elk Grove Village, IL: American Academy of Pediatrics.
American Academy of Pediatrics, Shelov, S., & Hannemann, R. (Eds.). (2014). *Caring for your baby and young child: Birth to age 5* (5th ed.). Elk Grove Village, IL: American Academy of Pediatrics.
American College of Nurse-Midwives: Parent Education Materials http://www.midwife.org/
    Share-With-Women
    Circumcision
    Newborn Screening and Hearing Test
    Promoting Skin-to-Skin Contact
    Umbilical Cord Clamping After Birth

Breastfeeding and Birth Control

Breastfeeding and Working

Bringing your Baby to Breast: Positioning and Latch

Brazelton, T. B. (2004). *Baby basics* [video] and *Home before you know it* [video]. Cambridge, MA: Vida Health Communications.

Brimdyr, K. (2011). *The magical hour: Holding your baby skin-to-skin in the first hour after birth* [DVD]. East Sandwich, MA: Healthy Children Project.

Davis, D., & Stein, M. T. (2004). *Parenting your premature baby and child: The emotional journey.* Golden, CO: Fulcrum.

Flushman, B., & Gale, G. (1999). *My special start: A guide for parents in the neonatal intensive care unit.* Palo Alto, CA: VORT.

Gale, G., & Brooks, A. (2006). A parent's guide to palliative care. *Advances in Neonatal Care, 6*(1), 54. Directed to parents, this article describes what palliative care is, who it may benefit, and where and for how long it may be provided for babies.

Harrison, H. (1983). *The premature baby book.* New York, NY: St. Martin's Press.

Healy, T. (1988). *Guiding your child through preterm development.* Alexandria, VA: Parent Care.

Hormann, E. (2007). *Breastfeeding an adopted baby and relactation.* Schaumburg, IL: La Leche League International.

Huggins, K. (2007). *The nursing mother's companion* (6th ed.). Boston, MA: Harvard Common Press.

Hussey, B. (1988). *Understanding my signals.* Palo Alto, CA: VORT.

Ibarra, B., & Goodstein, M. (2011). A parent's guide to a safe sleep environment. *Advances in Neonatal Care, 11,* 27.

Jana, L. A., & Shu, J. (2011). *Heading home with your newborn.* Elk Grove Village, IL: American Academy of Pediatrics.

Karp, H. (2003). *Happiest baby on the block.* New York, NY: Bantam Books.

Kenner, C., & McGrath, J. (Eds.). (2004). *Developmental care of newborns and infants.* St. Louis, MO: Mosby.

Klaus, M. (2000). *Your amazing newborn.* Boston, MA: DaCapo Press.

La Leche League International. (2010). *The womanly art of breastfeeding* (8th ed.). Schaumburg, IL: Author.

Lauwers, J., & Swisher, A. (2010). *Counseling the nursing mother.* (5th ed.). Sudbury, MA: Jones and Bartlett.

Ludington-Hoe, S., & Golant, S. (1993). *Kangaroo care: The best you can do to help your preterm infant.* New York, NY: Bantam Books.

Meek, J. Y. (Ed.). (2011). *New mother's guide to breastfeeding* (2nd ed.). Elk Grove Village, IL: American Academy of Pediatrics.

Meier, P. (2003). *Breast feeding multiple babies.* Columbus, OH: Ross Products Division Abbott Laboratories. (Available in English and Spanish.)

Meier, P. (2003). *Breast feeding your premature baby.* Columbus, OH: Ross Products Division Abbott Laboratories. (Available in English and Spanish.)

Meier, P. (2003). *Expressing milk for your premature baby; Breast feeding your premature baby with a nipple shield; Troubleshooting milk volume problems in the NICU; Choosing a correctly fitting breast shield.* McHenry, IL: Medela.

Mohrbacher, N., Stock, J., & Newton, E. (2003). *The breastfeeding answer book* (3rd ed.). Schaumburg, IL: La Leche League.

Olds, S., Marks, L., & Eiger, M. (2010). *The complete book of breast feeding* (4th ed.). New York, NY: Workman Publishing.

Pryor, G., & Huggins, K. (2007). *Nursing mother, working mother: The essential guide to breastfeeding your baby before and after returning to work.* Boston, MA: Harvard Commons Press.

Sears, R. (2011). *The vaccine book.* New York, NY: Little Brown and Company.

Stokowski, L. A. (2005). Family teaching toolbox: A parents' guide to understanding apnea. *Advances in Neonatal Care, 5,* 175.

VandenBerg, K., Browne, J., Perez, L., & Newstetter, A. (2003). *Getting to know your baby: A developmental guide for community service providers and parents of NICU graduates.* Oakland, CA: Special Start Training Program, Mills College, Department of Education. www.specialstart.ucsf.edu.

Vergara, E., & Bigsby, R. (2004). *Developmental and therapeutic interventions in the NICU.* Baltimore, MD: Brooks Publishing.

When children die: Improving palliative and end-of-life care for children and their families. (2003). Washington, DC: National Academies Press.

Wolf, N. (2003). *Misconceptions: Truth, lies, and the unexpected on the journey to motherhood.* New York, NY: Anchor Books.

Internet Resources

A place to remember: www.aplacetoremember.com

American Heart Association: *Children with congenital or acquired heart disease:* www.americanheart.org

Association for Death Education and Counseling: www.adec.org

Baby's First Test: www.babysfirsttest.org. Information and resources for parents about newborn screening.

Bereaved Parents of the USA: www.bereavedparentsusa.org

Center for Loss in Multiple Birth, Inc.: www.climb-support.org

Centering Corporation and *Grief Digest*: www.centering.org

The Compassionate Friends: www.compassionatefriends.org

CongenitalHeartDefects.com, sponsored by Baby Hearts Press: www.congenitalheartdefects.com

Congenital Heart Information Network: www.tchin.org

Depression After Delivery (D.A.D.): www.communityresources.net/postpartumdepression.html

Developmental and Behavioral Pediatrics: www.dbpeds.org. Information on pediatrics and developmental screening.

DLD Productions: www.breastmilksolutions.com/index.html

Epilepsy Foundation of America: www.epilepsyfoundation.org

Genetic Alliance: www.geneticalliance.org

Genetics Home Reference: http://ghr.nlm.nih.gov

Grieving for Babies: www.grievingforbabies.org

Happiest Baby on the Block: https://happiestbaby.com

Hydrocephalus Association: www.hydroassoc.org

Hygeia Foundation: www.hygeia.org

Individuals with Disabilities Education Act (IDEA): http://idea.ed.gov

Initiative for Pediatric Palliative Care: www.ippcweb.org

International Hip and Dysplasia Institute: Hip-healthy swaddling: Are you swaddling your baby properly? www.hipdysplasia.org

Kids with Heart, National Association for Children's Heart Disorders: www.kidswithheart.org

Lact-Aid International. PO Box 1066, Athens, TN 37303; 1-866-866-1239. www.lact-aid.com

LaLeche League International: http://www.llli.org

LaRocca, J., & Powers, D. Family-centered developmental care in the NICU. PowerPoint Presentati-on at http://www.powershow.com/view/14e6d6-NGMyN/FAMILY_CENTERED_DEVELOPMENTAL

Little Hearts, Inc.: www.littlehearts.org

March of Dimes: www.marchofdimes.com/catalog

    Brain development card and/or flyer

    Breastfeeding: A how-to guide

    Loss and grief in the childbearing period

    My 9 months: Guide to a healthy pregnancy

    Premature birth: Reducing your risks

    Signs of preterm labor

    Why the last weeks of pregnancy count

Mothers in Support and Sympathy (MISS) Foundation: www.missfoundation.org

National Hydrocephalus Foundation: www.nhfonline.org

National Organization for Rare Disorders (NORD): www.rarediseases.org

Newborn Channel: www.thenewbornchannel.com

Online PPMD Support Group: www.ppdsupportpage.com

Partners for Understanding Pain: https://theacpa.org/PARTNERS-for-Understanding-Pain

Pediheart Organization: http://www.golneo.org

Perinatal Hospice and Palliative Care: www.perinatalhospice.org

Postpartum Support International: www.postpartum.net

Pregnancy Loss and Infant Death Alliance: www.plida.org

Remember When: www.rememberwhenvideo.com. Video and DVD tributes.

Renfrew, M., Fischer, C., & Arms, S. (2004). *Breast feeding: Getting breast feeding right for you.* Berkeley, CA: Celestial Arts.

SHARE Pregnancy and Infant Loss Support, Inc.: www.nationalshare.org

Spina Bifida Association of America: www.spinabifidaassociation.org

U.S. Department of Health and Human Services, Office on Women's Health: www. womenshealth.gov/breastfeeding

Videos

Bergman, N. (2000). *Kangaroo mother care: Restoring the original paradigm for infant care and breast feeding* [Video]. Cape Town, South Africa. www.kangaroomothercare.com

Colorado Collective for Medical Decisions, Neonatal Care Subcommittee. (1998). *You are not alone.* Denver, CO: Nickel's Worth Productions.

Dorner, A. (1983). *Prematurely yours* [Video]. Boston, MA: Polymorph Films.

Institute for Family-Centered Care. (1996). *Newborn intensive care: Changing practice, changing attitude* [Video]. Bethesda, MD: Author.

Jonas-Simpson, C. (Producer). (2010). *Why did baby die? Mothering children living with the loss, love and continuing presence of a baby sibling* [DVD].

Jonas-Simpson, C. (Producer). (2011). *Enduring love: Transforming loss* [DVD]. https://vimeo.com/20017892

Morton, J. (2001). *A premie needs his mother: First steps to breast feeding your premature baby* [Video]. Palo Alto, CA.

Rosenberg, S. (1996). *Kangaroo care: A parent's touch* [Video]. Chicago, IL: Prentice Women's Hospital.

Rush Mothers' Milk Club. (2010). *In your hands: The importance of mother's milk for premature babies* [DVD]. Chicago, IL.

Resource Materials for Parents Dealing with Grief

Balter, L. (1991). *A funeral for Whiskers.* New York, NY: Barron's Educational Services.

Berezin, N. (1982). *After a loss in pregnancy.* New York, NY: Fireside Books.

Borg, S., & Lasker, J. (1981). *When pregnancy fails.* Boston, MA: Beacon Press.

Boyle, F. (1997). *Mothers bereaved by stillbirth, neonatal death, or sudden infant death syndrome.* Ashgate, UK: Aldershot.

Brown, L., & Brown, M. (1996): *When dinosaurs die: A guide to understanding death.* Boston, MA: Little, Brown.

Burns, L., & Ilse, S. (2000). *Miscarriage: A shattered dream.* Maple Plain, MN: Wintergreen Press.

Buscaglia, L. (1982). *The fall of Freddie the leaf.* Thorofare, NJ: Slack.

Cardin, N. (2001). *Tears of sorrow, seeds of hope: A Jewish spiritual companion for infertility and pregnancy loss.* Woodstock, VT: Jewish Light Publishing.

Case, B. (2001). *Living without your twin.* Portland, OR: Tibbutt.

Cirulli, C. (1999). *Pregnancy after loss: A guide to pregnancy after a miscarriage, stillbirth, or infant death.* New York, NY: Berkeley Books.

Davis, D. (2000). *Empty cradle, broken heart.* Golden, CO: Fulcrum Publishing.

Davis, D., & Stein, M. (2004). *Parenting your premature baby and child: The emotional journey.* Golden, CO: Fulcrum Books.

Dyer, K. A. (n.d.). Journey of hearts. www.journeyofhearts.org

Eckl, C. (2010). *A beautiful death.* Littleton, CO: Flying Crane Press.

Eckl, C. (2012). *A beautiful grief.* Littleton, CO: Flying Crane Press.

Eddy, M. L., & Raydo, L. (1990). *Making loving memories: A gentle guide to what you can do when your baby dies.* Omaha, NE: Centering Corporation.

Eldon, K., & Eldon, A. (1998). *Angel catcher: A journal of loss and remembrance.* San Francisco, CA: Chronicle Books.

Emswiler, M., & Emswiler, J. (2000). *Guiding your child through grief.* New York, NY: Bantam Trade.

Griffin, T., & Celenza, J. (2014). *Family-centered care for the newborn: The delivery room and beyond.* New York, NY: Springer.

Grollman, E. (1990). *Talking about death: A dialogue between parent and child.* Boston, MA: Beacon Press.

Grollman, E. (1993). *Straight talk about death to teenagers.* Boston, MA: Beacon Press.

Isle, S. (1996). *Empty arms.* Maple Plain, MN: Wintergreen Press.

Jonas-Simpson, C. (Producer). (2010). *Why did baby die? Mothering children living with the loss, love and continuing presence of a baby sibling* [DVD]. https://vimeo.com/20017892

Jonas-Simpson, C. (Producer). (2011). *Enduring love: Transforming loss* [DVD]. www.bereavementdocumentaries.ca/enduring_love.html

Leon, I. C. (1990). *When a baby dies: Psychotherapy for pregnancy and newborn loss.* New Haven, CT: Yale University Press.

Limbo, R., & Wheeler, S. (1998). *When a baby dies: A handbook for healing and helping.* La Crosse, WI: Lutheran Hospital–La Crosse.

Linden, D., Paroli, E., & Doron, M. (2000). *The essential guide for parents of premature babies.* New York, NY: Pocket Books.

March of Dimes: www.marchofdimes.com/catalog

   From hurt to healing: Dealing with the death of your baby

   What can you do? Helping loved ones deal with the death of their baby

   When you want to try again: Thinking about pregnancy

Miller, S. (1999). *Finding hope when a child dies.* New York, NY: Simon & Schuster.

Mundy, M. (1999). *Sad isn't bad: A good-grief guidebook for kids dealing with loss* (Elf-Help Books for Kids). St. Meinrad, IN: Abbey Press.

Pector, E. (n.d.). Multiplicity: Resources for loss, prematurity and special needs. www.synspectrum.com/multiplicity.html

Read, B., Bryan, E., & Hallett, F. (1997). *When a twin or triplet dies.* London, UK: Multiple Births Foundation.

Shriver, M. (1999). *What's heaven?* New York, NY: Golden Books.

Standucher, C. (1991). *Men and grief.* Oakland, CA: New Harbinger Publications.

Thomas, P. (2001). *I miss you: A first look at death.* Hauppauge, NY: Barron's Educational Series.

Tracy, A., & Maroney, D. (1999). *Your premature baby and child.* New York, NY: Berkley Books.

Woodward, J. (1998). *The lone twin: Understanding twin bereavement and loss.* London, UK: Free Association Books.

Zaichkin, J. (2009). *Newborn intensive care: What every parent needs to know* (3rd ed.). Petaluma, CA: NICU Inc.

Index

Note: Page numbers followed by *b*, *f*, or *t* indicate material in boxes, figures, or tables, respectively.

A

abaissement, 195
abnormal central nervous system
    (CNS) signs, 299
abnormal findings
    back, hips and extremities,
        126*t*–130*t*
    cardiac examination, 108*t*
    common murmurs, 109*t*
    genitalia, 123*t*–124*t*
    head, eye, ear, nose and
        throat (HEENT), 114*t*,
        116*t*, 118*t*
    respiratory examination, 107*t*
    skin, 112*t*
    thorax and abdomen, 121*t*–122*t*
abnormal transition, 83*t*, 84*b*
    history, 82
    newborn competencies and
        behaviors, 86–88
    physical examination, 86
    signs and symptoms, 82–86
Academy of Breastfeeding
    Medicine, 23*t*
acquired neonatal infections,
    viral, bacterial, and fungal,
    283*t*–295*t*
acute hypoglycemia
    management, 91*f*
acute-phase reactant tests, 301
adequate milk supply/intake,
    neonatal signs, 152*b*
alcohol consumption, pregnant
    woman and, 51
American Academy of Pediatrics
    (AAP), 19*t*, 21*t*–22*t*, 29
    on breastfeeding, 140
    discharge of healthy term
        infants, 236*b*
    hospital setting, 223–225
    minimum postpartum stays, 220
American Association of Birth
    Centers (AABC), 92
    on discharge timing, 225
    interdependence
        postpartum, 226

American Heart Association
    (AHA), 21*t*
American Nurses Association
    (ANA)
    Code of Ethics for Nurses, 2
    nursing, definition (1980), 1
American Society of Pain
    Management Nurses, 21*t*
amino acid formulas, 169, 174
Anand and International Evidence-
    Based Group for Neonatal
    Pain, 22*t*
anatomic/physiologic difference,
    newborn, 3*t*–15*t*
anthropometric measurements, 104
anti-regurgitation formula
    (AR-formula), 177
antiviral therapies, 303
Apgar Score, 60, 101–103, 300
    expanded, 102*f*
appropriate for gestational age
    (AGA), 104
Association of Women's Health,
    Obstetric, and Neonatal
    Nurses (AWHONN),
    19*t*, 22*t*

B

baby blues, 209–211
back, hips, and extremities
    abnormalities, 126*t*–129*t*
bacterial sepsis, 300
bad air *(mal aire)*, 304
Ballard scale, 102, 104
Barlow's test, 326*f*
    maneuver, developmental
        dysplasia of the hip, 130*b*
bathing, 243
beats per minute (BPM), 106
behavioral phases of term newborns,
    first hour of life, 72*t*
bilirubin
    adult metabolism, 256
    clinical significance, 253
    enterohepatic factors, 256–258
    hematologic metabolism, 256

incidence, 255
intestinal flora, 258
metabolism, 257*f*–258*f*
number of feeding, 163*t*
phototherapy initiation, 266*f*
TcB and TSB results, 264*f*
blood culture, bacteremia
    detection, 300
blood glucose, routine
    monitoring, 90*b*
blood poisoning, 276
breastfeeding, 70–72, 80, 90, 93
    cessation, 207
    co-regulation, 205–206
    contradictions, 146
    initiation, hospital policies, 137
    intrapartal promotion, 138
    maternal problems
        candidiasis, 152, 153*b*, 154*t*
        engorgement, 148–149, 151*b*
        flat/inverted nipples, 148, 150*b*
        insufficient milk supply,
            149–150, 151*b*
        mastitis, 153
        sore nipples, 147
    newborn/neonatal conditions
        ankyloglossia (tongue-tie),
            157, 159, 160*f*
        feeding refusal, 155, 155*t*
        hyperbilirubinemia, 163
        hypoglycemia, 159–163
        jaundice, 163
        late-preterm infants (LPIs),
            155–157
        palate abnormality, 159
        poor weight gain, 163–164
    physiology and pathophysiology
        AAP recommendations, 140
        contradictions, 146
        lactation, 140
        nutritional composition of
            breastmilk, 140–145
    postpartal promotion, 138–139
    prenatal promotion, 137–138
    standards of care, 164–165
    teaching and counseling, 165

breastmilk
  lactogenesis, 141
  nutritional composition, 140–141

C
candidiasis
  incidence, 152
  symptoms, 152b
  traditional and complementary
    therapies, 154t
capillary refill time (CRT), 299
cardiac examination, 108t
  abnormal findings, 108t–109t
  structural complications,
    323–324
caregiving considerations, 87t–88t
Centers for Disease Control and
    Prevention (CDC), 23t, 93
central nervous system (CNS),
    4t–5t
  circadian rhythms, 7t–8t
  neurologic conditions/
    presentations, 8t–10t
  pain, 5t–6t
  sensory, 6t
certified midwives (CMs), 2,
    29–30, 225
certified nurse-midwives (CNMs),
    1–2, 29–30, 225
certified professional midwives
    (CPM), 1–2, 29–30, 225
cesarean birth, 57
cessation, breastfeeding, 207
childbirth, cultural
    consideration, 60, 61b
chronic hypertension, 44, 48
circulatory pattern before birth, 75f
circumcision, male infant, 244–245
  clinical estimation,
    expanded, 103f
clinical nurse specialists (CNS), 1–2
clinical supervision, 211–212
cluster feeding, 207
co-regulation
  behavioral perspective, 203
  breastfeeding dyad, 205–206
  lactogenesis, 206–207
  newborn's sleep, 201, 208
  regulation, definition, 202
  sleep–wake cycle, 207–209
  staged interventions, 203
  stooling pattern, 207
  three-hour cycles, 206
colic, 180–181, 181f
colostrum (first milk), 141–142,
    144, 163

Committee on Fetus and Newborn,
    21t, 23, 29
common murmurs of the
    newborn, 109t
congenital anomalies, 322t
congenital heart disease, 323t
congenital hypothyroidism, 44
constipation or diarrhea
  definition, 179
  gastrointestinal symptoms, 179t
  regurgitation management, 178f
  stool consistency, 178–179
cord care, 244
cow's-milk protein allergy (CMPA),
    169, 177, 180
cow's milk–based formulas, 168,
    170t–171t
CRAFFT substance abuse screen
    (adolescents and young
    adults), 55t
cranial and facial, structural
    complications, 325
C-reactive protein (CRP) levels, 301
critical congenital heart disease
    (CCHD), 106, 110, 226,
    230, 302
crying periods, 209–210
  sharing strategies, 211
cultural and ethical variations in
    infants, common factors,
    349b–350b
cultural considerations
  celebrations of newborn, 94
  childbirth, 60–61
  discharge timing, 228–229
  health maintenance visit, 348–350
  infections, 304–306
culturally sensitive communication
    data, 61b
curandero, 304
cyanosis, 299

D
dehydration, 16
delivery complications
  intracranial hemorrhage, 320
  predisposing factors, 319–320
  shoulder dystocia, 320
developmental care approach.
    See also neonatal behavioral
    transition
  biological nurturing, 197
  breastfeeding process, 200, 206
  clinical supervision, 211–212
  co-regulation and maternal–
    newborn wellness, 192

conceptual foundation, 192–197
  ethical dimension, 192
  first behavioral cues, 203
  first period of sleep, 201
  holding phase, 195–197
  optimal nutrition, 212
  parental anxieties, 208–209
  psychodynamic, 191–192
  regression concept, 193
  touchpoints approach, 194
developmental competencies of
    newborns and neonates,
    333b–334b
developmental immaturity, 3t–15t
diapering, 243–244
discharge preparations
  circumcision procedure, 244–245
  feeding, 241–242
  immunizations, 242–243
  infant care, 243–244
  infection control, 242
  newborn screen, 238–241
  safety, 245–247
discharge teaching. See also
    discharge preparations
  individualized instruction, 235
  newborn screens, 238–241
  standards of care, 236–238
  timing of discharge, 235–236
discharge timing
  birth center, 225–226
  cultural considerations, 228–229
  ethical considerations, 220
  general criteria, 224t
  historical perspectives, 220
  home setting, 225–226
  hospital setting, 223–225
  newborn screening, 222
  physical examination, 221–222
  prenatal history, 221
  readmission risk, 226–228
  routine medication, 222
  teaching and counseling,
    222–223

E
early-onset infections, 277b, 297
Edinburgh Postnatal Depression
    Scale, 342t–343t
Eighth Joint National Committee
    (JNC-8), hypertension
    management guidelines, 44
elimination
  bowel movements, 242
  parental concerns, 209
  urination patterns, 242

Engle, Tomashek, Wallman, and Committee on Fetus and Newborn, 23
engorgement, 151*b*
epigenetics, 70–71
eustress, 70, 76
evidence appraisal, 26*f*
Ewing's Four P's screening tool, 55*t*
exterogestational period, 71
extracorporeal membrane oxygenation (ECMO) treatment., 78–79, 86
extreme preterm (EPT) infants, 102

F
fallen fontanel *(mallera caida)*, 304
family history
   chronic health conditions, 36–38, 37*t*
   genetic conditions, 38*t*–43*t*
   and risk of selected diseases and chronic health conditions, 37*t*
febrile infants, 303
feeding
   behaviors, 16
   breastfeeding, 241–242
   formula feeding, 165–167, 166*b*, 242
   refusal, 155, 155*t*
first hour of life
   behavioral phases, 72–74
   physiology and pathophysiology, 75–81
first to second week of life visit, 346*b*
   observation, 345–346
   physical examination, 346
flat/inverted nipples, 150*b*
follow-up care, 247–248, 248*b*
formula choices
   amino acid, 169, 174
   composition, 168
   cow's milk–based, 168, 170*t*–171*t*
   hydrolyzed, 169, 172*t*–173*t*
   nutritional composition, 170*t*–171*t*
   preparation, unsafe practices, 167*t*
   prethickened, 174
   reduced-lactose, 174–175
   soy protein–based, 168–169
formula-fed infants
   colic management, 181*f*
   constipation management, 180*f*
   gassiness management, 175*f*
   regurgitation management, 178*f*

formula feeding, 165–167, 166*b*
formula intolerance, 175–176
fourth trimester, 71
full term (FT) infants, 102
functional residual capacity (FRC), 76, 78–79

G
gastroesophageal reflux (GER), 174, 176, 180
gastroesophageal reflux disease (GERD), 177, 179*t*, 180
genetic complications
   congenital anomalies, 322*t*
   morphologies, 321*t*
genetic conditions, newborn, 39*t*–43*t*
   genetic disorders, classification, 38*t*
genitalia abnormalities, 123*t*–124*t*
genomics, 38
gestational age, 101–104, 130
gestational diabetes mellitus (GDM), 47–48
gestational hypertension, 47–48
glucose support considerations, 89*f*
Golden Minute, 59
Guidelines for Perinatal Care, 93

H
head, eye, ear, nose, and throat (HEENT) examination, 114*t*–118*t*
health education, 94–95
health maintenance visit
   core concept, 333*b*
   cultural considerations, 348–350
   first to second week of life visit, 345–346
   national guidelines for care, 348
   one month, 347
   outpatient, 332–333
   postpartum psychosis, mother, 336–337
   standards of care, 348
   three-day-old visit, 337, 341
healthcare provider's practice
   evidence-based practice (EBP), 25–26
   legal issues, 26–29
   medical professionals, 24
   neonatal care, 29–30
   professional nursing and midwifery practice, 17

scope of practice (nurses and midwives), 23–24, 24*t*
   standards of care and practice, 18*t*–23*t*
healthy infants
   breastmilk storage guidelines, 166*t*
   colic, 180–181, 181*f*
   constipation or diarrhea, 178–179, 180*f*
   gastroesophageal reflux (GER), 176–177
   gastroesophageal reflux disease (GERD), 177, 179*t*
   plasma glucose concentrations, 161*f*
   regurgitation, 176–177, 176*b*, 177*b*, 178*f*
   supplemental feedings, 145
healthy people 2020 objectives, 348*b*
hearing screening, auditory brain stem responses and otoacoustic emissions, 240*b*
hip developmental dysplasia, 130*b*
Hirschsprung's disease, 179
hydrolyzed formulas, 169, 172*t*–173*t*
hyperbilirubinemia, 16
   adequate breastfeeding, 163, 163*t*
   clinical guidelines, 259*b*
   conjugated, 268–269
   exchange transfusion, 267–268
   guidelines for management
     AAP recommendation, discharge time, 268
     adequate breastfeeding, 259–260
     bilirubin measurement, 263
     clinical guidelines, 259*b*
     nursery protocols, 260
     systematic assessment, 260–263
     visual inspection, 263
   identification protocols and evaluation, 260
   incidence, 255–256
   isoimmunization, 269
   phototherapy, 265–268
   predictable stages, 253, 254*f*
   risk assessment, 260–261, 261*b*, 262*t*
   terminologies, 254*b*
   visual inspection, 263
hypoglycemia, 16, 299
   clinical signs, 91*b*
   risk factors, 162*t*
   transient, 159

hypothyroidism, 44
hypoxia, 299

I

immunizations, 242–243
infant care, 94–95
  bathing, 243
  cord care, 244
  diapering, 243–244
  parenting, 243
  skin, 244
infants of diabetic mothers (IDMs),
    318–319
infection control, 242
infections. *See also* perinatal
    infectious diseases
  causative agents, 277*b*
  cultural considerations, 304–306
  definition, 275–276
  diagnostic evaluation,
      299–301, 300*b*
  differential diagnoses, 301–302
  etiology, 275–276
  mortality rates, 275
  parent education, 305
  physical examinations, 297–299
  prevention and control
      strategies, 278
  risk factors, 276*b*
  signs and symptoms, 279*t*,
      296*b*–297*b*, 296*f*
  standard of care, 302–304
  TORCH, 279*t*–282*t*
insufficient milk supply, 149–150
  etiology, 151*b*
  neonatal signs, 151*b*
International Consensus on
    Cardiopulmonary
    Resuscitation
    and Emergency
    Cardiovascular Care
    Science with Treatment
    Recommendations Task
    Force, 58
intracranial hemorrhage, 320
intrapartum history
  Apgar score, 60
  cesarean birth, 57–58
  cultural considerations, 60–61
  neonatal resuscitation, 58–59
  normal physiologic childbirth, 56
intrauterine growth, 101, 104,
    118, 121
  restriction, 316–317

J

jaundice
  adequate breastfeeding, 163, 163*t*
  definition, 268
  erythrocyte destruction, 269–270
  infection, 270
  isoimmunization, 269
  vitamin K administration, 92
  management, 270–271
  parental education, 268–269
  sequestered blood, 270
  structural abnormalities, 270

L

labor and birth in water, 81–82
lactation specialist
  consultation, 164*b*
lactogenesis, 140, 145, 148, 163
large for gestational age (LGA),
    104, 318
late-onset infections, 276, 277*b*, 301
late-preterm infants (LPIs), 102
  AAP's discharge criteria, 255*b*
  brain growth, 156
  breastfeeding difficulties, 156
  hydration and caloric intake, 159*t*
  nutritional support, 157
  preterm discharge formulas, 158*t*
  strategies to facilitate
      breastfeeding, 157*b*
legal issues, professional
  professional negligence, 27–29
  statute of limitations, 26–27
levels of evidence, 25*t*

M

mastitis, 153
maternal fatigue, 210
maternal medical history
  diabetes mellitus, 43–44
  gestational diabetes, 47–48
  hypertensive disorders, 44
  hypertensive disorders of
      pregnancy, 48–49
  obstetric history, 45–47
  thyroid disorders, 44
maternal problems, breastfeeding
  candidiasis, 152, 153*b*, 154*t*
  engorgement, 148–149, 151*b*
  flat/inverted nipples, 148, 150*b*
  insufficient milk supply,
      149–150, 150*b*
  mastitis, 153
  sore nipples, 147

maternal substance abuse, 51
mature milk, 141, 144
meconium ileus or plug, 179
meningitis, 301
metabolic acidosis, 299
Midwives' Alliance of North
    America, 227
moderate-severe preterm
    (MSPT), 102
modified Finnegan scoring
    system, 54
multicultural health care, 350*b*
musculoskeletal, structural
    complications, 325–326

N

National Association of Certified
    Professional Midwives
    (NACPM), 225
National Association of Neonatal
    Nurses (NANN), 18*t*, 20*t*, 21*t*
National Association of Pediatric
    Nurse Practitioners
    (NAPNAP), 21*t*
National Birth Center Study II, 227
National Family History Day, 36
national guidelines for care
  health maintenance visit, 348
  hospital discharge, 236–237
National Institute for Health Care
    and Excellence (NICE),
    guidelines for breastfeeding,
    164–165
National Survey on Drug Use and
    Health (NSDUH), 51
nature knows best, physiologic
    birth, 70–71
neonatal abstinence syndrome
    (NAS), 53–54
Neonatal Behavioral Assessment
    Scale (NBAS), 132, 203
neonatal behavioral transition
  brain at birth, 198–199
  extrauterine life, 198
  predictable behavioral sequence,
      199–201
  reticular activating system
      (RAS), 199
neonatal deaths, 36, 43
neonatal hyperbilirubinemia, 262*t*
neonatal hypoglycemia, 43, 47
neonatal infection/sepsis, 16–17
neonatal injuries from operative
    delivery, 57*t*

neonatal intensive care unit (NICU), 227
neonatal period, saying goodbye
 colic, 209–210
 crying period, 209–211
 distress and fatigue, 210
Neonatal Resuscitation Program (NRP), 92–93
 guidelines, 58
neonatal transition period, 73*f*, 74*b*
neonate/newborns
 anatomic/physiologic difference, 3*t*–15*t*
 cardiac system, 4*t*
 central nervous system (CNS), 4*t*–6*t*
 circadian rhythm/sleep–wake cycles, 7*t*–8*t*
 common murmurs, 109*t*
 definition, 2
 developmental immaturity, 3*t*–15*t*
 difference between, 3*t*–15*t*
 first developmental task, 202
 gastrointestinal (GI) system, 12*t*–13*t*
 glucose homeostasis, 13*t*–14*t*
 hematologic system, 11*t*
 hormonal system, 15*t*
 immune system, 10*t*
 nephrology/renal, 14*t*
 neurologic conditions, 8*t*–10*t*
 professional practice, 29–30
 respiratory system, 3*t*–4*t*
 skin sytem, 15*t*
neonatology, 2
neuromuscular maturity, Ballard scale, 103*f*
newborn care
 advanced practice providers, 1, 15
 neonatal assessment principles, 16–17
 routine care, 1
newborn development
 developmental task, 335
 physical, 333–335, 341, 344, 346–347
 safety, 336
 social/cognitive, 335
newborn, genetic condition, 39*t*–43*t*
newborn scale of sepsis (SOS), 298*f*

newborn screens
 critical congenital heart disease (CCHD), 240–241
 hearing, 239
 hyperbilirubinemia/jaundice, 239–240
 metabolic, 238–239
 newborn visit, follow-up components, 248*b*
newborn with complications
 delivery, 319–320
 infants of diabetic mothers (IDMs), 318–319
 intrauterine growth restriction, 316–317
 large for gestational age (LGA), 318
 multifetal pregnancy, 315–316, 315*t*, 316*f*
 placental, 313, 314*t*
 small for gestational age (SGA), 317–318
 structural, 323–326
nurse practitioners, 1, 29–30

O

omphalitis, 299
one month visit, 347*b*
 observation, 347
 physical examination, 347
operative delivery. *See also* cesarean birth
 potential injuries, 57*t*
opioid-based therapies
 buprenorphine, 54
 methadone, 54
optimality principle, perinatal outcomes, 70
Ortolani's test, 326*f*
 maneuver, developmental dysplasia of the hip, 130*b*

P

parental education
 formula intolerance, 175–176
 infections, 305
 jaundice, 268–269
pediatric health maintenance visit, 332*b*
pediatrics, 2
perinatal health record
 family history, 36–43
 intrapartum history, 56–61
 maternal medical history, 43–49

perinatally acquired infections, 49–50
 substance abuse, 51–55
perinatal history and related neonatal outcomes, 45*t*–47*t*
perinatal infectious diseases, 49*t*–50*t*
perinatal substance abuse
 opioid use during pregnancy, 51–53
 screening, 55
 transfer of substances (fetus and newborn), 53–54
perinatal substance exposure on infant, 52*t*
perinatally acquired infections, 49–50
persistent pulmonary hypertension (PPHN), 78–79, 85–86
phototherapy
 adverse effects, 267
 discontinuation, 266
 illumination, 267
 indications, 265
 safety and protective measures, 267
 technical features, 265
physical examination, 105*b*
 abnormal transition, 86
 Brazelton exam, 132
 cardiac exam, 106
 cranial nerves
  abducens, 131
  auditory, 132
  facial, 131–132
  glossopharyngeal, 131
  hypoglossal, 131
  oculomotor, 131
  olfactory, 131
  optic, 131
  trigeminal, 131
  trochlear, 131
 critical congenital heart defect (CCHD), 106–110
 discharge timing, 221–222
 first to second week of life visit, 346
 genitalia assessment
  male and female, 120
 handling and caring, 104–105
 head assessment
  abdomen, 120
  caput succedaneum, 113
  cephalohematoma, 113
  chest, 120

physical examination (*continued*)
 ears, 119
 eye examination, 113–119
 mouth, 119
 neck, 119
 nose, 119
 infections, 297–299
 neurologic, reflexes
  Babinski, 131
  galant, 130
  moro, 130–131
  palmar grasp, 130
  plantar grasp, 131
  rooting, 125
  tonic neck, 130
 one month visit, 145
 respiratory rate and rhythm, 106
 skin assessment, 110–112
 spine, 120–125
 upper and lower extremities, 125
 vital signs, 105
physical examination of
 newborn, 344*b*
physical maturity, Ballard scale, 103*f*
physician assistants, 1, 24, 29–30
physicians, 1, 23–24, 30
physiological birth
 evolutionary eustress, 70
 fetal pulmonary system, 75–76
 intrapartum hydrotherapy, 81
 "nature knows best" concept,
  70–71
 pathophysiologic process
  versus, 69
 recent research, 71
placental complications, 313, 314*t*
point of maximal impulse (PMI), 106
post-term (PoT) infants, 102
postpartum depression predictors
 inventory (PDPI), 339*t*–341*t*
postpartum mood disorders, 337*b*
predictable behavioral sequence
 first period of reactivity, 199–200
 newborn–maternal
  exploration, 200
 post-birth sleep period, 200–201
 second period of reactivity, 201
predictable sleep–wake–feed–satiety
 cycles, 207
predisposing factors, delivery
 complications, 319–320
preeclampsia, 43–44, 47–49
pregnant women
 alcohol consumption, 51
 substance abuse, screening, 55
 use of illicit opioid drugs, 52

preterm (PT) infants, 102
prethickened formulas, 174
primordial emotion, 196
professional negligence, 27–29
professional nursing care providers
 certified midwives (CMs), 2,
  29–30, 225
 certified nurse-midwives
  (CNMs), 1–2, 29–30, 225
 certified professional midwives
  (CPMs), 1–2, 29–30, 225
 evidence-based practice (EBP),
  25–26
 legal issues, 26–29
 medical practice, 24
 professional practice, 29–30
 scope of practice, 23–24
 standards of care and practice,
  17, 18*t*–23*t*
professional nursing practice,
 scope, 24*t*
pulmonary diseases, 324–325

R
readmission, risk factors, 227*b*
reduced-lactose formulas, 174–175
regurgitation in healthy infants, 176*b*
respiratory distress
 common causes, 78*t*–79*t*
 symptoms, 77*b*
 syndrome, 77*b*
respiratory examination, 107*t*
resuscitation at birth
 risk factors, 59*t*
 updated recommendations, 58*b*
routine care, transition
 eye prophylaxis, 92
 glucose screening, 89,
  90*b*–91*b*, 91*f*
 vitamin K administration, 92
Rubarth Newborn Scale of Sepsis
 (RNSOS), 297

S
safe sleep environment, 247*b*
safety
 in home, 245*t*–246*t*
 newborns and neonates, 336*b*
 recommendation, 245*t*–246*t*
self-regulatory *versus* stress
 behaviors, 204*t*
sepsis
 antibiotics, 303
 blood culture, 300
 diagnostic evaluation, 297, 299
 laboratory tests, 301

newborn scale of sepsis
 (SOS), 298*f*
 signs and symptoms, 296
 skin changes, 299
sexually transmitted infections, 45*t*,
 50*t*, 51, 53
shaken-baby syndrome, 211
shoulder dystocia, 320
sick baby, recognizing, 247
skin
 care, 244
 changes, 299
 variations, 110*t*, 112*t*
sleep environment, 246–247, 247*b*
small for gestational age (SGA),
 104, 317–318
soy protein–based formulas, 168–169
standards of care
 AAFP recommendation for
  hospital discharge,
  236–237
 breastfeeding, 164–165
 discharge teaching, 236–238
 discharge timing, 223–225
 health maintenance visit, 348
 healthcare provider's practice,
  18*t*–23*t*
 infections, 302–304
 routine newborn, 92–94
 specialty care providers, 18*t*–22*t*
stillbirth, 35, 43
structural abnormalies, infant's
 tongue
 ankyloglossia (tongue-tie), 157,
  159, 160f
 palate, 159
structural abnormalities, breast
 engorgement, 148–149
 flat/inverted nipple, 148
structural complications
 Barlow's test, 326*f*
 cardiac, 323–324
 congenital heart disease, 323*t*
 cranial and facial, 325
 musculoskeletal, 325–326
 Ortolani's test, 326*f*
 pulmonary diseases, 324–325
Substance Abuse and Mental
 Health Services
 Administration (SAMHSA),
 51–53
substance abuse, screening
 CRAFFT (for adolescents and
  young adults), 55*t*
 Ewing's Four P's screening
  tool, 55*t*

substances cross mechanisms, placenta, 53*t*
Surgeon General's Family Health Initiative (2004), 36

T
Task Force on Sudden Infant Death Syndrome, 22*t*
teaching and counseling
  breastfeeding, 165
  discharge timing, 222–223
thorax and abdomen in the newborn examination, 121*t*–122*t*
three-day-old visit, 345*b*
  history, 337, 341
  physical examination, 341, 344
total serum bilirubin (TSB), 262–268, 270
traditional midwives, 225
transient congenital hypothyroidism, 44
transitional milk, 141, 144
transitional period. *See also* abnormal transition

acute hypoglycemia management, 90*b*–91*b*, 91*f*
cardiac system, 75–77
cultural consideration, 94
first hour of life (behavioral phases), 72*t*
heat loss, 77–81
  conductive, 80
  evaporative, 80
  labor and birth in water, 81–82
pulmonary system, 75–77
routine care
  eye prophylaxis, 92
  glucose screening, 89–91
  vitamin K administration, 92
skin-to-skin (kangaroo) care, 70–72, 80–82, 93, 96
stages, 73*f*, 74*b*
standards of care, 92–93
states and considerations for caregiving, 87*t*–88*t*
thermoregulation, 77–81
troublesome regurgitation, 177*f*

W
wake–sleep cycle, 208
well newborn. *See also* developmental care approach
biological nurturing, 197
breastfeeding process, 200, 206
clinical supervision, 211–212
co-regulation and maternal–newborn wellness, 192
conceptual foundation, 192–197
ethical dimension, 192
first behavioral cues, 203
first period of sleep, 201
holding phase, 195–197
optimal nutrition, 212
parental anxieties, 208–209
psychodynamic, 191–192
regression concept, 193
touchpoints approach, 194
Winnicott's theory, clinical supervision, 191–193, 195–196, 199–200, 202, 210–212